Devinder Kumar and
John Alexander-Williams

Crohn's Disease and Ulcerative Colitis

Surgical Management

With 141 figures

Springer-Verlag
London Berlin Heidelberg New York
Paris Tokyo Hong Kong
Barcelona Budapest

Devinder Kumar, PhD, FRCS
Senior Lecturer, Department of Surgery, Queen Elizabeth Hospital,
Birmingham B15 2TH, UK

John Alexander-Williams, MD, FRCS
Professor of Gastrointestinal Surgery, The General Hospital,
Birmingham B4 6NH, UK

With contributions from:
R.N. Allan, MD, FRCP
Consultant Physician, The Queen Elizabeth Hospital, Edgbaston,
Birmingham B15 2TH, UK

Cover illustration: Ch. 12, Fig. 12. A long strictureplasty in Crohn's disease. The incised gut is bent over in a loop and the posterior wall is sutured with a continuous seromuscular stitch. Ch. 23, Fig. 16. The steps in pouch construction. The beginning of the suture line for the anterior layer of a pouch; a small hole is made in the proximal limb of the pouch; completed pouch-anal stapled anastomosis.

ISBN 3-540-19730-3 Springer-Verlag Berlin Heidelberg New York
ISBN 0-387-19730-3 Springer-Verlag New York Berlin Heidelberg

British Library Cataloguing in Publication Data
Kumar, Devinder
Surgical Management of Crohn's Disease
and Ulcerative Colitis
I. Title II. Alexander-Williams, John
617.5
ISBN 3-540-19730-3

Library of Congress Cataloging-in-Publication Data
Kumar, Devinder.
The Surgical management of Crohn's disease and ulcerative colitis
/ Devinder Kumar and John Alexander-Williams; [with contributions fron R.N. Allan].
p. cm.
Includes bibliographical references and index.
ISBN 3-540-19730-3 (alk. paper) : $112.50 (est.). – ISBN
0-387-19730-3 (alk. paper) : $112.50 (est.)
1. Enteritis, Regional – Surgery. 2. Ulcerative colitis – Surgery.
I. Alexander-Williams, John. II. Allan, R.N. (Robert Norman)
III. Title.
[DNLM: 1. Crohn Disease – surgery. 2. Colitis, Ulcerative – surgery. WI 512 K96s 1993]
RD541.K85 1993
617.5'541059–dc20
DNLM/DLC
for Library of Congress 93-4186
CIP

Typeset by Expo Holdings Sdn. Bhd.
12/3830-543210 Printed on acid-free paper

Foreword

As with most chronic diseases having a low mortality but high morbidity, the inflammatory bowel diseases (IBD) are distressing for patients and for their physicians. The frustrations and fears of our patients should be readily understood, though they are perhaps not as well appreciated by doctors as they should be. My own training in IBD was with W.E. King and "Bill" Hughes in Melbourne, Avery Jones in London and in the Mayo model of J. Arnold Bargen; these teachers impressed upon me that patients with ulcerative colitis and Crohn's disease deserve and require special education as to the nature of their illnesses, and that the expectations, options and uncertainties of their diseases must be addressed. Though lay organizations have done much to address these concerns, my experience in consultative practice has been disappointing. Too often, patients have been given little or no appreciation of the relative roles of medical as against surgical management or they have unrealistic expectations of one form of therapy versus the other.

As doctors, we all share the responsibility. Medical gastroenterologists appear at times to regard the surgical options of IBD as impugning their therapeutic skills, and to interpret these as indicating their failure as "medicine men". One has seen many errors of judgement based on this false tenet; in the right patient, at the right time, surgery for ulcerative colitis and Crohn's disease is imperative! Certainly, ill-judged or excessive surgery has also created many intestinal cripples. A useful philosophy might be that those with IBD should have an aggressive and secure gastroenterologist and a thoughtful and conservative surgeon!

Concepts of the IBDs are currently undergoing much change. Crohn's disease, which was once considered almost as a malignant equivalent – "let us remove all the disease, even by radical excision" – is now accepted as a pathological condition that can involve the gut from mouth to anus. We now accept the inevitability of its expression and, thanks in large measure to John Alexander-Williams, the medico-surgical philosophy has changed. Surgery will never be curative, and operative philosophies need to be focused on specific indications and expectations. To move to ulcerative colitis: it is thanks largely to Nils Kock, Alan Parks and others, that the less attractive consequences of proctocolectomy have been addressed and, in part, corrected. Surgical treatment of stubborn colitis is much better accepted by patients and doctors; the sphincter-saving operations have altered our thinking dramatically. We may even be seeing a swing of the pendulum to the other extreme – perhaps the ileo-anal anastomosis offers too easy a "fix" for colitis. Patients are now often referred too soon for colectomy; patients, that is, with maximal symptoms and minimal disease. These are individuals unable to deal with the symptoms of the disease and sometimes unwilling to deal with the consequences of colectomy, even after successful pouch procedures. Thus, even though better medical options may be offered by 5-ASA and cortico-steroids without major systemic side effects and even though the more rational surgical options engender optimism, we all know that the IBDs still represent major dilemmas.

This monograph therefore is timely, and both authors are well placed to evaluate the current and future practice of surgery in IBD. John Alexander-Williams brought continued fame to the chair he inherited from his mentor, Bryan Brooke. He has been acclaimed for three decades as a teacher, by gastroenterologists and fellow surgeons alike. Devinder Kumar is also a physician's surgeon, his extensive training and record in gastrointestinal physiology is well suited to a surgical discipline that alters so dramatically the overall functions of the gut.

Until major etiological breakthroughs enable us to prevent or cure the (probable) multiple forms of inflammatory bowel disease, surgical intervention will be needed. In the interim, we must apply the surgical arts rationally, conservatively and wisely. This text examines the options and provides much for further thought. We should read and think seriously about all that is written here.

Gastroenterology Unit
Mayo Clinic
Rochester, MN, USA

Sidney F. Phillips, MD

Preface

Since the 1940s the Birmingham School, where medical/surgical collaboration has always been strong, has been in the forefront of the treatment of inflammatory bowel disease. We have been privileged to practise in a tertiary referral centre to which many complex intestinal problems have been referred.

We decided to collaborate to produce this book for a variety of reasons. We came to work together as colleagues in Birmingham when one of us was coming to the end of his surgical career and the other was just beginning. The senior author was completing over 30 years' experience in the surgical management of Crohn's disease and the other was on the threshold of a specialist career in colorectal surgery having had a background of clinical and research experience in colorectal physiology. We were each impressed by what the other had to offer from the opposite ends of their surgical careers. We also had in common our research training in Minnesota, USA.

We have aimed the presentation at a wide audience. We feel that this book will interest specialist colorectal surgeons who will wish to compare our technique and results with their own. In addition, surgical trainees will find a comprehensive description of the rationale for, as well as technique and results of, an operative approach based on a sound pathophysiological basis. Furthermore, the book has important messages for our medical gastroenterologist colleagues, who should understand the rationale behind the essential surgical approaches to these diseases and also learn from us what they can reasonably expect from their surgical collaborators.

Medico-surgical collaboration is the very essence of these diseases whose cause is still elusive and whose natural history is still little influenced by medical manipulation. Both Crohn's disease and ulcerative colitis are conditions in which surgical intervention does nothing to alter the natural history, but simply alleviates the discomfort and distress of the inevitable complications.

The section on ulcerative colitis bases its approach firmly on the study of the physiology of the large bowel, particularly the physiology of defaecation. It is based also on the careful assessment of the patient with a view to predicting the outcome of surgical intervention. There is particular emphasis on predicting the likelihood of malignant change and the chances of a successful outcome after sphincter-saving surgery. It appropriately concludes with precise details of our techniques for performing the different surgical options of panproctocolectomy, ileo-rectal anastomosis and the continent ileo-anal pouch.

The section on Crohn's disease is based on an understanding of the pathophysiological progression of the disease with a natural history that is relentless, although often intermittent. The role of surgical intervention is simply to overcome the consequences of the fibrotic stenoses that follow chronic gut ulceration. We stress the detection and management of these stenoses, preferably before they lead to complications such as abscess and fistula. The essential theme throughout the management of Crohn's disease of the small bowel, large bowel and ano-rectum is one of timely intervention and a conservative operative approach. As we anticipate that many of the chapters will be referred to in isolation when advice is sought about a problem case, we have deliberately repeated some of the technical advice and even some of the illustrations.

We feel a compelling need to record what we have learned about these fascinating diseases. At the same time, we are conscious that the details of the various management options are constantly changing, yet feel that, until the underlying cause is found and can be eradicated, the present principles of management will prevail.

Birmingham 1993

D. Kumar
J. Alexander-Williams

Acknowledgement

Permission to reproduce MRI pictures
Department of Surgery, Tuebingen

Contents

Section III

Section I

1 History

J. Alexander-Williams

The history of Crohn's disease

The disease up to 1932

Although it was the workers from the Mount Sinai Hospital in New York who put the disease that we now call Crohn's disease on the medical map, others had clearly recognised its occurrence as a distinct disease entity for at least a century before the most quoted paper of Crohn et al. (1932). Historical surveys have revealed descriptions of apparent cases of Crohn's disease going back as far as Morgagni in 1769. In 1813 Coombe and Saunders reported the clinical history and autopsy finding in a young man who died of intestinal obstruction after many years of abdominal pain; the distal ileum was described as thickened and narrowed. In 1828 Abercrombie described a similar case and, according to Kirsner (1991), later in the same century, Moore in 1882 and Fenwick in 1889 produced further single case reports. Fenwick's patient was a young female who had an intestinal fistula complicating a stenosis. An often quoted but little read paper by Lesniowski (1904) was written in Polish and not apparently cited in English language reviews until it was quoted by Lindhargen in 1982. The English-speaking world however cannot really be forgiven for disregarding the paper by Dalziel published in the *British Medical Journal* of 1913. Dalziel described nine cases, the first one of which was a doctor who was operated on in 1901 (Fig. 1.1). Of the nine cases, six almost certainly had what we now call Crohn's disease. In Dalziel's paper the macroscopical appearance of the distal ileum was graphically described as "an eel in a state of rigor mortis".

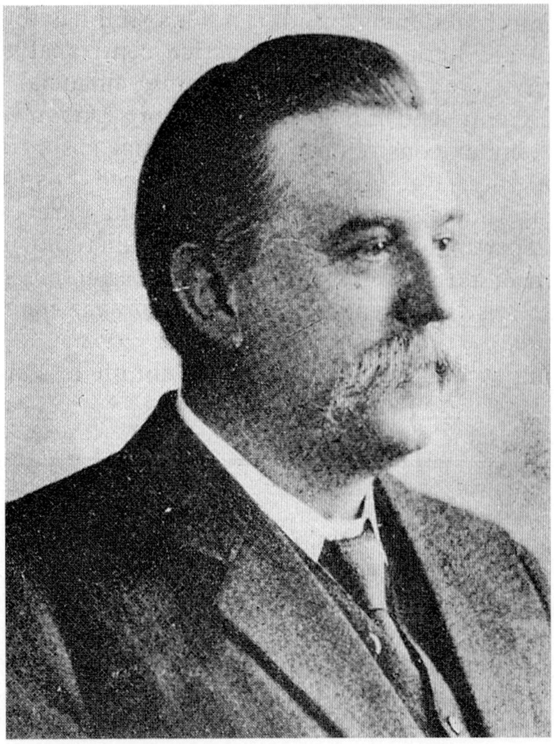

Fig. 1.1. Mr. (later Sir) T. Kennedy Dalziel. A surgeon from Glasgow, Scotland.

In an overview entitled *The road to Crohn's disease,* Janowitz (1985) quoted Wilks and Moxon who produced a textbook and lectures of pathological anatomy in 1875 in which they describe the case of a young man with a lesion of the ileum that was so narrow that a quill could not be passed through it. Janowitz also states that Braum described several cases of non-specific enteritis.

In the Netherlands a thesis by De Groot written in Dutch described three cases of stenotic lesions of the small intestine in which tubercle bacilli and spirochetes were excluded (van Coevorden 1989). At operation this patient showed dilatation proximal to two stenotic areas in the terminal ileum. The mesentery was thickened and encroached on the ileal wall. There were nodules like tuberculosis on the serosa and the ileal wall was rigid and the mucosa ulcerated. Microscopically the inflammation was transmural with lymphocytes and plasma cells, gross fibrosis and giant cells.

It was in 1932 that there occurred what Janowitz (1985) described as a "quantum leap" with the presentation of two papers from the group of physicians, surgeons and pathologists from Mount Sinai Hospital. Even before then the pathologists Willenski and Moschowitz (Janowitz 1985) had reported granulomatous lesions of the small bowel. These had been found in the patients that were to make up the 14 patient series presented to two learned societies in the United States. In 1932 Ginsberg and Oppenheimer presented a paper to the American Gastroenterological Association entitled "Non-specific granulomata of the intestines (inflammatory tumor and strictures of the bowel)" which was later published in 1933 in the *Annals of Surgery*. In the same month Crohn presented a paper by himself and Drs Oppenheimer and Ginsberg to the American Medical Association. In its original presentation the paper by Crohn and his colleagues referred only to localised ileitis which they called "terminal ileitis". However, during the discussion Dr. Bargen from the Mayo Clinic suggested that the term terminal ileitis had agonal connotations and suggested that the term regional ileitis would be more appropriate and such was the title when the classic paper was first published in the same year in the *Journal of the American Medical Association* (Crohn et al. 1932).

Even before this paper was published, the Dutch medical literature carried a paper by Nuboer (1932) describing two patients with chronic phlegmonous ileitis, a condition that was obviously the same as that described by Crohn and his colleagues later in the same year.

1932 onwards: which part of the gut is affected?

Although the work of Ginsberg and Oppenheimer, finally published in 1933, had been concerned with a total of 52 cases presenting with abdominal masses and obstruction, all of whom they felt had been described erroneously as tuberculosis or carcinoma, the 1932 paper by Crohn, Oppenheimer and Ginsberg concentrated only on those 14 cases from the same series that affected the terminal ileum. This paper concentrated people's minds on the concept of a specific terminal ileal disease.

Ginsberg and Oppenheimer's larger series had included cases of sealed-off perforations of the bowel, strictures secondary to ischaemic disease and hypertrophic ulcerative stenosis with skip lesions. They also described a fourth group of patients with what they called localised hypertrophic colitis. Ginsberg later presented radiographic evidence in films taken in 1925 showing obvious granulomatous disease of the right side of the colon.

Even before the classic 1932 paper, pathologists under Dr. Paul Klemperer at the Mount Sinai Hospital had recognised that this same non-tuberculous, non-caseating granulomatous disease could affect several parts of the intestine (Janowitz 1985). It is perhaps surprising, therefore, that it took so many years before the disease, as we now recognise it, was acknowledged as affecting all parts of the alimentary tract. The recognition of chronic granulomatous ulcerative disease of the colon masquerading as carcinoma or tuberculosis but pathologically distinct from them is attributed to Moynihan (1907) and Mayo-Robson (1908) both from Leeds. Obviously the Mount Sinai pathologists had recognised the colonic involvement in the 1920s but it was 1934 before Dr. Colp, a surgeon of that institution, described the disease affecting the colon. In 1933 Harris and colleagues had described a similar granulomatous disease affecting the duodenum and had suggested that the name should be changed from regional ileitis to regional enteritis, while in 1934 Brown and his colleagues recognised that the disease could occur throughout the alimentary tract. In 1936 Crohn and Rosenak described nine cases in which regional enteritis was associated with a chronic granulomatous disease of the colon. They felt that the disease in the colon was a form of ulcerative colitis and that its association with regional enteritis was interesting and possibly coincidental.

The disease was recognised as affecting the stomach by Bartstra and Kooreman (1939), the oesophagus by Maden and his colleagues in 1969 and the duodenum by our unit (Fielding 1985). In the 1970s many investigators were using the new discovery of the Crosby capsule to obtain mucosal biopsies from throughout the alimentary tract. They used it to investigate the mucosa in patients who apparently had a localised area only affected by Crohn's disease. It was found that, in these patients, some histological abnormality could be detected in the. mouth, oesophagus, stomach, duodenum, jejunum and in the rectum and anus. It was recognised that the disease was pan-intestinal in its manifestations. It even occurred in the mouth and pharynx (Croft and Wilkinson 1972; Basu and Asquith 1980; Sculley et al. 1982).

Although it is relatively easy to understand the pathology of a disease that affects any part of the alimentary tract, it becomes difficult to understand when manifestations of the disease appear to occur outside the mucous membrane of the alimentary tract. Typical histological manifestations of the disease have been described in the submammary skin (Mountain 1970), the umbilical skin (Phillips and Glazer 1981) and even in the scrotum and prepuce (Atherton et al. 1978). These cutaneous and subcutaneous manifestations became known as metastatic Crohn's disease, so making it even more difficult to fit the various propounded theories of aetiology. It has been estimated that the overall frequencies of extra intestinal manifestations is about 35% (Present 1983) occurring principally in the joints, skin, eye and mouth.

What are we to call the disease?

As we have seen Crohn, Oppenheimer and Ginsberg originally wanted to call the disease they were describing "terminal ileitis" but this was soon changed to "regional ileitis", only to be changed to "regional enteritis" once it was realised that other parts of the small bowel could be affected (Fig. 1.2). It is now still known as regional enteritis in much of the United States. Serious problems of nomenclature arose when other parts of the alimentary tract were seen to be affected; initially purely anatomical names were used to describe the depth of penetration of the inflammation such as "transmural colitis" or terms that described some of the characteristic histological manifestations, such as "granulomatous colitis". As it became clear that these alimentary manifestations as well as many of the extra alimentary manifestations such as in the joints and skin and eyes were all part of the same disease, some sort of global terminology was required; accepting the fact that it was still a disease of unknown aetiology. In Europe and in

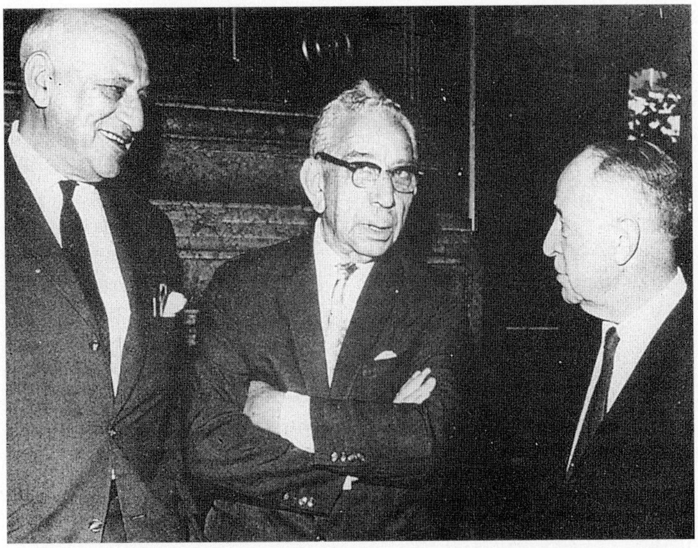

Fig. 1.2. Drs. Oppenheimer, Crohn and Ginsberg.

Scandinavia the term Crohn's disease was accepted quite readily, as most physicians accepted the 1932 Mount Sinai paper as the classical description of the disease. The physicians in the United States were much less ready to accept this eponymous name, principally because it was realised that this was not a disease discovered by Dr. Crohn. He was first author of a paper done, principally, at the Mount Sinai Hospital by a group of distinguished physicians, surgeons and pathologists. American physicians in general and those from Mount Sinai in particular considered that it would be invidious to single out one name to describe a disease that would perhaps have better been termed "Berg's disease", "Klemperer's disease" or "The Mount Sinai disease".

In the English language we accept what can be termed the law of common usage. Whenever a word is commonly used by a body of people communicating in that language and when the word is well understood without ambiguity then that word becomes accepted. Eventually, after what could be described as a "decent interval", it becomes incorporated in the standard dictionaries of the English language. According to the law of common usage, it appears that after 50 years have passed and after the death of Dr. Burrell Crohn it would be reasonable to accept the term Crohn's disease, at least until such time as the aetiology of the disease is known. For this reason in this chapter, as in most other current English language contributions, the term Crohn's disease will be used.

Crohn had collected his 14 resected cases of ileitis with his surgical colleague Dr. A.A. Berg. Crohn presented his paper at the New Orleans meeting of the American Medical Association, Berg having modestly declined to include his name in favour of his younger staff members. The fact that many different terms are used to describe the disease suggests that no-one is ideal, which is probably why the eponymous term Crohn's disease is still the most popular. Granulomatous enteritis or colitis seems to be attractive pathologically but in 25% to 40% of cases granulomata cannot be demonstrated. Regional or segmental can be a misleading term as many cases have the whole of the colon involved and many others simply isolate one segment of the terminal ileum. Transmural colitis seemed a useful term to differentiate Crohn's colitis from mucosal ulcerative colitis; however, severe ulcerative colitis can affect all layers of the gut.

Milestones in medical management

Medical management is considered in detail in Chapter 2. It is summarised here from an historical perspective seen through surgical eyes. Before and around 1932 the disease was studied rather than treated; the only definitive treatment at that time was surgical. Medical management consisted of what was euphemistically called general management. It usually consisted of bed rest, nourishing high protein, liquid or semi-solid diet and replacement of any specific detected deficiencies such as those of iron, vitamin B_{12} and folic acid.

It was not until the early 1940s that sulphasalazine was used on an entirely empirical basis. In the mid-1970s it was determined that the active ingredient of sulphasalazine was 5-aminosalicylic acid (5-ASA) and at about the same time controlled trials began to be used in the elucidation of its place in the management of Crohn's disease.

Cortico-steroids were first used in the management of Crohn's disease in the 1950s but there are few clinical trials and almost as many people condemned the drug as advocated it. The gastroenterologist Dr. W. Trevor Cooke who was the leading force in the management of inflammatory bowel disease was an eloquent if dogmatic critic of steroid therapy. He was largely responsible for directing so many patients towards early surgical therapy when fashion dictated that prolonged steroid therapy should be tried and surgery only used as a last desperate resort (Allan et al. 1977) (Fig 1.3).

Case reports of the use of immunosuppressive agents such as 6-mercaptopurine and azathioprine appeared in the late 1960s and early 1970s and by the late 1970s a few controlled clinical trials showed some significant benefit from immunosuppressive therapy. Since then cyclosporin A and disodium cromoglycate have been introduced, tried and found to be of limited use (Lennard-Jones 1990).

Antibiotics have been used in the management of Crohn's disease from the time of their discovery, particularly to treat the septic complications. Many physicians were using broad spectrum antibiotics in 1960 and some were reporting early improvement. However, long-term benefit was not reported until the introduction of metronidazole to the antimicrobial armamentarium (Gitnick 1991).

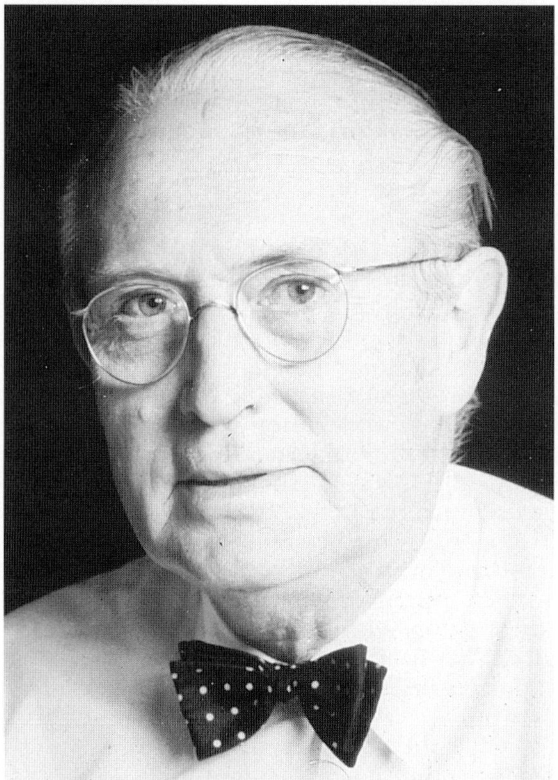

Fig. 1.3. Dr. W. Trevor Cooke, gastroenterologist and founder of the inflammatory bowel disease unit at the Birmingham General Hospital.

Milestones in surgical management

Dalziel (1913) treated chronic inflammatory disease of the terminal ileum by resection as did Dr. A.A. Berg, the pioneer surgeon working with the team at Mount Sinai Hospital, New York. It soon became clear that the serious complications of terminal ileal Crohn's disease such as fistula and abscess were too complicated to be treated by simple surgical excision and in the early series of patients from Mount Sinai Hospital a mortality of 16% led to the concept of bypass rather than excision for complicated phlegmonous masses (Garlock & Crohn 1945). The principal advantage of bypass over excision was lower operative risk; however, after improvements in anaesthesia and pre- and post-operative management the surgical mortality was reduced and resection once again began to regain favour, particularly because the disease can still progress in the bypassed segment and lead to complications such as fistula, abscess or perforation. (Greenstein et al. 1974) with frequent reoperations. (Krause et al. 1971; Alexander-Williams et al. 1972).

In the 1940s the Mount Sinai Hospital surgeons, realising that the disease continues in the bypassed segment, advocated bypass with exclusion whereby the distal end of the ileum just short of the diseased segment was either brought out as a mucus fistula or closed. The dangers of closing it were that pressure could build up proximal to the remaining obstruction and, in some instances, perforation occurred. The principal reasons for the abandonment of bypass as a method of treating complicated terminal ileal Crohn's disease was the finding of carcinoma by Lightdale et al. (1975) and Greenstein et al. (1978). Both these reports showed a very high incidence of terminal ileal carcinoma occurring in bypassed Crohn's disease. For this reason bypass was largely abandoned, apart from the treatment of stenosing duodenal Crohn's disease.

With the return to resection there were many surgeons who took the original advice of Crohn and resected widely, removing all macroscopically diseased tissue with a wide excision of the root of the mesentery and all involved lymph nodes. Many of these surgeons advocated removal of 20–30 cm of normal bowel on either side of the lesion. Later reports showed that there was no great advantage of wide excision and always a high risk of recurrence. Surgeons then moved towards minimal excision (see Chapter 12). By the 1980s many of the stenotic small bowel lesions were being treated by strictureplasty and in recent years some of them even by dilatation without excision or operation.

The history of ulcerative colitis

Historians cannot resist the temptation to attribute diseases that have been recognised as specific only in modern times to some great historical writer. Obviously it is only those who have written most and whose works have been preserved who are most likely to be attributable. Although the disease of chronic mucosal ulcerative colitis can only have been differentiated from acute infectious colitis towards the end of the 19th century, once bacteriology was sufficient of a science to identify specific causes. Nevertheless in the writings of many of our past medical heroes can be found accounts that would do reasonably well for descriptions of chronic ulcerative colitis. These include Hippocrates of Cos, Aretaeus of Cappadocia and Soranus of Ephesus who between the years of 640 BC and AD 170 described the clinical details of those who suffered from one of other cause of chronic diarrhoea; usually with blood and an ulcerated bowel. Then came the Dark Ages and it was not until the 17th century that written descriptions of diarrhoea or dysenteric diseases were again recorded in graphic detail. It is possible, though never can it be proved that the "bloody flux", described by Sydenham in 1669 was the ulcerative colitis that we know today (Hawkins 1990; Kirsner 1991).

The end of the 19th century

Until recently it has been fashionable to attribute the first "modern" description of ulcerative colitis to Sir Samuel Wilks who wrote a letter to the *Medical Times and Gazette* in 1895; he refers to a death from idiopathic dysentery and suggested that the ulcerated bowel was caused by an abortifaciant. This opinion, when expressed in the criminal court, almost resulted in Dr. Thomas Smethurst MD being hanged for the murder of his mistress Isabella Banks. However, as Professor John Fielding of Dublin argued so convincingly in the *British Medical Journal* in 1985, Wilks was almost certainly describing a case of Crohn's disease rather than either ulcerative colitis or homicide. Miss Banks died in early pregnancy after a short illness. Wilks describes the autopsy as follows: "The intestines lay in a coil adherent by a thin layer of lymph indicative of recent inflammation; the ileum was inflamed for three feet from the ileo-caecal valve though otherwise the small intestine looked normal. The large intestine was ulcerated from end to end with ulcers of various sizes mostly *isolated* – though some had run together ... Inflammation was most marked at the proximal colon and the caecum appeared to be sloughing causing the peritonitis. Tuberculosis was excluded".

It was later that Wilks, writing this time with Walter Moxon (Wilks and Moxon 1875) in *Lectures on pathological anatomy*, made the first distinction of ulcerative colitis from specific forms of dysentery. His observations are astute and the arguments persuasive although there are little or no hard data with which they can be verified. In those days a doctor's reputation was based more on the quality of his prose and style rather than on scientifically verifiable data. It is easy to see how Wilks attracted the reader's attention when he wrote "the term colitis is sometimes used as though synonymous with dysentery. Our usual language has indeed been too indefinite, nay, incorrect, in speaking of all affections of the large intestine as dysenteric ... there is quite as much reason to regard febrile epidemic dysentery as a disease distinct from simple ulcerative colitis as there is to regard febrile epidemic diphtheria as a disease distinct from croup ...". It was perhaps unwise of him to have coined the phrase "simple ulcerative colitis" as most of the data were from patients coming to autopsy. Wilks and Moxon describe a severe, highly vascular inflammation of the entire colon with scattered minute points of ulceration in a young woman who died after experiencing severe bloody and mucoid diarrhoea.

S.O. Habershon writing in *Diseases of the abdomen*, published in London in 1862, was probably the first to describe intestinal pseudo-polyps in ulcerative colitis. He wrote "in the third stage we find ulceration, sometimes merely as minute circular ulcers but generally of a more extensive character; the ulcers are often oval in form, and based in the transverse axis of the intestine, and their edges are raised and injected, irregular and undermined; and their base is formed by the cellular or muscular coats. These ulcerations gradually extend so as to coalesce till at last nearly the whole of the mucous surface is destroyed, except here and there prominent isolated portions which become intensely congested, and resemble polypoid growths". Sir William Allchin (1885) from the Westminster Hospital in London reported on the autopsy of a young woman who died after an acute illness following her fifth confinement, and described gross ulceration of mucosa of the colon. Allchin comments she experienced relatively little pain, an observation that we can confirm today in patients with fulminant ulcerative colitis. In discussion he states "it is to be regretted that the term dysentery is not restricted to the true tropical malady and it should not at once be applied in an adjective form to any diarrhoea dependent upon ulceration of the colon when the factors for the production of the specific disease are, as far as can be recongised, wanting".

As was so common in the 19th century, serious diseases tended only to be described by pathologists and cogitated over by physicians. However, at the end of the 19th century we see the first surgical "break-through". It probably was that great surgical pioneer from Leeds, A.W. Mayo-Robson who performed the first definitive operation for ulceration. He created a temporary colostomy in 1893. The colitis was then treated, we know not how, and the colostomy later closed (Kirsner 1991).

The first half of the 20th century

With the increasing use of anaesthesia, antisepsis and asepsis it is not surprising that this new century heralded the entry of surgeons into the management of colitis. In 1909 J.P. Lockhart-Mummery described the use of sigmoidoscopy in ulcerative colitis and emphasised its value in the detection of large bowel cancer. In the same year there was a major symposium at the Royal Society of Medicine (1909) in London based on the collected findings from 307 patients observed between 1888 and 1907. Most of the cases reported were from autopsy reports with death occurring from colonic perforation, peritonitis, haemorrhage or sepsis. An important part of the discussion at this symposium concerned the possible value of surgical intervention. J.P. Lockhart-Mummery said that "the choice of operation lay between caecostomy and appendicostomy" whereas G.H. Makins expressed a preference for colostomy rather than appendicostomy. One of the other contributors to the symposium was H.P. Hawkins from St. Thomas' Hospital who wrote a separate article in the *British Medical Journal* in 1909 reporting patients treated with either colostomy or ileostomy. The problem with all surgical intervention in the early decades of the 20th century was that there were no stoma appliances to prevent skin excoriation. Nor did they appreciate that the exposed serosa of the gut would soon be covered in granulation tissue which would heal by fibrosis until it produced unmanageable stenosis.

At the Paris Congress of Medicine in 1913 there was another discussion on ulcerative colitis. It was largely a regurgitation of the ideas expressed four years earlier in London. However, in the same year J.Y. Brown of the United States proposed the operation of ileostomy "to rest the bowel" and allow its healing, as had been recommended by the British physicians earlier. This therapeutic approach was adopted briefly in the United States in the 1930s and soon discarded. It is not surprising that in those days surgical intervention had a bad name, it was regarded as "last ditch therapy"; the effects of the operation usually being considered worse than those of the disease. Therefore, it is not surprising that the first half of the 20th century saw an almost unlimited expansion of ingenious therapeutic regimens from diet to immune stimulation with hardly a mention of operation (Kirsner 1991).

The psychogenic basis for ulcerative colitis was proposed by a medical student C.D. Murray (1930). It rapidly gained favour and in the subsequent decades many patients were treated by psychotherapy and psychoanalysis. Sadly the approach was of little therapeutic benefit.

Despite what Brown (1913) had written, the early surgical procedures such as appendicostomy, caecostomy and colostomy were performed more to allow proximal installation of topical antiseptic agents than to "rest the bowel". Many litres of antibacterial solutions such as potassium permanganate and hypochloride were instilled to little effect. In hardly any patient was the success of Mayo-Robson's patient repeated. It was not until Koernig developed an adhesive rubber bag that the era of a successful permanent ileostomy arrived. Koernig was a chemistry student who had ileostomy for ulcerative colitis under the care of Dr. A.A. Strauss. Koernig was encouraged to create a rubber bag, cemented to the skin closely around the stoma to prevent contact between the intestinal effluent and skin. He eventually developed a cement that, in most patients, was relatively non-irritant. Largely as a result of this petrochemical breakthrough, Strauss and Strauss (1944) were able to publish 104 cases of ileostomy. In the following year Clarence Dennis (1945), working in Minneapolis with Wangensteen, emphasised the need for colectomy at the same time as ileostomy.

However, the world was still waiting for a manageable ileostomy stoma to be invented. The stomas at that time were either flush with the skin and had constant leakage onto the surrounding skin or were brought out as a spout but with exposed serosa with the disastrous consequences already described.

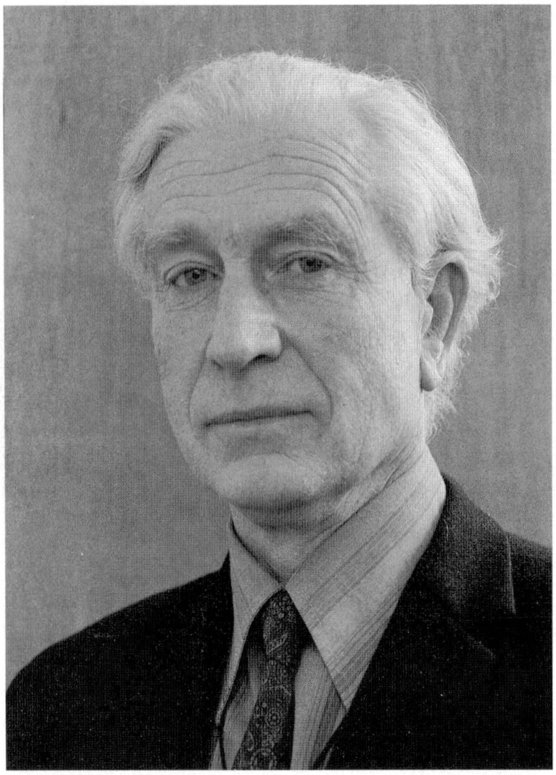

Fig. 1.4. Bryan N. Brooke. Emeritus Professor of Surgery, St. George's Hospital, London. Senior Lecture in Surgery, Birmingham University in the late 1940s when he perfected his ileostomy eversion.

At this time Lionel Hardy, the Professor of Gastroenterology at the University of Birmingham read with interest about the revolutionary rubber bags from the United States but despite all his charm and persuasion, was unable to obtain them for use on his patients. Therefore with the help of Dr. Clifford Hawkins and the research department at Fort Dunlop in Birmingham, they developed a bag similar to that of Koernig, stuck to the skin with a similar latex solution (Hawkins 1990). The conditions were then right to be exploited by the inventive genius of Bryan Brooke, then a young academic surgeon working closely with Hardy and Hawkins. He invented what is still known around the world as the "Brooke Ileostomy". Brooke's concepts were that:

1. If mucocutaneous apposition could be achieved there would be no granulation tissue to contract
2. If the mucosa of the ileum was everted, like a prepuce there would be a spout of ileum that could fit into the newly invented rubber bag.

Independently and at the same time Rupert Turnbull at the Cleveland Clinic in the United States developed the same hypothesis about the abolition of granulation tissue and a spout but he solved it by means of skin grafting the serosal aspect of the ileostomy. These two surgeons, Brooke and Turnbull, life-long friends and collaborators, are jointly credited with the birth of the era of successful permanent and ileostomy. It is, however, Brooke's technique of eversion that persists today, hence it is appropriate that it should be termed the "Brooke ileostomy". (Brooke 1952; Brooke 1954) (Fig. 1.4).

The second half of the 20th century

Since 1950 the modern history of surgical intervention in ulcerative colitis developed along three lines:

1. The perfection of the formation of an end ileostomy
2. The definition of the indications for and limitations of an ileo-rectal anastomosis
3. The endeavours to create a continent ileostomy by making a small bowel pouch as a neo-rectum and making it continent either with an inverted nipple valve or anastomosis to the anus with preservation or re-creation of a functioning anal sphincter.

End ileostomy

The original Brooke ileostomies, as he taught us to make them, were sited just outside the lateral edge of rectus abdominus muscle and were sufficiently long to be able to dangle into the large black rubber bags that were then the only relatively odour-free appliances. It was soon realised that ileostomy prolapse or retraction was common unless the stoma was brought out through the separated muscle fibres of the rectus abdominus. It was also soon realised that long stomas were both unsightly and easily traumatised. With the development of light odour-proof plastic bags and small effective seals to the skin it was no longer necessary to have a long spout and this was gradually replaced by the modern "bud" or "button" rarely more than 2 cm long. This refinement of the end ileostomy combined with proctocolectomy is arguably the most trouble-free surgical solution to dangerous or incapacitating chronic mucosal ulcerative colitis.

Ileo-rectal anastomosis

Because ulcerative colitis commonly begins in and predominantly affects the rectum it is rarely possible to salvage a functioning rectum if the colitis is sufficiently severe to warrant colectomy. However, there is a small proportion of cases (in our series under 10%) in which there is absolute or relative rectal sparing. It was Stanley Aylett in the 1950s who was the advocate of ileo-rectal anastomosis in Great Britain (Aylett 1960). He eventually accumulated over 300 cases of diffuse ulcerative colitis treated by total colectomy and ileo-rectal anastomosis (Aylett 1966, 1971).

Until the recent improvements in function following restorative proctocolectomy, ileo-rectal anastomosis had many advocates as it had a number of obvious advantages over the alternative of end ileostomy; however, it was not without its risks of anastomotic dehiscence post-operative intestinal obstruction (Jones et al. 1977) and risk of carcinoma developing in the residual rectal stump of about 5% at 20 years (Baker et al. 1978; Williams and Johnston 1985).

Continent ileostomy with abdominal stoma

It is Neils Koch who is the acknowledged pioneer of the continent abdominal pouch that usually bears his name. His work, pioneered in Gothenburg and developed during a sabbatical year in Zurich, was widely adopted until it was gradually replaced with restorative protocolectomy when pouch to anus anastomosis was developed. It is described further in the chapters on ulcerative colitis, where its complications and advantages and disadvantages are detailed (Koch 1969).

Ileo-anal anastomosis

Owen Wangensteen of Minneopolis (Fig. 1.5) is usually credited with the first ileo-anal anastomosis (Wangensteen 1943) although the result was so bad that it was revised to an ileostomy within weeks. Best (1948) and Goligher (1951) tried and abandoned the operation because of the high incidence of frequency, urgency and nocturnal incontinence. Even those moved to advocate the operation reported satisfactory function in less than 50% of patients (Devine and Webb 1951; Schneider 1955).

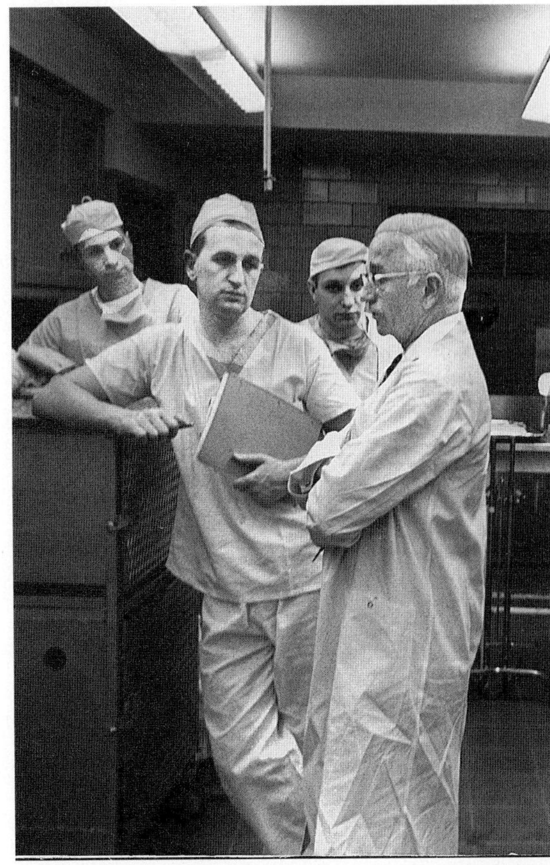

Fig. 1.5. John Alexander-Williams (holding folder) listening, possibly with ill-disguised boredom, to the words of wisdom of Owen H. Wangensteen in the experimental laboratories at the University of Minnesota in 1959.

The first serious attempt to preserve the anal sphincter was made by separating the diseased mucosa from the muscle of the preserved upper anal canal. After successful experiments in dogs, Ravitch (1948) reported two young adults who were said to be continent and able to discriminate flatus from faeces. It has only been in children and young adults that the operation of "straight" ileo-anal anastomosis has had any success and even in the young has now largely been superseded by the pouch.

The concept of a total excision of the large bowel mucosa, the creation of large reservoir pouch that is anastomosed close to the anal verge is an operation that evolved rather than was invented. Many names have been associated with its early evolution, names frequently cited and all worthy of recognition include Ravitch (1948), Valiente and Bacon (1955), Peck and Allenbeck (1964) Glotzer and Phil (1969), Koch (1969); Fonkalsrud and Ament (1978); however, in the United Kingdom the credit is usually attributed to Parks and Nicholls (1978), whereas in Japan Utsunomiya and colleagues (1986) were the first major players in the field. Details of development and operative techniques are to be found in the section under ulcerative colitis.

References

Abercombie J (1828) Pathological and practical reseraches on disease of the stomach, the intestinal canal, the liver and other viscera of the abdomen. Waugh and Innes, Edinburgh

Alexander-Williams J (1972) Surgery and the management of Crohn's disease. Clin Gastroenterol 1:469

Allan R, Steinberg DM, Alexander-Williams J, Cooke WT (1977) Crohn's disease involving the colon: an audit of clinical management. Gastroenterology 73:723–

Allchin WH (1885) Case of acute extensive ulceration of the colon. Trans Pathol Soc Lond 37:199–202

Atherton DJ, Massam M, Wells RS, Harries JT, Pincott TR (1978) Genital Crohn's disease in a 6-year-old boy. Br Med J iv:552

Aylett SO (1960) Diffuse ulcerative colitis and its treatment by ileorectal anastomosis. Ann R Coll Surg Engl 27:260–265

Aylett SO (1966) Three hundred cases of diffuse ulcerative colitis treatment by total colectomy and ileorectal anastomosis. Br Med J i:1001–1005

Aylett SO Ileorectal anastomosis: review 1952 (1968). Proc R Soc Med 64:967–971

Baker WNW, Glass RE. Ritchie JK, Aylett SO (1978) Cancer o the rectum following colectomy and ileorectal anastomosis for ulcerative colitis. Br J Surg 65:862–868

Bartstra DS, Kooreman PJ (1939) Peculiar localisation of so-called regional ileitis. Ned Tijdschr v Gen 83:2069–2072

Basu MK, Asquith P (1980) Oral manifestation of inflammatory bowel disease. Clin Gastroenterol 65:390–397

Best RR (1948) Anastomosis of the ileum to the lower part of the rectum and anus. A reporrt on experience with ileorectostomy and ileoproctostomy with special reference to polyposis. Arch Surg 57:276–285

Brooke BN (1952) The management of an ileostomy including its complications. Lancet ii:102–104

Brooke BN (1954) Ulcerative colitis and its surgical treatment. Livingstone, Edinburgh

Brooke BN, Cave Dr, Kind DW (1976) Place of azathioprine for Crohn's disease. Lancet i:1041–1042

Brown JY (1913) The value of complete physiological rest of the large bowel in the treatment of obstructive lesions of this organ, with description of operative technique and report of cases. Surg Gynecol Obstet 16:610–613

Colp R (1934) Case of nonspecific granuloma of terminal ileum and cecum. Surg Clin North Am 14:443–449

Coombe C, Saunders W (1813) A singular case of stricture and thickening of the ileum. Med Trans Coll Physicians Lond 4:16–18

Croft CB, Wilkinson AR (1972) Ulceration of the mouth, pharynx and larynx in Crohn's disease of the intestine. Br J Surg 59:249–252

Crohn BB, Ginsberg L, Oppenheimer GD (1932) Regional ileitis: a pathologic and clinical entity. JAMA 99:1323–1329

Crohn BB, Rosenak BD (1936) A combined form of ileitis and colitis. JAMA 106:1

Dalziel TK (1913) Chronic interstitial enteritis. Br Med J ii:1068–1070

Dennis C (1945) Ileostomy and colectomy in chronic ulcerative colitis. Surgery 18:435–452

Devine J, Webb R (1951) Resection of the rectal mucosa; colectomy and anal ileostomy with normal continence. Surg Gynecol Obstet 92:437–442

Fielding J (1985) Inflammatory bowel disease. Br Med J 290:47–48

Fonkalsrud EW, Ament ME (1978) Endorectal mucosal resection without protocolectomy as an adjunct for abdominoperineal resection for non-malignant conditions: clinical experience with five patients. Ann Surg 188:245–248

Garlock JH, Crohn BB (1945) An appraisal of the results of surgery in treatment of regional ileitis. JAMA 127:205–211

Gitnick G (1991) Inflammatory bowel disease: diagnosis and treatment. Igaku-Shoin, New York

Glotzer PG, Phil BG (1969) Preservation of continence after mucosal graft in the rectum and its feasibility in man. Am J Surg 117:403–409

Goligher JC (1951) The functional results after sphincter-saving resection of the rectum. Ann R Coll Surg Engl 8:421–439

Greenstein AJ, Kark AE, Dreiling DA (1974) Crohn's disease of the colon. I. Fistula in Crohn's disease of the colon, classification presenting features and management in 63 patients. Am J Gastroenterol 62:419

Greenstein AJ, Sachar D, Pucillo A (1978) Cancer in Crohn's disease after diversionary surgery. A report of seven carcinomas occurring in excluded bowel. Am J Surg 135: 86–90

Habershon SO (1862) Diseases of the abdomen, London, p 384

Harris FI, Bell GH, Brunn H (1933) Chronic cicatrizing enteritis. Surg Gynecol Obstet 57:637–645

Hawkins CFH (1990) Historical review. In Allan RN, Keighley MRB, Alexander-Williams J, Hawkins CF (eds) Inflammatory bowel diseases. Churchill Livingstone, Edinburgh

Hawkins HP (1909) Natural history of ulcerative colitis and its bearing on treatment. Br Med J i:765–770

Janowitz HD (1985) Inflammatory bowel disease. A personal view. Field, Rich and Associates, New York

Jones PF, Munro A, Ewen SWB (1977) Colectomy and ileorectal anastomosis for ulcerative colitis: report on a personal series with a critical review. Br J Surg 64:615–623

Kirsner JB (1991) Historical aspects in inflammatory bowel disease. J Clin Gastroenterol 10:286–297

Koch NG (1969) Intra-abdominal reservoir in patients with permanent ileostomy. Arch Surg 99:223–231

Krause KU, Bergman L, Norlen BJ (1971) Crohn's disease, a clinical study based on 186 patients. Scand J Gastroenterol 6:97–108

Lennard-Jones JE. Corticosteroids and immunosuppressive drugs in inflammatory bowel disease. In: Allan RN, Keighley MRB, Alexander-Williams J, Hawkins

CF (eds) Inflammatory bowel diseases. Churchill Livingstone, Edinburgh
Lesniowski A (1904) Towarzystwa lekarskiego II; 630
Lightdale CJ, Sternberg SS, Psner G, Sherlock P (1975) Carcinoma complicating Crohn's disease. Report of seven cases and review of the literature. Am J Med 59:262–268
Lockhart-Mummery JP (1909) In discussion on ulcerative colits. Proc R Soc (Medical Section) 2:92
Mayo-Robson AW (1908) Some abdominal tumours simulating malignant disease and their teatment. Br Med J i:425
Morgagni JB (1769) De sedibu et causis morborum. Remondini, Venice
Mountain JC (1970) Cutaneous ulceration in Crohn's disease. Gut 11:18
Moynihan BGA (1907) The mimicry of malignant disease in the large intestine. Edin Med J 21:228
Murray CD (1930) Psychogenic factors in etiology of ulcerative colitis and bloody diarrhoea. Am J Med Ser 180:239–248
Nuboer FJ (1932) Chronische phlegnone van hit ileum. Ned T Geneesk 76:2989
Parks AG, Nicholls RJ (1978) Proctocolectomy without ileostomy for ulcerative colitis. Br Med J ii:85–88
Peck PA, Allenbeck GA (1964) Fecal continence in the dog after replacement of rectal mucosa with ileal mucosa. Surg Gynecol Obstet 119:1312–1317.
Phillips RKS, Glazer G (1981) Metastatic Crohn's disease of the umbilicus. Br Med J 283:287
Present DH (1983) Crohn's disease; extraintestinal manifestations. Mount Sinai J Med 50:126–132
Ravitch MM (1948) Anal ileostomy with sphincter preservation in patients requiring total colectomy for benign conditions. Surgery 24:170–187
Royal Society of Medicine (1909) Symposium on ulcerative colitis. Proc R Soc Med 2:59–156
Sculley C. Cochran KM, Russell RI et al. (1982) Crohn's disease of the mouth: an indicator of intestinal involvement. Gut 23:198
Schneider S (1955) Anal ileostomy: experiences with a new three-stage procedure. Arch Surg 70:539–544
Strauss AA, Strauss SF (1944) Surgical treatment of ulcerative colitis. Surg Clin North Am 24:211–224
Utsunomiya J (1986) In; Symposium on restorative proctocolectomy for ileal reservoir. Int J Colorectal Dis 1:2–19
Valiente MA, Bacon HE (1955) Construction of a pouch using 'pantaloon' technique for pullthrough of ileum following total colectomy. Am J Surg 90:742–750
van Coevorden F (1989) Surgical aspects of Crohn's disease. Amsterdam Doctorate Thesis
Wangensteen OH (1943) Primary resection (closed anastomosis) of the colon and rectosigmoid. Surgery 14:403–432
Wilks S, Moxon W (1875) Lectures on pathological anatomy, 2nd edn. Lindsay and Blakiston, Philadelphia, pp 408–409
Williams NS, Johnston D (1985) The current status of mucosal proctectomy and ileo-anal anastomosis in the surgical treatment of ulcerative colitis and adenomatous polyposis. Br J Surg 72:159–168

2 Aetiopathology and Natural History

R.N. Allan

Definition

A strict definition of the natural history of a disease is its course and outcome without medical or surgical intervention. It is only possible to follow the true natural history of inflammatory bowel disease in a few patients at the benign end of the spectrum since perforce in practice the course is modified in nearly all patients by medical or surgical treatment.

The object of this chapter is to define the natural history and the modifications that are possible with medical treatment and to identify those patients with persistent symptoms who should be considered for appropriate surgical treatment.

Pathogenesis

Pursuit of the underlying causes of inflammatory bowel disease remain the most important goal (Allan and Hodgson 1992) since our understanding of these factors should enable modification of the natural history so that medical and surgical treatment are no longer needed. There are two developments in pathogenesis which may allow the natural history to be modified.

The possibility that mycobacteria may play a role is still under active consideration and has led recently to the introduction of anti-tuberculous therapy for Crohn's disease. However, it may be that the early benefit derived from this treatment results from treatment of secondary non-mycobacterial invaders to antibiotics rather than a specific anti-mycobacterial effect (Sanderson and Hermon-Taylor 1992).

The second development is that a large number of inflammatory mediators have been identified which perpetuate the inflammatory response, albeit initiated by agents as yet unknown. New drugs are likely to be available shortly which block inflammatory mediator responses and thus modify the natural history (Manzano et al. 1992).

One disease or two?

Clinically, ulcerative colitis and Crohn's disease seem to be distinct conditions. However, their age and sex distribution, genetics and immunology are similar. There is evidence of overlap between the two conditions, particularly among patients undergoing pouch surgery for what ostensibly seems to be ulcerative colitis which subsequently proves to be Crohn's disease.

In practical terms the two conditions can be considered separately for evaluating the natural history and its modification by medical treatment.

Ulcerative colitis

The distribution of disease according to extent depends on factors influencing the selection of patients, so that hospital series tend to have a higher proportion of patients with extensive colitis than an unselected population-based group. In an unselected group of patients the disease will be confined to the rectum or sigmoid colon in two thirds of the patients, 10% having extensive disease (up to and including the hepatic flexure) and 15% having total disease (Hendriksen et al. 1985).

Proctitis

Proctitis is the commonest form of disease giving rise to troublesome intermittent symptoms of diarrhoea, bleeding and particularly urgency. General health remains good. The underlying inflammatory change can usually be readily suppressed with short courses of steroid enemas, often combined with oral sulphasalazine (consisting of the carrier sulphapyridine which delivers the active ingredient, 5-aminosalicylate (5-ASA), to the colon). For most patients, short-term treatment for exacerbations is all that is required. For those individuals subject to frequent or severe exacerbations, maintenance therapy with oral sulphasalazine reduces the number of relapses. The 5-ASA may now be delivered in a number of different vehicles, including pH-dependent release capsules or two 5-ASA molecules linked by a diazobond, similar to the parent compound.

All the newer compounds eliminate sulphapyridine, which is responsible for many of the side effects including headache, nausea and vomiting, skin rashes and infertility in men (Allan and Hodgson 1992).

The newer preparations, (Editorial 1990) particularly those released in the small bowel may occasionally cause renal problems, whereas those preparations still containing a diazobond, (for example olsalazine), may in the first few days of treatment induce watery diarrhoea which can be minimised by gradually increasing the dose.

An analysis of patients with proctitis for at least 10 years shows that half remain asymptomatic, a third have local extension of the disease to the sigmoid colon and 10% have developed extensive colitis (Powell-Tuck et al. 1977).

Severe attacks of proctitis may require short courses of oral prednisolone to resolve symptoms, and occasionally symptoms may persist and be so troublesome that surgery has to be considered. Proctitis alone remains a rare indication for surgical treatment.

Left-sided disease

Left-sided disease may be identified at diagnosis or develop during follow-up as an extension of proctitis. Liquid steroid preparations (rather than foam preparations) may be appropriate since they spread more proximally in the colon. Oral prednisolone in short courses is also needed more commonly than in patients with proctitis alone because the attacks tend to be more severe or persistent. The pattern and modification of the natural history is otherwise similar to that seen in proctitis.

Extensive or total colitis

Extensive and total colitis can be grouped together when considering natural history. Patients can be grouped into four categories: severe acute colitis, intermittent symptoms, chronic persistent symptoms and asymptomatic (Hang et al. 1988).

Severe acute colitis

This is usually diagnosed at first presentation or as a recurrence of previously severe disease. Rarely, severe exacerbations may follow previously mild episodes of the disease.

Severe acute colitis is characterised by diarrhoea, abdominal pain, bleeding and urgency with systemic symptoms of anorexia and weight loss. The diagnosis is confirmed on examination by fever, tachycardia, abdominal tenderness and severe mucosal changes on sigmoidoscopy, with evidence of extensive disease on radiographs of the abdomen. The severity can be confirmed by the presence of anaemia, depressed serum albumin and elevated acute phase proteins.

A careful history and repeated stool cultures will usually identify or exclude specific pathogens. Untreated, the natural history of severe acute colitis is increasingly severe symptoms followed by toxic dilatation and colonic perforation. This adverse natural history can be rapidly and readily reversed by intensive treatment with intravenous corticosteroids and intravenous fluids with dramatic improvement of symptoms often within a few hours.

Failure to respond to intensive therapy with evidence of impending toxic dilatation or failure of rapid resolution within a few days are indications for surgical intervention. Sometimes there is some, but incomplete improvement. In this situation the treatment may be continued beyond the five days recommended in the Oxford regime. The observation that individuals presenting with a severe acute attack, tend to have severe recurrent attacks provides a sound basis for recommending earlier rather than delayed surgical intervention.

Intermittent symptoms

Most patients have intermittent symptoms with exacerbations once or twice a year. These exacerbations are usually treated with oral prednisolone with rapid resolution of symptoms. Mild to moderate attacks may respond to oral sulphasalazine or the new derivatives, together with corticosteroid enemas. Occasional severe acute attacks will require intravenous steroid therapy.

If the attacks are frequent or severe then the natural history can be modified by regular maintenance therapy, either with sulphasalazine or the new salicylates which reduce the frequency of attacks. This treatment is one of the few examples where long-term therapy can modify the natural history of disease.

Chronic persistent disease

A few patients have chronic persistent symptoms, despite maintenance therapy with sulphasalazine and intermittent use of corticosteroids, either orally or locally. There is some, but not very convincing, evidence that immunosuppressive therapy may alter the natural history in these patients by controlling symptoms and thus reducing the need for surgical intervention (Hawthorne and Hawkey 1989; Hodgson 1991). However, chronic persistent symptoms are still the commonest indication for surgical intervention.

Asymptomatic disease

Many patients with radiological evidence of total colitis have few or no symptoms either because of the benign nature of the disease, or the use of effective maintenance therapy.

There is no need to consider surgical intervention in this group except in the context of the risk of developing colorectal cancer. There is little or no risk of developing dysplasia or colorectal cancer in the first ten years from diagnosis of extensive colitis, but the risk thereafter is 0.5%–1% per year (Gyde et al. 1988). This adverse feature in the natural history can be minimised, but not excluded, by some form of regular surveillance, either by colonoscopy or flexible sigmoidoscopy with multiple biopsies combined with annual clinical symptomatic review and appropriate laboratory investigations of haemoglobin, acute phase proteins and serum albumin. The object of the surveillance programme is to identify severe dysplasia before colorectal cancer has developed and thus recommend surgical treatment at this early stage. In this way surgical treatment can be confined to those who develop these adverse features, leaving the majority of asymptomatic patients with the colon intact (Lennard-Jones et al. 1990).

Ulcerative colitis: extra-intestinal manifestations

Arthropathy

The peripheral arthritis associated with ulcerative colitis is usually worse during exacerbations of the disease. Severe arthropathy is occasionally an additional factor for considering surgical treatment.

Ankylosing spondylitis is also associated with ulcerative colitis, but the course is independent of the underlying colitis and is therefore not affected by colectomy.

Liver disease

Sclerosing cholangitis is an uncommon, but well-recognised complication of ulcerative colitis. It is genetically predetermined and is unaffected by colectomy and is not therefore an indication for surgical treatment (Sachar 1991).

Pyoderma gangrenosum

Originally pyoderma gangrenosum was thought to occur during severe exacerbations of disease and was an additional reason for considering surgical treatment. More commonly, pyoderma gangrenosum in a much milder form is associated with all types of colitis but is rarely an indication for surgical intervention (Levitt et al. 1991).

Crohn's disease

Crohn's disease encompasses a wide variety of disorders, masquerading under the one name. It is a diffuse lesion with microscopic evidence of the disease throughout the gastrointestinal tract. However, symptoms which are the key feature in clinical practice are largely determined and arise from sites of macroscopic disease, identified either radiologically, endoscopically or at laparotomy.

Distal ileal disease with or without right colonic involvement

Two thirds of patients with Crohn's disease have macroscopic disease in the terminal ileum. While the disease probably starts with mucosal inflammatory change, by the time patients have symptoms sufficiently severe to consult their doctor, most have already developed a fibrous stricture and the original mucosal inflammatory change has largely resolved (Andrews et al. 1991).

There is good clinical evidence in some patients to suggest that their disease has been present for many years, before the symptoms became severe enough to warrant initial investigation.

Fibrous stricture formation

The distinction between inflammatory mucosal change and fibrous stricture is not always clearcut. Recurrent attacks of intestinal obstruction in an otherwise healthy individual who is well between episodes and in whom the symptoms settle either spontaneously or with intravenous fluids for a few days, suggests that the predominant problem is one of fibrous stricture formation. Most such patients, once the diagnosis is established, usually have recurrent attacks of sub-acute intestinal obstruction and if they recur on more than three or four occasions they are advised to undergo either local resection or strictureplasty if the strictures are short (<6 cm).

About 10% of patients have radiological evidence of distal ileal fibrous stricture and yet have little in the way of recurrent symptoms despite prolonged follow-up. This benign outcome in some patients provides the basis for not advising immediate resection for a single obstructive episode, but they should be under review and surgical treatment advised for those with recurrent obstructive episodes.

Abscess formation

Local complications include abscess formation which usually complicates either a focal deep Crohn's ulcer, or arises proximal to a fibrous stricture. They should be treated by drainage and local resection. The distinction between an inflammatory mass and an abscess requiring local resection may be difficult. In cases of doubt, treatment with antibiotics and subsequent radiological assessment once the acute phase is settled usually resolves the dilemma. The presence of a local abscess can also be confirmed by a leucocyte scan. Laparotomy is no longer needed to distinguish between these two groups.

Fistula formation

Enterocutaneous fistula as a primary presentation of Crohn's disease is rare, but may complicate recurrent disease when the track usually originates from a point immediately above a stricture due to recurrent Crohn's disease. Medical treatment does not alter the long-term natural history of enterocutaneous fistula associated with underlying macroscopic Crohn's disease. Parenteral or enteral nutrition may achieve temporary improvement. There is no evidence that medical therapy (including metronidazole and immunosuppressive therapy) induces permanent healing of enterocutaneous fistula associated with underlying macroscopic Crohn's disease.

Non-obstructive disease

Mucosal inflammatory disease in the ileum and right colon is often asymptomatic. It may induce diarrhoea following interruption of the entero-hepatic cycling of bile salts so that bile salts pass into the large intestine where they induce colonic mucosal secretion of water and electrolytes.

Cholestyramine which binds bile salts will often relieve such symptoms. If the mucosal inflammatory disease is associated with malaise, anorexia and weight loss, then short courses of oral sulphasalazine or the new 5-aminosalicylates are superior to placebo. Short courses of oral prednisolone are also effective, but do not modify the outcome in the medium term. Much of the mucosal inflammatory change heals with time, often with residual stricture formation. Patients then develop intermittent sub-acute obstructive symptoms which, if they recur or persist, are an indication for further local resection.

Distal and left-sided colonic disease

Distal and left-sided colonic disease is particularly common in the older patient with Crohn's disease, most of whom experience a benign course with few symptoms which can be readily relieved by oral sulphasalazine or 5-aminosalicylates, together with local steroids.

Short courses of oral prednisolone are sometimes needed. Because the course is usually benign few require surgical treatment. Nearly 40% of patients with disease at this site require minimal treatment over a long period of time (Fabricius et al. 1985).

However, occasional patients present with severe fulminating left-sided disease with systemic disturbance including fever, tachycardia, weight loss, anorexia, severe left lower quadrant tenderness, with anaemia, low serum albumin and elevated acute phase proteins. This small sub-group, particularly in the elderly, may need emergency surgical treatment, usually colectomy and ileostomy.

Extensive or total colitis

Patients with extensive or total colitis usually present acutely as young adults with diarrhoea, urgency, bleeding, lower abdominal pain and marked systemic disturbance with fever, tachycardia and abdominal tenderness. There is laboratory evidence of active disease with anaemia, low serum albumin and elevated acute phase proteins.

This adverse natural history can be reversed in the short term by intravenous fluids, and corticosteroids with intravenous antibiotics in the presence of positive blood cultures or other signs of systemic disturbance. Patients usually go into remission, but unfortunately the benefit of oral corticosteroids is short-lived and recurrent attacks usually respond less well to intensive medical therapy.

The addition of immunosuppressive therapy to oral prednisolone may be helpful, but there is no good evidence for prolonged benefit with either steroids or immunosuppressive therapy.

Except for 10% of patients who experience a benign course, most patients with extensive or total Crohn's colitis have persistent or recurrent symptoms and need to be considered for surgical treatment relatively early in the course of their disease. This is often and understandably delayed because patients and their families are loath to accept a permanent stoma.

Nearly half the patients with extensive Crohn's colitis have rectal sparing and are thus suitable for colectomy and ileorectal anastomosis. The remainder have rectal involvement and their only surgical option is pan proctocolectomy. Loop ileostomy alone may induce remission for 1–2 years.

Recurrent disease after colectomy and ileorectal anastomosis, either in the ileum immediately proximal to the anastomosis or extensive disease in the rectum, is well recognised, although half the patients still have an intact ileorectal anastomosis ten years after their initial resection. It is often possible to undertake local ileal resection so that the ileorectal anastomosis remains intact. However, protectomy and permanent stoma is often required for those with severe disease of the rectum.

The long-term outcome of extensive or total Crohn's colitis is good, except that some 40% will require a permanent stoma. The incidence of recurrent disease after pan proctocolectomy is low (about 30% at 10 years) and is usually confined to a short segment of the ileum immediately proximal to the stoma which can be readily resected with minimum morbidity, should the individual experience recurrent obstructive symptoms (Andrews et al. 1989a).

Peri-anal disease

Peri-anal disease is a common feature of Crohn's disease and a useful diagnostic hallmark.

It is usually asymptomatic except when complicated by local abscess formation which may respond to antibiotic therapy, but more commonly requires surgical drainage. Examination under anaesthetic is often indicated for painful peri-anal disease when there is no obvious abscess formation since an occasional deep abscess, not obvious on the surface, may explain the symptoms, and require drainage.

Peri-anal disease itself is an uncommon primary indication for resection of the colon, but is an additional feature in some people with distal colonic Crohn's disease (Williams and Hughes 1990).

Crohn's disease at other sites

Extensive diffuse small bowel disease poses major problems in management and it is among these patients that medium- or long-term corticosteroid therapy, with or without immunosuppressive therapy, may suppress disease activity. Patients often have considerable short-term morbidity, but the long-term outlook is good, as much of the inflammatory mucosal change will heal with time, although often with fibrous stricture formation. Recurrent obstructive symptoms in such patients require either local resection or, more commonly, multiple strictureplasties to relieve their symptoms.

Gastroduodenal disease

Gastroduodenal disease is an uncommon, but well-recognised site for Crohn's disease. Incidental mucosal aphthoid ulcers may be identified radiologically. Less commonly, there is stricture formation at the gastroduodenal junction with gastric outlet obstruction. If symptoms persist or recur, bypass surgery is needed to relieve the problem.

Recurrent disease

Recurrent Crohn's disease is a feature of the natural history, but its importance has perhaps been overemphasised and induces more anxiety than is necessary. Recurrent disease after distal ileal resection or after extensive resection of the colon is uncommon, occurs at or around the anastomosis over a short segment of gut and gives rise to clearcut symptoms in an individual with established Crohn's disease. The symptoms, if they persist or fail to respond to short-term medical therapy, can be resolved by further local resection.

There is a small group of patients, perhaps <1% of the total group, in whom recurrent disease is more frequent or more extensive. The occasional patient undergoing pan proctocolectomy for Crohn's colitis develops diffuse small bowel Crohn's disease. Some patients undergoing ileal resection may develop recurrent disease every few years. However, these patients constitute a very small proportion of the total group.

Mortality

Until recently there was an excess mortality among patients with Crohn's disease, related to either sepsis associated with underlying disease or complicating the post-operative period. The occasional patient died of fluid or electrolyte imbalance, or from complications of corticosteroid therapy.

Recently peri-operative sepsis has been minimised by pre-operative antibiotic prophylaxis and the vigorous treatment of sepsis complicating the underlying disease so that sepsis is now rarely a cause of death. Because the evidence suggests that corticosteroids should only be used in the short-term; the long-term sequelae of corticosteroid therapy are uncommon.

The occasional patient still develops colorectal cancer complicating Crohn's disease, but the absolute numbers are small. In some series there is no excess mortality from Crohn's disease, but this outcome can only be achieved in specialised units, particularly where surgical treatment is undertaken by experienced surgeons (Andrews et al. 1989b).

Prognosis for disease in remission of after resection

Medical treatment to reduce the chances of relapse or the development of recurrent disease is an attractive proposition for Crohn's disease in remission of after resection. Sulphasalazine or oral prednisolone and immunosuppressive therapy have not proved superior to placebo treatment. The new 5-aminosalicylates are currently being evaluated, but since sulphasalazine has not proved superior to placebo it is unlikely that they will exert a dramatic effect. Locally active corticosteroids (for example, budesonide) are also under evaluation. A dramatic benefit is again unlikely since the parent compound, oral prednisolone, has not proved beneficial.

Summary

The combination of medical and surgical treatment in inflammatory bowel disease can usually produce a good outcome, although there is an associated morbidity with medical treatment and an inevitable morbidity associated with surgical treatment. A permanent stoma, particularly in patients undergoing surgical resection for extensive colonic Crohn's disease, is often required.

The occasional patient with major sequelae requiring long-term in-patient management and the resolution of complex problems often masks the fact that most patients have a good long-term prognosis and that their problems can be readily resolved by appropriate medical and surgical management.

An understanding of the pathogenesis would greatly improve the lot of a predominantly young adult population unlucky enough to develop these diseases at a time when most of their peers are fit and well.

References

Allan RN, Hodgson HJF (1992) Recent advances in inflammatory bowel disease. In: Pounder RE (ed) Recent advances in gastroenterology 9. Churchill Livingstone, Edinburgh

Andrews HA, Lewis PJ, Allan RN (1989a) Prognosis after surgery for colonic Crohn's disease. Br J Surg 76:1184–1190

Andrews HA, Lewis PJ, Allan RN (1989b) Mortality in Crohn's disease – a clinical analysis. QJM 71:399–405

Andrews HA, Keighley MRB, Alexander-Williams J, Allan RN (1991) Strategy for management of distal ileal Crohn's disease. Br J Surg 78:679–682

Editorial (1990) Current problems. Committee on Safety of Medicines, 30 December 1990 HMSO, London

Fabricius PJ, Gyde SN, Shorter P et al. (1985) Crohn's disease in the elderly. Gut 26:461–465

Gyde SN, Prior P, Allan RN et al. (1988) Colorectal cancer in ulcerative colitis: a cohort study of primary referral from three centres. Gut 29:332–335

Hang K. Schrumpf E, Barstad S et al. (1988) Epidemiology of ulcerative colitis in western Norway. Scand J Gastroenterol 23:517–522

Hawthorne AB, Hawkey CJ (1989) Immunosuppressive drugs in inflammatory bowel disease. Drugs 38:267–288

Hendriksen C, Kreiner S, Binder V (1985) Long-term prognosis in ulcerative colitis – based on a regional patient group from the county of Copenhagen. Gut 26:158–163

Hodgson HJF (1991) Cyclosporin in inflammatory bowel disease. Alim Pharmacol Ther 5:343–350

Lennard-Jones JE, Melville DM, Morson BC et al. (1990) Pre-cancer and cancer in extensive colitis. Gut 31:800–806

Levitt MD, Ritchie JK, Lennard-Jones JE, Phillips RK (1991) Pyoderma gangrenosum in inflammatory bowel disease. Br J Surg 78:676–678

Manzano L, Alvarez-Mon M, Abreu L et al. (1992) Mycobacterial disease of the gut: some impact from molecular biology. Gut 33:145–147

Powell-Tuck J, Ritchie JK, Lennard-Jones JE (1977) The prognosis of idiopathic proctitis. Scand J Gastroenterol 12:727–732

Sachar DB (1991) Ulcerative colitis and sclerosing cholangitis. Gastroenterology 100:1469–1470

Sanderson JD, Hermon-Taylor J (1992) Mycobacterial diseases of the gut: some impact from molecular biology. Gut 33:145–147

Williams JG, Hughes LE (1990) Abdomino-perineal resection for severe perianal Crohn's disease. Dis Col Rectum 33:402–407

3 Nutrition in Inflammatory Bowel Disease

D. Kumar

In this chapter the term inflammatory bowel disease (IBD) will be used to include both Crohn's disease and ulcerative colitis. The nutritional aspects described here are common to both ulcerative colitis and Crohn's disease, although malnutrition is more severe in patients with Crohn's disease.

The majority of patients with inflammatory bowel disease show signs of malnutrition before they start medical or surgical therapy. Often the severity of malnutrition in patients with IBD is underestimated by the attending physicians and surgeons. A careful assessment of malnutrition must be made and replacement therapy designed accordingly. It is now well established that nutritional therapy has little to offer in the management of fistulae or obstruction. It is also known that nutritional support has little impact on the long-term natural history of IBD. However, the main role of nutritional support in IBD is to maintain nutrition to support medical and/or surgical treatment.

A combination of diarrhoea, abdominal pain, bleeding and pyrexia and specific complications such as fistulae and abscesses lend to either reduced intake of nutrients or increased catabolism resulting in malnutrition in inflammatory bowel disease.

Table 3.1 shows the prevalence of some of the malnutrition indicators in hospital patients with IBD (Depew 1990). However, in one study from our unit pre-operative weight loss in adult IBD patients undergoing elective surgery did not appear to have an adverse effect on post-operative outcome (Higgens et al. 1984). In particular, this study showed that pre-operative weight loss was not associated with a higher incidence of post-operative sepsis.

Table 3.1. Prevalence (%) of malnutrition in patients with Crohn's disease and ulcerative colitis

	Crohn's disease	Ulcerative colitis
Variable		
Weight loss	60–75	20–60
Hypoalbuminaemia	25–80	25–50
Negative nitrogen balance	65–70	—
Anaemia	60–80	60
Iron	40	80
Deficiencies		
Vitamin B_{12}	50	5
Folic acid	40–50	30–40
Vitamin D	25–75	35
Zinc	20–40	—
Calcium	13	—
Magnesium	15–30	—
Potassium	5–20	—

— Observed but prevalence not calculated.
Adapted from Depew (1990).

Specific nutritional problems in IBD

Nitrogen balance

In active disease, a negative nitrogen balance is common in malnourished patients. Nitrogen intake is reduced because of loss of appetite and also there is loss of protein into the intestinal lumen. When demands are increased to respond to inflammation and to promote repair there may be consumption of protein stores as energy substrates, especially when intake and absorption are compromised. In severely ill patients as much as 6–12 g of nitrogen may be lost into the intestinal lumen daily (Dickenson et al. 1980). Similarly protein breakdown rates are elevated as well (Powell-Tuck et al. 1984). The rate of protein breakdown appears to be related to disease activity determined clinically. However, pyrexia or steroid use have no effect on protein breakdown (Powell-Tuck et al. 1984). Neither enteral nor parenteral nutritional support affects the rate of protein synthesis and breakdown. Supplementation of protein and energy in adequate quantities via an appropriate route does reverse the negative nitrogen balance and the associated loss of lean body mass.

Energy balance

Patients with no signs of sepsis or fever do not have increased energy expenditure. Contrary to the popular belief that active mucosal inflammation increases energy requirements contributing to malnutrition, the hypothesis has not been supported by careful studies of energy balance (Barot et al. 1982; Chan et al. 1986). Resting energy expenditure in patients with active mucosal disease who are not malnourished (21.2 kcal/kg/day) is slightly less than in patients whose body weight is less than 90% of ideal weight (26.4 kcal/kg/day) (Barot et al. 1982). In malnourished patients the daily administration of 40–45 kcal/kg will result in a positive nitrogen balance and a weight gain of approximately 0.4 kg daily (Fleming 1987). In the presence of sepsis and fever the calorie requirements will increase accordingly.

Zinc deficiency

Poor food intake and excessive enteric losses of minerals result in zinc deficiency in IBD (Rosenberg et al. 1985). Active inflammation and increased metabolism also lead to hyperzincuria, which further aggravates the deficiency. Furthermore since there is a close correlation between plasma zinc and albumin concentrations, hypoalbuminaemia may be associated with low plasma zinc values in the absence of total body zinc depletion (Wolman et al. 1979). Zinc depletion has also been found to be associated with a negative nitrogen balance and zinc supplements appear to result in increased nitrogen retention. A rough practical guide to zinc replacement is the presence or absence of diarrhoea. Patients with excessive gastrointestinal fluid losses have approximately 12 to 17 mg of zinc/kg of faecal output daily whereas those without excessive loss require approximately 3 mg daily (Wolman et al. 1979).

Magnesium deficiency

Magnesium deficiency is particularly common in patients with advanced Crohn's disease. As with zinc the deficiency is commonly related to inadequate intake, malabsorption and excessive gastrointestinal losses (Depew 1990).

Folic acid

Folic acid depletion in IBD is usually secondary to malabsorption due to diseased small intestinal mucosa in Crohn's disease, inadequate intake and drug related malabsorption (Rosenberg et al. 1985). Folate uptake is dependent on a carrier-mediated process which may be inhibited by sulphasalazine. However, at higher luminal concentrations this competitive inhibition is overcome and folate uptake occurs passively. In the absence of excessive demand states such as pregnancy and/or malabsorption due to small bowel disease the administration of 2 grams or less of sulphasalazine daily rarely produces clinically obvious folate deficiency. At higher drug doses, oral supplementation of 2 mg of folic acid daily is often enough to offset the inhibitory potential of sulphasalazine.

Nutrition problems following restorative proctocolectomy

Following restorative proctocolectomy, long-term nutritional assessment has shown normal absorption of fat and normal serum folate concentrations (Mortensen 1988). Some have reported a mild microcytic anaemia in approximately 30% of patients and others found low serum iron concentrations (Nicholls et al. 1981; O'Connell et al. 1986). Marginal deficiencies of vitamin B_{12} have been reported and so levels should be checked regularly. When abnormalities of liver function are present before operation they tend to persist postoperatively (O'Connell et al. 1986). Protein and calorie malnutrition does not occur after restorative proctocolectomy.

Perioperative nutritional support

Loss of appetite is a common feature in an acute exacerbation of inflammatory bowel disease. This results in poor intake of food which together with excessive luminal losses of protein from inflamed mucosa manifests as protein calorie malnutrition. Enteral nutritional supplementation is ideal, particularly in patients with ulcerative colitis where the small bowel is normal. Due to persistent nausea most patients are reluctant to take nutrients orally and in them fine-bore tube feeding may be the solution. However, the placement of the feeding tube and maintenance of its position can be a problem. Tubes are best introduced into the duodenum by means of a gastroscope. Even so the majority of these tubes will become pulled back into the stomach unless the end of the tube is anchored past the duodenojejunal flexure. Occasionally in patients with Crohn's disease a feeding gastrostomy or jejunostomy may be an acceptable alternative and is preferable to total parenteral nutrition. When enteral feeding is not possible, for example, in the immediate perioperative period, parenteral feeding via either a central or peripheral route may be necessary. Enteral feeding can be resumed after the ileus has settled and it is safe to give oral nutrients.

Nutritional support in the treatment for IBD

In addition to the role of nutritional supplementation in the management of malnutrition in IBD, it has been suggested that specific forms of nutritional support may be effective in achieving remission of the disease itself. This suggestion is based on the assumption that specific types of food antigens may be responsible for perpetuation of the primarily immune-mediated inflammatory process and that by providing specific forms of nutritional support it may be possible to reduce the antigenic load (Rhodes and Rose 1986) and also that by reducing the food antigens the mucosal inflammatory response is suppressed (Levi 1985). The "bowel rest" achieved by reducing the antigenic load and avoiding complex lumimal nutrients produces clinical remission. Some of these hypotheses have been tested clinically but the results have failed to provide a satisfactory answer to most of these controversies. Parenteral and enteral feeding regimes have been used in clinical trials. However, the lack of clearly defined end-points and specific entery criteria make interpretation of results exceedingly difficult.

The response to enteral feeding in Crohn's disease parallels that seen with total parenteral nutrition. Approximately two thirds of patients have a good response and improvement in nutritional status. Rigaud et al. (1991) found that in a prospective randomised clinical trial of 30 patients with active Crohn's disease, an elemental diet was no better than a polymeric defined formula in the treatment of Crohn's disease. The treatment with the elemental diet or polymeric defined formula was continued for 4–6 weeks and two thirds of the patients in each group showed clinical remission but most patients relapsed within 12 months (Rigaud et al. 1991). In another study, 34 patients with active Crohn's disease were treated with an elemental diet for four weeks; approximately 80% showed signs of clinical remission within a week (Teahon et al. 1991). None of the trials cited report significant complications and all have employed relatively short courses of enteral feeding. One study compares enteral and parenteral feeding (Greenberg et al. 1988); at one year both showed a similar remission and relapse rate. However, in this study the control patients on a normal diet showed similar remission and relapse rates to those on enteral or parenteral feeding. This observation raises serious doubts about the concept of bowel rest in therapy for Crohn's disease.

There is little doubt that nutritional support therapy is valuable in the treatment of malnutrition in inflammatory bowel disease. The most important role of nutritional therapy is to support patients so that they are well prepared if surgery becomes necessary. There is no evidence that any form of nutritional treatment therapy changes the long-term natural history of either Crohn's disease or ulcerative colitis.

Patients with chronic colitis require a high-protein diet with iron and vitamin supplements. In severely metabolically deficient patients who have lost a significant amount of weight, enteral feeding with dietary supplements should be considered.

References

Barot LR, Rombeau JL, Feurer ID, Mullen JL (1982) Caloric requirements in patients with inflammatory bowel disease. Ann Surg 195:214–218

Chan ATH, Fleming CR, O'Fallon WM, Huizenga KA (1986) Estimated versus measured basal energy requirements in patients with Crohn's disease. Gastroenterology 91:75–78

Depew WT (1990) The role of nutritional support in inflammatory bowel disease. Can J Gastroenterol 4:30–36

Dickenson RJ, Ashton MG, Axon ATR, Smith RC, Yeung CK, Hill GL (1980) Controlled trial of intravenous hyperalimentation and total bowel rest as adjunct to the routine therapy of acute colitis. Gastroenterology 79:1199–1204

Fleming CR (1987) Nutritional considerations in inflammatory bowel disease. In: Nutrition in gastroenterology. American Association of Gastroenterology, postgraduate course, May 1987, pp 1–10

Greenberg GR, Fleming CR, Jeejeebhoy KN, Rosenberg IH, Sales D, Tremaine WJ (1988) Controlled trial of bowel rest and nutritional support in the management of Crohn's disease. Gut 29:1309–1315

Higgens CS, Keighley MRB, Allan RN (1984) Impact of preoperative weight loss and body composition changes on postoperative outcome in surgery for inflammatory bowel disease. Gut 25:732–736

Levi AJ (1985) Diet in the management of Crohn's disease. Gut 26:985–988

Mortensen N (1988) Progress with the pouch – restorative proctocolectomy for ulcerative colitis. Gut 29:561–565

Nicholls RJ, Belliveau P, Neill M, Wilks M, Tabaqhali S (1981) Restorative proctocolectomy with ileal reservoir: a pathophysiological assessment. Gut 22:462–468

O'Connell PR, Rankin DR, Weiland LH, Kelly KA (1986) Enteric bacteriology, absorption, morphology, and emptying after ileal pouch anal anastomosis. Br J Surg 73:909–914

Powell-Tuck J, Garlick PJ, Lennard-Jones JE, Waterlow JC (1984) Rates of whole body protein synthesis and breakdown increase with the severity of inflammatory bowel disease. Gut 25:460–464

Rhodes J, Rose J (1986) Does food affect acute inflammatory bowel disease? The role of parenteral nutrition, elemental and exclusion diets. Gut 27:471–474

Rosenberg IH, Bengoa JM, Sityin MD (1985) Nutritional aspects of inflammatory bowel disease. Annu Rev Nutr 5:463–484

Rigaud D, Cosnes J, Le Quintrec Y, Rene E, Gendre JP, Mignon M (1991) Controlled trial comparing two types of enteral nutrition in treatment of active Crohn's disease: elemental v. polymeric diet. Gut 32:1492–1497

Teahon K, Smethhurst P, Pearson M, Levi AJ, Bjarnason I (1991) The effect of elemental diet on intestinal permeability and inflammation in Crohn's disease. Gastroenterology 101:84–89

Wolman SL, Anderson GH, Marliss EB, Jeejeebhoy KN (1979) Zinc in total parenteral nutrition: requirements and metabolic effects. Gastroenterology 76:458–467

4 Psychosis, Psychology, Stress and Counselling

J. Alexander-Williams

Relationship of psychiatric and psychological disorders

Helzer et al. (1984) have reported a 56% incidence of psychiatric disorders in patients with Crohn's disease compared with a 30% incidence in a group of medically ill controls without Crohn's disease. However, there was no evidence that the two disease syndromes have any consistent relationship to each other. Other studies have suggested an increased prevalence in depression in patients with Crohn's disease (Gerbert 1980). Nevertheless, psychiatric illnesses are even more prevalent in patients with functional gastrointestinal disorders than they are in Crohn's disease. Alpers and Clouse (1986) stress that the detection of psychiatric disease in a patient who also has inflammatory bowel disease will not resolve all the symptoms that cannot be attributed directly to the inflammatory bowel disease. However, it will clarify many difficulties. They felt that physicians treating patients with Crohn's disease should learn to seek and recognise symptoms of psychiatric disorder and that it was well worthwhile to treat active psychiatric symptoms; especially affective and anxiety disorders (Alpers and Clouse 1986). There seems to be little firm evidence to suggest that psychiatric disease can have an adverse effect on the natural history of Crohn's disease, but it is not surprising that, with the onset of recrudescence of symptoms in a chronic bowel disease, there is likely to be worsening of any inherent psychiatric illness.

Smoking has a less obvious connection with the incidence of Crohn's disease than it has in ulcerative colitis. The smoking habits of patients with Crohn's disease appear to differ insignificantly from those of controls.

Stress

Anecdotal evidence led some physicians to believe that there was some connection between episodes of stress and at least the exacerbations if not the initiation of Crohn's disease. Recent studies indicate that there is no such connection nor is there any evidence that there is greater stress in families affected by Crohn's disease than in controls. However, it is natural that exacerbations of any incapacitating disease are likely to have an effect on the apparent family stress. In any population there are classes of patients who are less able to cope with stressful situations and it takes little imagination to understand why less resilient patients will become upset, depressed and withdrawn as soon as they realise that their dreaded chronic disease is beginning to exacerbate. There is evidence of no specific personality characteristic disposing to the onset of the disease and probably no evidence to relate personality characteristics or emotional stress to relapse (Feldman et al. 1967; Whybrow et al. 1968; Goldberg 1970).

The effect of the diagnosis

I find that it is difficult to make an instant or rapid assessment of the effect of the diagnosis of Crohn's disease on the patient and the family. Much depends on their level of education and their ability to understand what is Crohn's disease and what are its effects. Their reaction is most likely to be affected by their knowledge of someone else who is known to have the disease and as Crohn's disease has a familial tendency this is quite often someone close to them. It is important to determine immediately how much they know about Crohn's disease and how they acquired that knowledge. As Crohn's disease is frequently diagnosed in young people, I find it helpful to have early consultations with the whole immediate family unit. With children this will include the parents and with young adults the spouse. The key note initially is optimism rather than a catalogue of potential complications. It is important never to tell untruths to the patient but optimistic stories of how well comparable patients have done can raise comfort and hope much better than do the cold statistics of mortality rates and complications.

Another important point in obtaining a psychological base line to provide helpful psychological counselling is to arrange repeated visits and to make it clear that you are always available to answer questions and to give support. I believe that it does not harm to overindulge a patient in the early stages of establishing a relationship with the caring team. Rarely do patients take advantage of this and become excessively demanding. I find that there is no group of patients with whom I am more likely to form a personal friendly relationship than those with Crohn's disease. This is probably because over the years I see them more often than I do most patients but also it is because they have a strong need to feel that I have their interests at heart.

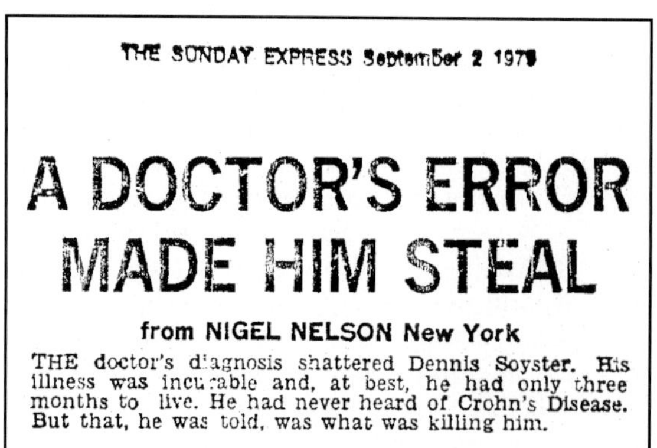
THE SUNDAY EXPRESS September 2 1978

A DOCTOR'S ERROR MADE HIM STEAL

from NIGEL NELSON New York

THE doctor's diagnosis shattered Dennis Soyster. His illness was incurable and, at best, he had only three months to live. He had never heard of Crohn's Disease. But that, he was told, was what was killing him.

Fig. 4.1. Misinformation. A misleading newspaper column.

Psychological counselling of patients with Crohn's disease

When patients with Crohn's disease first know of their diagnosis many are bewildered and some are depressed. Perhaps rather surprisingly the majority are relieved to know the diagnosis, presumably because they had feared worse. Almost all tend to look for further information and guidance; initially to the person who informed them of the diagnosis.

Aims of counselling

I believe that the purpose of counselling patients with Crohn's disease is to give them information and strength to live with the disease.

I believe also that the keynote of counselling should be optimism; it is important not to overwhelm them with information, particularly information that can be misconstrued. An article from the *Sunday Express* in 1978 (Fig. 4.1) indicates the degree of ignorance with which many members of the public regard Crohn's disease; ignorance that is sometimes shared by some members of the medical and nursing profession. I believe that, for patients with Crohn's disease, health education is as important as is sex education for children. It deserves as much careful thought in planning and care in execution as does sex education yet it is something that is rarely considered deeply and seldom taught. These personal views expressed above are born of instinct and nurtured by commonsense. However, my views have been matured by information obtained by distributing a questionnaire among 81 patients with a known diagnosis of Crohn's disease attending our Crohn's disease follow-up clinic. The sample may not be representative of the nationwide or worldwide views of patients with Crohn's disease because the patients sampled are attending a long-established structured Crohn's disease follow-up clinic in a gastrointestinal unit. (Table 4.1)

Table 4.1. Questionnaire to assess patient information about Crohn's disease

We are interested in investigating your knowledge about Crohn's disease to try to improve the quality of the information that we give to our patients. To help us we would like you to complete this questionnaire; your answers will be considered as strictly confidential.

Who first informed you about the disease? When was this done?
Doctor in hospital 72 (89%) Nurse 0 GP 7 (9%)
Anybody else 2 (2%)

Did you know anything about Crohn's disease before you were told of your diagnosis?
No 75 (93%) Yes 6 (7%)

Did you know anyone else suffering from it?
No 69 (85%) Yes 12 (15%)

As soon as you knew the diagnosis, were you given a satisfactory explanation about your condition?
No 37 (45%) Yes 44 (55%)

What did you think of the information you were given?
Too superficial or limited 43 (53%) Adequate 35 (43%) too detailed or complex? 3 (4%)

Do you think that any of the following could have been useful in explaining to you more about the disease? Please tick where appropriate.
Yes 76 (34%) No 5 (6%)
A short article or pamphlet 33 (40%) a book explaining the disease 50 (62%) a video film 13 (16%) speaking with other patients suffering of the same disease 31 (38%)

What was your reaction on knowing the diagnosis? (Tick more than one if relevant.)
Relief 38 (47%) Depression 21 (26%) Interest 22 (27%) Horror 8 (10%) Bewilderment 30 (37%)

Was a member of your family present at the time of the first explanation?
No 46 (57%) Yes 34 (42%) (1 patient did not answer)

If no, do you think they should have been?
No 25 (31%) Yes 56 (69%)

If they were not present did you immediately tell your family about the name and nature of your disease?
No 11 (14%) Yes 70 (86%)

After knowing about your disease, did you make any further enquiries such as asking your doctor, reading papers or books?
No 31 (38%) Yes 50 (62%)

Since the beginning of your disease, have you discovered any important problems or new developments related to the disease that you were not made aware of initially?
No 49 (60%) Yes 32 (40%)

Are you satisfied with the way you were instructed by your medical attendants?
No 19 (23%) Yes 60 (75%) (2 patients did not answer)

Do you belong to any patients associations?
No 67 (82%) Yes 14 (18%)

Should you have been given more information about patients associations when you were first told about your disease?
No 21 (26%) Yes 60 (74%)

Eighty-one patients answered (45 females); data are given as numbers of answers received with percentages in brackets.

What the patients know already

As Crohn's disease is an uncommon disease it is unlikely that patients will know something about it before they are diagnosed as suffering from the disease unless they have a friend or relative similarly affected. Such information is likely to be unduly pessimistic because they are more likely to be aware of the worst problems and the more dramatic complications. In our survey 75 (93%) of our patients knew nothing about Crohn's disease before they were told of the diagnosis, although 12 (15%) said that they knew of somebody else who was suffering from it. Therefore it seems wisest to assume that patients will be in total ignorance of the disease when first they discover the diagnosis and that, even if they know people who have the disease, this is unlikely to mean that they are adequately informed about it.

How much patients are able to comprehend

From my experience in giving patients comprehensive books written principally for a North American patient population, I am certain that most sufferers are capable of assimilating a lot of information and achieving some understanding about the disease. So much so that their thirst for knowledge can rarely be satisfied by a brief personal consultation lasting less than half an hour. At the end of such an interview most patients are still anxious to receive further information and, if not satisfied, many will seek it from medical and surgical textbooks that are written for a sophisticated medical readership.

How much to tell them

The doctor informing the patient about their disease has a difficult task. The patient has to be informed without being confused or frightened. It is sometimes difficult for a doctor to understand the limited concept that the lay public has initially about the disease and its consequences. If he speaks to patients as he would speak to other members of the medical profession he may refer to such concepts as the risk of the development of cancer. While medical colleagues will understand it in statistical terms, to the patient the emotive words of cancer and risk will be heard entirely out of context. I believe that in our present state of knowledge we are wise if we dismiss or play down the risk of cancer developing in Crohn's disease. We are all impressed by and tend to quote to each other the evidence from Mount Sinai Hospital in New York indicating the greatly increased risk of cancer developing in bypassed small bowel (Greenstein et al. 1978). Fascinating though this information may be to researchers in the field, I believe that this information should not be given to patients simply to cover ourselves against the risk of litigation. I believe that we should tell patients that Crohn's disease is not a form of cancer and will to develop into it. Any form of chronic epithelial inflammation in the body may produce a slight risk of malignant disease occurring but this risk is minute and much less than the risk of developing lung cancer if you smoke or cervical cancer if you have more than one partner. To try to explain disease processes to someone without scientific knowledge, particularly someone with only a limited ability and comprehension, may create more problems than it solves. The saying "a little knowledge is a dangerous thing" could well have been coined to describe the patient's awareness of their chronic disease. However, our survey showed that a small majority (53%) of the patients thought that the initial explanation they were given about their disease was too superficial or too limited; 43% thought that the explanation they were given was adequate and 4% only considered that it was too detailed or too complex for them to understand. The large majority (94%) considered that they would like to have had more information about their disease than they received. Sixty-two per cent of them felt that they would like to have read a book giving further details about the disease from which they were suffering. (see Table 4.1)

When should patients be told and who should tell them?

As the diagnosis of Crohn's disease almost always results from a hospital investigation usually including radiography and histological examination of biopsies, it is usually the hospital doctor who is the first person to confront the patient with the final definitive diagnosis although Crohn's disease may have been suggested as a possible diagnosis before then. In our survey 89% of those questioned had their first information about the diagnosis and the disease from a doctor in a hospital, only 9% were informed by their general practitioner.

There seems to be no reason why patients with Crohn's disease should not be told the diagnosis immediately it is confirmed and so it will usually be the Consultant Physician or Surgeon in the office or out-patient clinic who will break the news, although in public hospital practice it may well be a junior member of the medical team. Anyone who has to impart the information to the patient has to be well aware of what the news may mean to the patient and to be in a position to give a satisfactory and comprehensive explanation of the implications of the disease. The doctor has to be prepared to assume the role of a counsellor and should remember the three precepts of giving information, hope and strength.

The patient's initial reaction

Our patients were asked to recall what was their reaction on first knowing the diagnosis and were given the opportunity of expressing more than one reaction. The commonest was relief (47%), followed by bewilderment (37%), interest (27%), depression (26%), and horror (10%). It is probably those who were afraid that they were suffering from cancer who were relieved (see Table 4.1).

I think that it is particularly important to realise that 37% were bewildered, principally because of lack of knowledge of the disease. To some patients the diagnosis of Crohn's disease may sound as serious as the diagnosis of cancer, indeed it may even seem so to some ill-informed members of the medical profession. It is important for those of us who are breaking the news to patients that they have Crohn's disease to realise that the impact of the diagnosis could have a serious and disturbing emotional impact on the patient. We should take care as to where and when the news is given. It is generally inappropriate that the diagnosis should be imparted to the patient over the telephone or even in writing. Eyeball-to-eyeball contact is undoubtedly the best environment. It is probably best during or after physical contact by doctor and patient, either in the form of a handshake or a physical examination. First impressions are probably of paramount importance and so it is advisable to give patients some information and explanation at the moment of imparting the diagnosis. Therefore it is important to have some time available for the patient and preferably in the presence of a close and supportive relative or friend. Our survey showed that 57% of our patients had no other member of the family present at the time of the first explanation and 69% felt that a relative should have been present, although 14% felt that they did not wish anybody else to know about the diagnosis. For doctors inexperienced in the art of imparting such information it is important that they consider it beforehand, have a plan before starting, do not just plunge into an explanation that may confuse rather than inform and lead to questions that cannot be answered satisfactorily.

Where to counsel and who should be present

As the information will usually be first imparted in the out-patient environment, some privacy is desirable rather than an environment with telephones ringing, typewriters chattering or with other patients or medical staff nearby. There is a lot to recommend a team approach to the first imparting of information. In teaching hospitals the consultation is often conducted in the presence of one or two students and a stoma care or specialist gastroenterological nurse. Although relatively few patients are going to require an intestinal stoma, stoma care nurses are usually specially trained in imparting information about inflammatory bowel disease and well trained in understanding the anxieties of patients with this condition. I believe that it is best if possible to have the spouse, or with children the parents, present at the first interview. If this is impractical it might be sensible to arrange a special consultation in order to discuss at some length with the patient and relatives the implication of the disease. I believe it is better to have an initial interview before the patient is given any books or manuals because I think it is only the interview that can impart the vital air of optimism that is so important with the first impression.

Should we tell all?

When we decide how much we are going to tell a patient initially, we have to judge their background, character and power of comprehension. If that is not a difficult enough task we also have to make a decision about how much science, how much analogy and how much poetic licence will be appropriate for the particular patient. Perhaps the most important attribute of the counsellor is empathy. Attitudes have changed. The issue is no longer "to tell or not to tell" but rather what information is appropriate for the particular patient. The full details of diagnosis and prognosis as required by many American trial protocols are as inappropriate as is bland reassurance. Although a degree of paternalism may be an ingredient of compassionate care, if it is associated with lack of empathy then it becomes destructive arrogance. I think that the tone of the first interview should be light on science, heavy on analogy and rich in sympathy.

Optimistic analogies

I explain to patients that they have a chronic inflammatory disease that is usually not particularly severe and one with which most patients can live through a normal span of life without a great inconvenience. The two analogies that I commonly use are chronic sinusitis and chronic eczema. I use them because the patient usually knows of someone suffering from one of these common afflictions. I explain that chronic sinusitis is a combination of infection and nasal blockage which may give many patients a persistent purulent runny nose. However, for most of the time it is relatively easy to live with; although they would rather be without it. Only occasionally does it flare up with an acute symptomatic exacerbation that requires drugs and time off work and only occasionally does it require any surgical intervention.

When I use the analogy of eczema, I explain that much of the time the disease is quiescent. Occasionally for some reason, which we understand better with dermatitis than we do with Crohn's disease, it will flare up and become inflamed. It may then require antibiotics to combat secondary infection or cortisone to suppress the inflammatory response. I tell them that most patients with chronic eczema can live a long and useful life with few limitations. I say that in many patients the eczema becomes totally quiescent even if once having been almost incapacitating. I find that one or both of these analogies is easily comprehended by a patient and puts their own disease into perspective.

I explain to them that, in our inflammatory bowel disease clinic, we have in our care about 500 patients with Crohn's disease and that, for most of the time, some 425 are having little trouble, requiring only a little dietary management and vitamin supplementation. At any one time, some 60 are undergoing exacerbations of the disease sufficiently severe to warrant powerful drug therapy with such things as steroids, other anti-inflammatory drugs or antibiotics. There are only about 15 of the 500 patients whose disease is causing any concern, enough to require weekly supervision or even in-patient treatment. Most of these 15 have some complication of the disease that warrants consideration of surgical treatment or temporary complete bowel rest. I explain that when this complication has been dealt with we expect all 15 to go back and join the 425 with minimal inconvenience. I realise that these statistics may have to be protected by the heading "poetic licence" but I make no apology for tinging the initial consultation with optimism.

The role of patient societies or clubs

In most countries of Northern Europe and North America where Crohn's disease is relatively common, associations or societies have been formed. In Great Britain the National Association for Colitis and Crohn's disease was founded in 1980 and by 1986 had a membership of 5018. They produce a twice yearly newsletter which acts as an "agony column" for those with problems, anecdotes or the need to write letters to an Editor. Not all patients wish to join societies or self-help organisations and a few are not prepared to spend the very small annual membership dues. However, for a large number of sufferers the NACC in Great Britain can provide great help and support. It also provides a particularly helpful booklet, *Crohn's Disease*, which gives about the right sort of information for most patients to take in after their first interview. In Canada, the Canadian Foundation of Ileitis and Colitis is a similar organisation producing a quarterly journal, useful brochures in English or French with an annual membership of $15. I believe that such organisations fulfil an important role and that it is the duty of the doctor in charge of a patient once diagnosed as having Crohn's disease to give them some information about the national associations or foundations. I was rather surprised and a little shamed by the response to our questionnaire that indicated that 82% of those questioned did not belong to a patient association and 74% who felt that they should have been given more information about the patient association when they were first told of their disease.

Assessment of the quality of life

The quality of life of patients with Crohn's disease is determined partly by the presence or absence of symptoms and partly by the effect of the disease on the patient's ability to achieve goals. Such goals are usually easily understandable and definable, such as the ability to perform a normal day's work, to be able to enjoy a social life in addition to work, to be able to play sport, to realise an achievable educational standard, to be able to study for examinations and to be able to develop their full potential.

Clinical indices of severity of the disease have largely focused on illness and includes subjective elements. In the 1970s attempts were made to quantify the severity of Crohn's disease and to create a disease activity index. The simple scale of severity of de Dombal (1974), the complex Crohn's disease activity index (CDAI) of Best and colleagues (1976) are summarised in Tables 4.2 and 4.3.

Table 4.2. de Dombal's scale of severity of Crohn's disease (de Dombal 1974)

	Mild	Severe
Local features		
Bowel actions	2–3/day	>5 per day
Pain	Occasional/mild	Continuous/severe
Rectal bleeding	Negligible	Visible blood
Systemic features		
Pulse	<90/min	>100/min
Temperature	<99°F	>100°F
Haemoglobin	>80%	<70%
Weight loss	<3.2 kg	>6.6 kg

Moderate attacks are intermediate between Mild and Severe.

Table 4.3. Crohn's disease activity index (CDAI) (Best et al. 1976)

Item	Multiplied by
Number liquid/very soft stools per week	2
Sum of 7 daily ratings of abdominal pain (0 = none to 3 = severe)	5
Sum of 7 daily rating of well being (0 = well to 4 = terrible)	7
Number of associated symptoms or findings (arthritis/arthralgia, skin/mouth lesions, iritis or uveitis, anal fissure/fistula/abscess, other external fistula, fever >100°F during week)	20
Taking opiate antidiarrhoeal (0 = no, 1 = yes)	30
Abdominal mass (0 = no, 2 = indefinite, 5 = yes)	10
Haematocrit deficit (males: 47 – Hct, females: 42 – Hct)	6
Body weight (% below standard)	1

Values below 150 indicate remission, over 400 severe disease.

The CDAI is both complex and heavily subjective. Nevertheless it is the index still most commonly used in clinical studies. In an attempt to create a more objective measure than the CDAI, which relies heavily on symptoms, van Heese and colleagues (1980) developed another complex index which largely disregards symptoms and signs (Table 4.4). While a much simplified index by Harvey and Bradshaw in 1980 relies entirely on the symptoms derived from a week's diary card and correlates highly with the CDAI ($r = 0.93$) (Table 4.5). These indices of activity means little in themselves but if strict criteria are used then they provide a good basis for studying the longitudinal course of the disease and for comparing the results of different therapy or of comparing therapy with placebo management. I think that for clinical studies a combination of both objective findings and symptomatic indices are best.

For an initial assessment of the effect of the disease on a patient's life. I prefer to encourage the patient to define their principal objectives in life in such aspects as work, play, social life and achievement aims and then to define whether, in their opinion, the present state of their disease affects those goals (1) not at all; (2) moderately; or (3) severely. Any number of goals can be chosen so that if a longitudinal comparative survey is intended the score will be divided by the number of activities measured. (See Perianal Crohn's Disease index of activity, Chapter 18.)

Table 4.4. Van Heese index (Van Heese et al. 1980)

Item	Multiplied by
Serum albumin (g/l)	– 5.48
Erythrocyte sedimentation rate (mm/hr)	0.29
Quetelet index (10 × weight/height2)	– 0.22
Abdominal mass (1 = none, 5 = >12 cm)	7.83
Sex (1 = male, 2 = female)	– 12.3
Temperature (°C)	16.4
Stool consistency (1 = formed to 3 = watery)	8.46
Previous resection (1 = no, 2 = yes)	– 9.17
Extraintestinal lesions (1 = no, 2 = yes)	10.7

From the sum of above products, subtract constant of 209 to get index value.
Values below 100 indicate inactive disease, above 210 indicate severe inflammatory activity.

Table 4.5. Harvey–Bradshaw index (simplified CDAI) (Harvey and Bradshaw 1980)

Item	Scoring
General well being	0 = very well to 4 = terrible
Abdominal pain	0 = none to 3 = severe
Liquid stools	Number/day
Abdominal mass	0 = none to 3 = present, tender
Complications[a]	1 point for each

[a] arthralgia, uveitis, erythema nodosum, aphthous ulcers, pyoderma gangrenosum, anal fissure, new fistula, abscess

Longitudinal surveillance (a surgical perspective)

Although the initial assessment of activity and its effect on life is important in planning the philosophy of management, it is more important to have an agreed series of indices that will be measured at each attendance. In our unit surveillance is the combined responsibility of the medical and surgical component of the gastroenterological team but the distribution of labour means that most of the follow-up documentation is performed by the medical team. Dr. Robert Allan is the gastroenterologist with whom I have worked closely for many decades. His perception of the role of follow-up clinics is outlined in Chapter 29. It is important to remember that, until we find a specific cure, Crohn's disease is for life and surveillance is forever. Crohn's disease varies in its course from a quiescent disease that is static for years to an active disease that is constantly changing throughout the patient's lifetime. Both quiescent and active phase may be predominant for months or years.

The recording of measurements at each attendance and the frequency of attendance is determined to some extent by the particular research interests of the team. It is also determined by the availability of resources and by our judgement of the extent to which the patient needs reassurance. Obviously we would not be advising MRI assessment at frequent intervals even though this is a non-invasive investigation, and we certainly would not suggest re-examination by X-ray or isotopes unless it was absolutely essential for the management of the disease.

In our unit we review patients with Crohn's disease regularly and as infrequently as is feasible dependent on the activity of their disease. All patients, even with quiescent disease, are reviewed annually. Patients with difficulties, but not severe enough to warrant admission to hospital, are usually reviewed at monthly intervals. As we live and work in a relatively small geographical area where the hospital is centrally located, most review is by personal attendance although we recognise that telephone or postal questionnaire follow-up is cost-effective in many parts of the world. At each review we routinely record weight and bowel frequency and on most visits simple blood screening tests are performed by the laboratory using auto-analyser programmes. The indices that we particularly regard as significant in longitudinal events are the haemoglobin, hematocrit, serum albumin and C-reactive proteins. I like also to include a survey of any aspects of goal achievement that are being affected by the disease.

References

Alpers DH, Clouse RE (1986) Psychiatric evaluation in inflammatory bowel disease – practical considerations. In: Rachmilewitz D (ed) Inflammatory bowel disease Martinus Nijhoff, Dordrecht

Best WR, Becktel JM, Singleton MD, Kearn F Jr (1976) Developments of a Crohn's disease activity index: national co-operative Crohn's disease study. Gastroenterology 70:439–444

de Dombal FR, Burton IL, Clamp SE, Goligher JC (1974) Short-term course and prognosis of Crohn's disease. Gut 15:435–443

Feldman F, Cantor D, Soll S, Bachrach W (1967) Psychiatric study of a consecutive series of 19 patients with regional ileitis. Br Med J iv:711

Gerbert B (1980) Psychological aspects of Crohn's disease. J Behav Med 3:41–48

Goldberg D (1970) A psychiatric study of patients with diseases of the small intestine. Gut 11:459

Greenstein AJ, Sachar D, Pucillo A et al. (1978) Cancer in Crohn's disease after diversionary surgery. A report of seven carcinomas occurring in excluded bowel. Am J Surg 135:86–90

Harvey RF, Bradshaw JM (1980) A simple index of Crohn's disease activity. Lancet i:514

Helzer JE, Schammas S, Norland CC, Stillings WA and Alpers DH (1984) A study of the association between Crohn's disease and psychiatric illness. Gastroenterology 86:324–330

van Heese PAM, van Elteren PH, van Lier HJJ, van Tongeren JHM (1980) An index of inflammatory activity in patients with Crohn's disease. Gut 21:279–286

Whybrow PC, Kane FJ, Lipton MA (1968) Regional ileitis and psychiatric disorder. Psychosom Med 30:209–221

Section II

5 Crohn's Disease: A Remaining Medical Enigma and Surgical Challenge

J. Alexander-Williams

Introduction

Because the place of surgery in the management of Crohn's disease is so different from that in the management of ulcerative colitis, these two diseases are described separately; therefore there will be a certain overlap between these two sections of the book. Many of the factors in the aetiology and epidemiology are so similar in the two diseases that many people consider that Crohn's disease and ulcerative colitis are different manifestations of the same disease. In many monographs on inflammatory bowel disease there is a tendency to consider the diseases under the one heading of idiopathic inflammatory bowel disease. However, we make no apology for separating them in this surgical textbook for reasons that will be obvious from reading the sections on the surgical treatment of the two diseases. Of the two, Crohn's disease is by far the more protean in its manifestations as will be seen; not only can it occur anywhere throughout the alimentary tract but also it can apparently affect the liver, skin, the eyes and joints. The number of complications produced by Crohn's disease include stenosis, bleeding, perforation, fistula and malignant change. Therefore, it is not surprising that there are many occasions when surgical intervention is required and a wide variety of different surgical manoeuvres may be needed.

No surgeon should contemplate undertaking operative treatment for Crohn's disease without some knowledge of the other aspects of the disease. We cannot condone the relegation of surgeons to the technical role of "craftsman" who are instructed by investigating, thinking gastroenterologists to cut here, resect there and join A sideways on to B. The surgeon playing a part in the management of Crohn's disease should know as much as his gastrointestinal colleague about the rival merits of different forms of non-operative management and evidence supporting the possible advantages of delaying surgical intervention until after a period of supplementary therapy or nutrition.

There is much less medical – surgical collaboration when managing ulcerative colitis than there is with Crohn's disease. The gastroenterologist treats ulcerative colitis until she/he or the patient decide that the quality of life is poorer or the perceived dangers greater with the medically managed disease than with the surgical options. Then care is transferred to the surgeon who decides what operation is best suited to that patient. Nevertheless the reputation of the surgeon for achieving safety and good function will affect significantly the gastroenterologist's threshold of surgical referral. In ulcerative colitis physicians choose to work with surgeons they trust.

There are specialist monographs on inflammatory bowel disease and general medical gastroenterological textbooks which provide detailed descriptions of the non-surgical aspects of the disease and we would expect interested surgeons to refer to these.

Demography

Incidence and prevalence: its geographical, secular, racial and social distribution

As the disease is so loosely defined it is obviously difficult to be certain of the incidence because many patients go undiagnosed and the disease is often unrecognised. It is possible that there are many patients whose minor perianal disease could be a manifestation of Crohn's disease and yet they do not necessarily complain to the medical profession or may not be referred to hospital, nor come to detailed post-mortem examination.

There are many parts of the world where the manifestations of Crohn's disease are mistaken for common diseases found in that part of the world such as tuberculosis, Bilharzia, Chagas' disease, etc. Patients with a gross manifestation of Crohn's disease that is easily recognised, such as stenotic terminal ileal disease, always have at least one admission to hospital and in western temperate society are usually diagnosed correctly. It is therefore from these parts of the world with presumably the highest incidence that we have most accurate demographic data. Fig. 5.1 shows the average annual incidence and prevalence rate for Crohn's disease per 100 000 population that have been reported since the 1950s; most from supposed high incidence areas. As will be seen from this figure most reports are from temperate regions although Baltimore may not always be so described (Calkins et al. 1984). The disease appears to be seen quite commonly in the southern United States. However, in the United States many patients seeking definitive medical treatment in the southern United States were born or grew up in the temperate or cold north. With such a movement of population as occurs in the United States it is difficult to give much epidemiological significance to these figures. From my own experience of lecturing about this disease in countries around the Mediterranean, I am convinced that the disease has a low incidence in Portugal, southern Spain, Italy, Greece, Iran and Egypt (Lanfranchi et al. 1976; Ruiz and Patel 1986). From the close association of our unit with experienced gastroenterologists from the Indian subcontinent I am persuaded also that the disease has a low incidence there compared with that in the United Kingdom. Although in any area where tuberculosis is

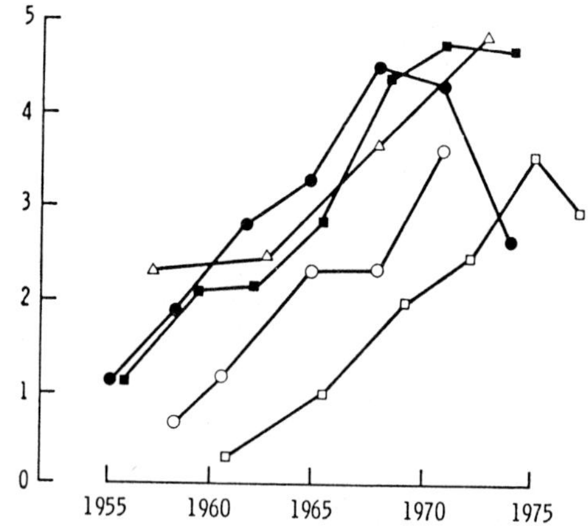

Fig. 5.1. The changing incidence of Crohn's disease. (Figures are average rates per 100 000 population per year.) △ Wales, Cardiff; ■ Sweden, Stockholm; ○ England, Nottingham; □ Denmark, Copenhagen, ● Scotland, Aberdeen.

endemic it must often be difficult to make a differentiation between these two diseases.

A small series of patients have been reported from gastroenterological centres in Czechoslovakia, Spain, Turkey, Uruguay, Southern Brazil and Colombia. Usually these series are related numerically more to the enthusiasm of the collectors of the series and their reputation in this particular field rather than to the true incidence of disease in the community they serve. However, I think that the evidence of geographical distribution is sufficiently clear to say that this is predominantly a disease of the colder or temperate parts of highly developed western civilisation. Such an observation may have some aetiological significance.

In the United States it was once believed that the disease occurred predominantly in Jews but this belief could have been due to the fact that in the early days much of the interest in the disease was at the Mount Sinai Hospital of New York and many of the medical pioneers in this field were Jews. Acheson (1960) demonstrated a four-fold incidence of the disease among service veterans of Jewish faith than among other non-black veterans. Monk et al. (1969) found a similar incidence differential of the disease in white males in Baltimore; Jews were affected more commonly than non-Jews. In Israel Crohn's disease among Jews seems to be less common than among the general population in Northern Europe or North America, but within Israel Israeli born and non-Ashkenazi Jews seem to be less susceptible to the disease than Jews in Europe or North America. These factors suggest that if Jews do have a higher incidence than non-Jews in some parts of the world the responsible factors are more likely to be environmental than racial. It has also been shown that, in the United States, non-Jewish whites had an incidence two and a half times higher than blacks. In New Zealand Maoris seem to be less likely to suffer from Crohn's disease than do whites and in South Africa whites seem to have a higher incidence than either blacks or those of Indian descent.

Monk et al. (1969) suggested that Crohn's disease is slightly commoner in people who have higher education than those in the lower social groups, and from Copenhagen Binder and Katz (1977) reported that the socioeconomic status of patients with Crohn's disease was higher than that of the control group. However, Kyle (1971) found the opposite tendency in Scotland. There appears to be a greater incidence of the disease in urban dwellers than in rural (Mendeloff et al. 1966; Kuiper et al. 1981) although some reports have denied this (Norlen et al. 1970; Hellers 1979). I doubt whether any aetiological significance can be read into such flimsy data.

Changes in the incidence

In the last 50 years there has been a striking increase in the frequency of the diagnosis of Crohn's disease; however, much of this rise could be due to increasing interest and better diagnostic facilities. Between 1955 and 1975, when good diagnostic facilities were generally available in the United Kingdom and Scandinavia, several reports (Fig. 5.1) have shown a gradual increase in the incidence of diagnosis of Crohn's disease. It will be interesting to see whether this increase continues over the next few decades or whether the incidence has already peaked, as might be suggested from the evidence depicted in Fig. 5.1. However, it is quite likely that the apparent sharp rise in incidence was due to better diagnostic facilities and greater awareness. These would result in patients being diagnosed sooner in the course of the disease than they had been in the former decades. Some years ago and even today, in some parts of the world where the disease is not particularly common, patients often achieve the final diagnosis of Crohn's disease only after decades of symptoms hitherto unexplained. Whereas in recent years in our rectal clinic I have seen patients, particularly the elderly, correctly diagnosed as having Crohn's disease on anal inspection at a time when they had no other intestinal symptoms. My interpretation of these apparently confusing data is that the incidence of Crohn's disease did increase during the middle decades of the 20th century but part of the increase was due to earlier diagnosis and in the latter decades of the 20th century the incidence of the disease has remained constant.

Age and sex incidence

Most reports indicate that Crohn's disease occurs roughly with equal frequency in the two sexes. Hospital series, as opposed to population series, tend to have unreliable bias because of referral patterns. The peak age incidence of the disease is between 20 and 49 although many series including our own show a small secondary peak in the early 60s. From Copenhagen the statistics of Binder et al. (1982) show that the sex ratio of Crohn's disease was 1.5 female to 1 male; the maximum incidence of Crohn's disease was between ages 20 and 35 with a late peak between 65 and 69.

Family incidence

Approximately 10% of patients with Crohn's disease have a positive family history of inflammatory bowel disease (Mayberry et al. 1979) which may include both ulcerative colitis and Crohn's disease. Several coincidences of Crohn's disease in identical twins have been recorded (McConnell 1971). Kirsner (1970) reported that cases of ulcerative colitis or Crohn's disease occur in approximately 25% of members of families with inflammatory bowel disease. Relatives of patients with Crohn's disease have an incidence of the disease about 30 times more common than in the general population. Patients who develop Crohn's disease at a younger age have a greater tendency to having a positive family history than those that develop the symptoms when they are older. McConnell (1971) also showed that relatives of patients with Crohn's disease, in addition to having inflammatory bowel disease more commonly, also had higher than expected incidence of ankylosing spondylitis. Ankylosing spondylitis is known to be associated with high incidence of HLA B27, an antigenic marker, in their serum. This marker is found in 5% of the general population, though few of them develop ankylosing spondylosis, whereas patients with inflammatory bowel disease with a positive HLA B27 marker have a 60% risk of having ankylosing spondylitis. Also there is evidence that there is a positive family history of eczema more so in the father (probability of difference from controls $P < 0.001$) than in the mother ($P < 0.005$) or siblings ($P < 0.01$) (McConnell 1971).

From these data it looks as if there is an important genetic factor in inflammatory bowel diseases and in Crohn's disease in particular. There is certainly not a simple mendelian inheritance; several genes are likely to be involved. It has been suggested that if a patient has many of the appropriate genes involved he or she is more likely to develop Crohn's disease, whereas if they have fewer of these genes positive then ulcerative colitis is more likely once stimulating factors are applied.

Environmental factors

From the evidence of geographical distribution of the disease it seems likely that climate plays some part in the initiation of the disease. It appears that it is more prevalent in a cold climate but there is nothing in the evidence to indicate whether it is temperature or humidity that is particularly important. Anecdotal evidence from the United States suggests that patients who have been born and brought up in the northern states are not necessarily protected from developing the disease if they move to warmer southern climates.

Diet

Diet may play some part in the aetiology of the disease. There is some evidence (Heaton 1979) that patients with Crohn's disease tend to eat less fibre than controls but from the evidence it is not clear whether this is as a result rather than the cause of the disease. The evidence tends to point towards their having consumed less fibre in the decades preceding the apparent onset of the disease. Patients with Crohn's disease are also said to eat less fruit than controls and the same arguments apply about the value of this evidence. There is no apparent difference between the sugar content of the diet of patients with Crohn's disease from that of controls.

References

Acheson ED (1960) The distribution of ulcerative colitis and regional enteritis in United States veterans with particular reference to the Jewish religion. Gut 1:291–293

Binder SE, Katz D (1977) Regional enteritis: and review of the literature. Ohio State Med J 73:661

Binder V, Both H, Kansen PK et al. (1982) Incidence and prevalence of ulcerative colitis and Crohn's disease in the County of Copenhagen 1962–1978. Gastroenterology 83:563–568

Calkins BM, Linfield AM, Garland CF, Mendeloff AI (1984) Trends in incidence rates of ulcerative colitis and Crohn's disease. Dig Dis Sci 29:913–920

Goligher JC (1972) Ileal recurrence after ileostomy and excision of the large bowel for Crohn's disease. Br J Surg 59:253–259

Heaton KW, Thornton JR, Emmett PM (1979) Treatment of Crohn's disease with an unrefined carbohydrate, fibre rich diet. Br Med J ii:764–766

Hellers G (1979) Crohn's disease in Stockholm County, 1955–1974. A study of epidemiology, results of surgical treatment and long term prognosis. Acta Chir Scand (Suppl) 490:1–84

Kirsner JB (1970) Some observations in familial inflammatory bowel disease. In: Weterman IT, Pena AS, Booth CC (eds) The management of Crohn's disease. Excerpta Medica, Amsterdam, pp 51–54

Kuiper I, Weterman IT, Biemond I et al. (1981) hymphocytotoxic antibodies in patients with Crohn's disease and family members. In: Pena AS et al. (eds) Recent advances in Crohn's disease. Martinus Nijhoff, Amsterdam, pp 341–347

Kyle J (1971) An epidemiological study of Crohn's disease in Northeast Scotland. Gastroenterology 61:826–833

Kyle J, Stark J (1980) Fall in the incidence of Crohn's disease. Gut 21:340–343

Lanfranchi GA, Michelin A, Brighola C (1976) Uno studio epidemiologico sulle malattie inflammatarie intestinali nella provinciade Bologna. G Clin Med 57:235–245

Lennard-Jones JE (1968) Medical aspects of Crohn's disease. Proc R Soc Med 61:81

Mayberry JF, Rhodes J, Hughes LE (1979) Incidence of Crohn's disease in Cardiff between 1934 and 1977. Gut 20:602–608

McConnell RB (1971) Genetics of Crohn's disease. Clin Gastroenterol 1:321

Mendeloff AI, Monk M, Siegel CI, Lilienfeld A (1966) Some epidemiological features of ulcerative colitis and regional enteritis – a preliminary report. Gastroenterology 51:748–756

Monk M, Mendeloff AI, Siegel CI, Lilienfeld A (1967) An epidemiological study of ulcerative colitis and regional enteritis among adults in Baltimore. I. Hospital incidence and prevalence, 1960–1963. Gastroenterology 53:198–210

Monk M, Mendeloff AI, Siegel CI, Lilienfeld A (1969) An epidemiological study of ulcerative colitis and regional enteritis among adults in Baltimore. II. Social and demographic factors. Gastroenterology 56:847–857

Norlen BJ, Krause U, Bergman L (1970) An epidemiological study of Crohn's disease. Scand J Gastroenterol 5:385–390

Ruiz V, Patel J (1986) Crohn's disease in Galicia, Spain 1968–1982. In McConnell R, Rosen P, Langman MJS, Gilat T. (eds) The genetics and epidemiology of inflammatory bowel disease. Karger, Basel

6 Surgical Management

J. Alexander-Williams

The general principles

The general principles of surgical management of Crohn's disease are determined by our concept of the present limitations of therapy. Our important management limitations are:

1. It is an incurable disease
2. It has panintestinal potential for involvement
3. Surgical intervention only overcomes the effects of complications of the disease and does not affect the disease itself.

These three limitations mean that the disease is relentlessly recrudescent. In many surveys there is a need for recurrent surgical intervention of about 3% and 6% per year (Ekelund and Linghagen 1989). I believe that there is a tendency for the recrudescence rate to be higher in young patients with multi-focal small bowel disease and to be lower in those who have had a proctocolectomy or a disease confined to the large bowel. However, no form of presentation of the disease is immune from the risk of recrudescence.

Because of the constant risk of recrudescence, there is usually a repeated need for surgical intervention. Therefore, I think that it is important to establish three overriding principles governing surgical intervention:

1. Make surgical intervention as safe as possible; have minimal morbidity and avoid mortality
2. Sacrifice as little gut as possible; repeated operations with wide margins of normal bowel on either side may mean that, by the time there have been three or four recrudescences of the disease, the patient will be becoming seriously short of bowel
3. Operate as soon as there are indications.

I believe that by delaying surgical intervention for stenosis we invite further complications such as abscess and fistula. These may result in there being a mass of bowel matted together. A mass of matted bowel is more likely to be resected en bloc than are a series of stenotic areas without secondary complications.

Overcoming the complications of Crohn's disease

The indications for surgical intervention and the immediate aims of the operation are to manage the complications of Crohn's disease, which are usually due to effects of mucosal ulceration. These are:

1. The fibrosis associated with the healing of ulcers
2. The access of micro-organisms, through the ulcers, into the tissue
3. Erosion of deep sepsis into adjacent organs causing a fistula or erosion of blood vessels.

Overcoming stenosis

This is the commonest initial complication of chronic ulceration, particularly of the small bowel. It is an inevitable consequence of Crohn's disease; by the time the patients with Crohn's disease have symptoms from small bowel disease, stenosis is inevitably present. Stenotic areas in the small bowel may be resected or made wider by strictureplasty or dilatation. The technical aspects of these procedures will be discussed in detail in Chapters 11 and 12.

Stricture dilatation is an attractive non-invasive option; the principle is similar to that employed when dilating peptic strictures of the lower oesophagus. There is no doubt that many Crohn's strictures are dilatable. We have successfully accomplished dilatation of four duodenal and eight ileo-colonic anastomotic strictures (see Chapter 11).

When the abdomen is opened at laparotomy, the tidiest option for small areas of recurrent Crohn's disease is resection of diseased tissue and end-to-end anastomosis. This gives the impression of having eradicated the disease and looks neat (see Chapter 10). Strictureplasty is aesthetically less pleasing but the diseased bowel is not sacrificed although the thickened, deformed bowel remains (see Chapter 12).

Drainage of sepsis

Any ulcer of the large and small intestine exposes the mesoderm to intestinal microflora, without the normal protection of healthy, active regenerating mucosa. Therefore, inevitably, all ulcers are infected. The body's ability to withstand such infection depends on the normal body defence mechanism, which is granulation tissue formation. Granulation tissue is comprised of loops of immature capillaries close to the interface between the gut lumen and the underlying mesoderm. The body's mobile defence mechanism, leucocytes, are immediately available for defence. Inevitably there is a loss of white cells and of serum through the intra-cellular spaces of the endothelium of the immature capillaries. Also, despite the presence of granulation tissue, there is some invasion of the tissues by micro-organisms. Trauma to the granulation tissue by intestinal contents is common, particularly when there is a tight stenosis through which they have to pass. The nature of the ulceration in Crohn's disease is typically that of deep, fissured ulcers penetrating the granulation tissue defence. Therefore, infection of the underlying tissues is common. The body has good defence mechanisms against infection. Even a large ulcerated area does not necessarily make the patient ill, although red cells, white cells and plasma may be leaking. It is undrained suppuration that makes the patient ill. Pus under tension separates tissue planes and is likely to be complicated by the entrance of micro-organisms into the venous system. This causes septicaemia with its associated fever, increased metabolism and, even, septicaemic shock. Once closed sepsis is suspected on clinical ground its presence must be confirmed as soon as possible by physical examination or by imaging. Pus under tension must then be drained either by percutaneous insertion of a drainage tube or by open surgical drainage (see Chapter 13).

In my experience the sepsis associated with neglected, complicated Crohn's disease is rarely simple or unilocular and is not readily drainable with a percutaneous catheter. Open drainage is often required and complete control of sepsis usually only follows the resection of the affected gut from which the sepsis is arising.

Management of fistula

I consider that an intestinal fistula in Crohn's disease arises from either (1) untreated stenotic disease, further complicated by deep penetrating ulceration and high intra-luminal pressure proximal to the stenosis; or (2) as a complication of leakage of an intestinal suture line after resection or strictureplasty. The first we term a "spontaneous" fistula and the second a "post-operative" fistula. A spontaneous fistula is always associated with a stenotic lesion and inevitably requires surgical management to overcome the stenosis. This is usually by resection. On two occasions in our series a fistula has been associated with such quiescent disease that it has been able to be cured by a simple strictureplasty of the stenotic segment. The management of Crohn's fistulae are discussed in further detail in Chapter 13. A post-operative fistula should heal if there is no residual distal obstructing stenosis.

Control of bleeding

Chronic ulceration anywhere in the alimentary tract may erode a major vessel. However, the chronic progression of ulceration in Crohn's disease rarely results in the acute breach of the wall of a significant vessel. As it progresses slowly the vessel usually first occludes by thrombosis as the inflammation progresses and the thrombosed blood vessel does not bleed. This is a general rule that applies to any chronic ulceration in the intestinal tract. The occasions on which gut ulceration produces acute or life-endangering bleeding is when the clot occluding the blood vessel is digested by proteolytic digestion as in the stomach or duodenum or in the Meckel's diverticulum. As there are usually no proteolytic enzymes active in the area of Crohn's disease ulceration, it is relatively rare that we are forced to operate because of acute intestinal bleeding.

Crohn's disease may be associated with ulcers in the duodenum and these may be subjected to the influence of acid/peptic digestive enzymes. It is then extremely difficult to differentiate a Crohn's disease ulcer, subjected to acid peptic ferments, from peptic ulcer occurring in someone with Crohn's disease. We have had to operate for the principal indication of continued intestinal bleeding on only four occasions in well over a 1000 operations for small bowel Crohn's disease in the past 25 years. However, chronic blood loss is a contributory indication in many patients who are deemed to require surgical intervention for colonic Crohn's disease (Chapter 14).

Provision of adequate nutrition

The commonest indication for surgical intervention in a patient with Crohn's disease is to improve the nutritional intake. This improvement occurs when chronic intestinal obstruction is overcome so that the patient can eat and take normal nutrients. Overcoming any of the complications of Crohn's disease and enabling the patient to return to an adequate diet can be considered as improving nutrition.

Many chronically ill patients with Crohn's disease do not feel like eating or drinking and it is often extremely difficult to persuade them to take an adequate oral intake. In most of these patients we use a fine bore nasogastric tube; often with nocturnal drip feeding. In a few patients this drip feeding is not well tolerated and in some of them we have placed a gastrostomy tube, particularly to facilitate nocturnal intra-gastric drip feeding (Fig. 6.1) (see also Chapter 3).

Although endoscopic placement of the gastrostomy feeding tube is feasible and practical we have experienced some difficulty with the technique; my two most successful long-term gastrostomy feeding endeavours have been achieved through a limited open operation.

When I have patients requiring complex operations for duodenal or upper jejunal Crohn's disease, particularly when these are associated with fistulae, I have placed an enterostomy feeding tube at the time of operation. I aim to place it 30–40 cm downstream from any anastomosis or fistula. This has

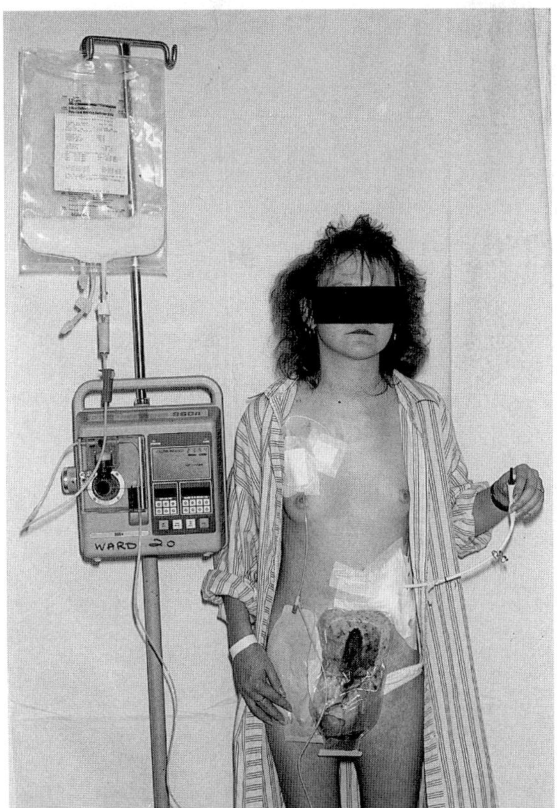

Fig. 6.1. Providing adequate nutrition. A patient with multifocal jejuno-ileal Crohn's disease with a juxtastomal complex fistula. She has persistent anorexia and intolerance of fine bore nasogastric feeding tubes. Total parenteral nutrition has been in progress for two weeks and she is now having supplemental nocturnal intra-gastric drip feeding via a Silastic gastrostomy tube.

proved both cost-effective and life-saving on three occasions. Jejunostomy feeding has proved to be a particularly effective form of long-term nutritional management in a patient with a duodeno-cutaneous fistula complicating Crohn's disease.

Reference

Ekelund GR, Lindhagen T (1989) Controversies in the surgical management of Crohn's disease. Pers Colon Rectal Surg 2:1–14

7 Indications for Surgical Intervention

J. Alexander-Williams

Emergency indications

Surgical emergencies are life-saving operations that have to be performed within a matter of hours, without time for comprehensive resuscitation. These are rare. More frequently in Crohn's disease an urgent operation is required after 12 to 24 hours of resuscitation to assure optimum operative conditions.

Perforation

Free intra-peritoneal perforation has occurred in only 12 of about 1000 of our operations for Crohn's disease and has only been seen once in the last ten years. It could be regarded as a sign of neglected disease as it has always occurred proximal to severely stenosed disease. It has occurred once in a patient who had an exclusion bypass operation, when it occurred in the loop of bowel just proximal to the bypassed stenosis (Fig. 7.1). The only recent free perforation that I have seen occurred in a grossly distended neo-terminal ileum above an ileo-rectal anastomosis in which we believed that the dilated pre-anastomotic small bowel had also undergone torsion.

Although free perforation is relatively rare it is more common to find that a once confined

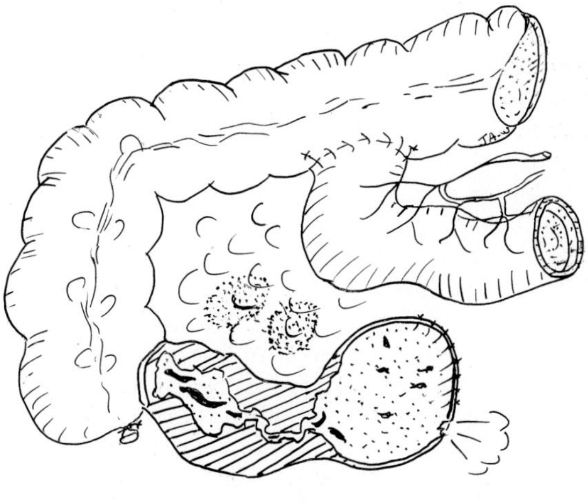

Fig. 7.1. Diagram of exclusion bypass showing end-to-side ileotransverse anastomosis. Excluded diseased ileum is cut open to show obstructing fibrotic disease with continued active ulceration. This ileum proximal to the obstruction has dilated and ruptured.

intra-abdominal abscess has discharged into the peritoneal cavity or part of it. The clinical picture is often one of a patient who was already suspected of harbouring an intra-abdominal abscess who suddenly deteriorated with signs of peritonitis. The sudden onset of peritonitis has been much less acute and dramatic than is normally associated with, for example, a perforated peptic ulcer. The abdomen is usually, but not inevitably, silent. In many of our patients this complication of intra-peritoneal rupture of the abscess has occurred when they have been on steroid therapy so that the inflammatory response and the signs of peritonitis are much less obvious than would normally be expected. There is usually radiographic evidence of gas outside the gut lumen. There is often no gas under the diaphragm because such patients often have frequent previous operations and there is not a complete peritoneal cavity.

Contrast radiology, apart from the normal air contrast already described, should not be necessary in the diagnosis of perforation. If the gas pattern on the plain radiograph is not sufficient to make a diagnosis, it is permissible to use water-soluble contrast. Ultrasound imaging may indicate free fluid in the peritoneal cavity but for reasons already discussed this is less common than are localised collections.

Clinical deterioration from peritonitis following perforation is usually rapid so that little time is available for resuscitation; the disadvantages of waiting will soon outweigh the advantages. Intravenous access is established to permit rapid infusion of physiological saline to counteract the rapid loss of fluid from the circulation into the peritoneal cavity and the intra-abdominal tissue places. The maintenance of blood pressure and the re-establishment of an adequate renal output are the best indices of the adequacy of the fluid replacement. Colloid replacement is not usually an immediate necessity.

A suitable stoma site is chosen and marked. Laparotomy is usually through a previous wound, as free perforation rarely occurs in a patient who has not already had one or more resections. If any previous wound seems inappropriate for a generalised laparotomy, a midline incision is usually chosen because this is the easiest to extend up or down or laterally once the site of the perforation is located. The preferred incisional sites for laparotomy in Crohn's disease are shown in Fig. 7.2.

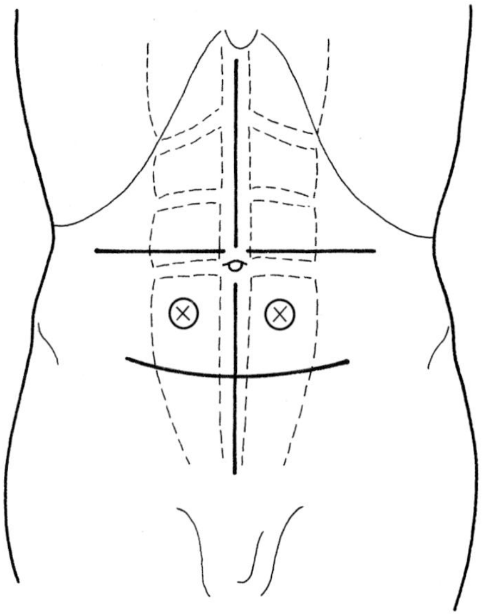

Fig. 7.2. Diagram of preferred incisions (bold lines) with optimal stoma sites.

In the small bowel it is usually easy to locate the site of perforation. It is usually within or proximal to an inflamed stenotic segment; the precise site of perforation being easily identified as it leaks intestinal contents. If there is any doubt about the site of the perforation the small bowel can be inflated with carbon dioxide, in the manner described below in the section on testing of anastomoses.

As the patient with peritonitis from perforation is usually ill and potentially septic it is unwise to attempt an anastomosis. The safest management is to resect the stenotic segment containing the perforation and to bring out a proximal end stoma in the first loop of gut that is sufficiently soft and pliable to permit a stoma to be everted. The stoma is best situated in the optimal stoma site in the left or right iliac fossa, depending on the ease of mobilising the gut. The distal end is best brought to the surface as a mucous fistula and this is usually simplest performed in the lower end of the laparotomy wound. As the defunctioned end will not be discharging intestinal contents there is no need for this stoma to be everted. The mucosa is usually sutured to the skin and the resulting stoma is termed a mucus fistula.

As a mucus fistula invariably discharges mucus and often pus, it usually requires subsequent management with an adhesive appliance. To avoid this some surgeons try not to produce a mucus fistula, by either closing the end of the bowel with staples or suture and either leaving it within the peritoneal cavity or fixing it in the lower part of the wound beneath the skin surface. In my opinion the safest manoeuvre is to create a properly defunctioned, draining mucus fistula. I advocate this because it is almost inevitably a short-term expedient that will be followed by restoration of intestinal continuity within 12 to 20 weeks.

Since we have kept accurate records on our unit over the past 40 years we have only encountered 12 instances of small bowel perforation. In some of these we have performed resection and primary anastomosis without serious complication but I would not recommend it as a safe option.

Free perforations of the large bowel usually occur as a complication of acute colitis, often with dilatation and sometimes with necrosis. This clinical picture is similar to that seen when perforation complicates toxic dilatation in ulcerative colitis. Perforation of the colon in acute colitis is something that I believe should never occur and I feel that it should be regarded as neglected disease. Nevertheless it can still occur, particularly in a patient in whom the physical signs of impending or definite perforation are suppressed under the influence of steroids or other immunosuppressive drugs.

Management is by immediate resuscitation and laparotomy in the manner described above for the small bowel. It should be regarded as an acute emergency and operation should not be delayed more than an hour or two. Before opening the abdomen an appropriate stoma site should be marked on the skin as described above and in the section under stoma.

In my experience the best operative management is total colectomy with end ileostomy in the right iliac fossa. Where possible the proximal end of the resection is in the sigmoid colon at the most distal level than can be brought to the lower end of the wound as a mucus fistula. On the rare occasions when there is perforation or necrosis of the sigmoid colon, resection can be taken down to the midrectum which is then closed as a Hartmann closure. This is sometimes necessary in elderly patients where perforated Crohn's disease is associated with extensive diverticular disease of the sigmoid colon when to bring up a mucous fistula is technically difficult. I imagine there could be some circumstances in which disease of the rectum is so severe that it is worth contemplating proctocolectomy; however, I have not yet seen such a case. I always recommend trying to leave the rectum for removal at a subsequent operation rather than trying to perform such an extensive operation as a pan-proctocolectomy on an ill patient.

Septicaemia

The sudden onset of unheralded septicaemia is uncommon in Crohn's disease. When it does occur it is usually associated with the rupture of a contained intra-abdominal abscess into all or part of the peritoneal cavity. The clinical picture is similar to that of perforation and like perforation it is usually associated with, and originates from, a stenotic area.

When septicaemia is established it is usually best, as in peritonitis, to remove the affected segment of Crohn's disease and bring out an ileostomy and mucus fistula. When septicaemia occurs as the result of an extensive abscess that has not ruptured freely into the peritoneal cavity, the clinical picture will be less acute; the patient will usually show signs of a swinging fever rather than a picture of septicaemic shock. The characteristic clinical picture of an abscess can often thus be detected on physical examination. However, scanning may be required to delineate accurately the size of the abscess. When the abscess is well localised, treatment by percutaneous tube drainage is a reasonable first move. It is usually best to assess the result of such draining before resorting to laparotomy.

In my experience large abscesses associated with Crohn's disease are often complicated and multi-loculated and are much less susceptible to percutaneous tube drainage than are abscesses associated with appendicitis or diverticular disease. Nevertheless I always attempt to use percutaneous drainage first and try to improve the patient's condition with appropriate antibiotics. After a few days I plan a definitive laparotomy to both drain the abscess and remove the acute area of Crohn's disease that is its source.

Bleeding

Bleeding is a rare indication for surgical intervention in Crohn's disease. Unless there is uncontrolled exsanguination it is better to transfuse, check the bleeding and clotting parameters, assess the whole disease and, if possible, try to localise the bleeding by endoscopy or angiography.

Our experience of this acute complication in Crohn's disease has been limited. In three patients in the last 10 years we have attempted to localise the bleeding by both angiography and endoscopy without success. In two patients bleeding continually from recurrent disease in the small bowel the problem was solved quite simply by resection of the affected area. The third patient, bleeding from a large ulcer in the second part of duodenum, continued to bleed despite two attempts at under-running the bleeding point and eventually died following breakdown of the duodenal suture line. On the basis of this experience I do not think it justifiable to propose codes of management.

Acute colitis

Emergency colectomy may be needed for acute colitis just as, but less commonly than, it is required for acute ulcerative colitis. The principal difference between the management of acute colitis in these two conditions is that in Crohn's disease we try to preserve the rectum wherever possible for subsequent ileo-rectal anastomosis after the acute episode has subsided, whereas in ulcerative colitis we are more inclined to preserve the rectum with a view to subsequently creating a restorative ileo-anal pouch procedure once the patient has recovered. In the past we have treated patients with acute Crohn's colitis by a primary colectomy and ileo-rectal anastomosis without a covering ileostomy. Although we have succeed in four patients, we have been criticised for attempting to restore continuity. I now feel sure that it is safest, when operating for acute Crohn's colitis, to perform a total colectomy and create an end ileostomy and mucus fistula. I then would wait until the patient has completely recovered and the histological diagnosis was established before considering restoration of continuity with an ileo-rectal or pouch-to-anus anastomosis.

Elective indications

Subacute obstruction

Most patients with Crohn's disease admitted to hospital as an emergency have subacute obstruction. This usually manifests as abdominal pain, distension and vomiting with total or incomplete constipation. Such episodes are more usually a manifestation of disease of small bowel rather than large bowel disease. The attack may be provoked by dietary indiscretion with the ingestion of indisgestible material such as uncooked fruit or vegetables. Sometimes it is due to an episode of acute exacerbation of inflammation causing inflammatory swelling of the gut wall and so critically narrowing already narrowed gut.

The clinical picture may be associated with abdominal tenderness but is usually clearly distinguishable from a closed-loop bowel obstruction. The large majority of such episodes settle on conservative management; usually by rest, restriction of oral intake, intravenous fluids and measures to reduce inflammation of the bowel wall such as steroids and/or antimicrobial agents.

Subacute obstruction is by far the commonest indication for operative intervention in small bowel Crohn's disease. In my experience it is four or five times more common an indication for surgical intervention than are the secondary complications of abscess or fistula. I believe that any series that does not have subacute food bolus obstruction as the commonest indication for surgical intervention is delaying operation for too long in too many people. I believe that you should not delay the surgical intervention for subacute food bolus obstruction for so long that it allows the development of secondary complication associated with penetrating ulceration of the gut. Nevertheless, we do not rush to operation on the first attack. All are given dietary advice. Many patients learn that they cannot tolerate some foods because these will precipitate colic and distension. However, some patients are much less observant than others and often they fail to appreciate that relationship between symptoms and food intake.

In many patients who come to operation for food bolus obstruction I find that proximal to the strictures there are numerous chunks of identifiable undigested food such as pineapple, cucumber, orange or apple that are known to have been ingested many days or even weeks before the operation. Some patients who are both perceptive and experienced, learn to avoid precipitating foods and are able to postpone operative intervention for months or even years by taking a "non-chunk" diet. This is either normal food that has been put through a blender or eating well-cooked food that they are able to mash with the back of a fork. As I have stated before, and I am in danger of repeating ad nauseam, I believe in the philosophy of not delaying so long in the management of strictures that secondary complications occur.

Radiographic confirmation is not essential in the assessment of strictures causing subacute obstruction. Neither is it essential to demonstrate proximal gut distension radiologically before entertaining such a diagnosis. It is quite common to find patients who are severely incapacitated by food bolus obstruction in whom it is not possible to demonstrate proximal gut distension radiologically. The radiological demonstration of stricture is sometimes clear but often adherent and overlapping loops of bowel make this difficult and when a stricture is demonstrated it is not clear how much of the narrowing is due to resolvable factors such as oedema. In my opinion the patient's history and perception of the problem is the principal guiding factor. On our unit we have a working rule relating to the number of emergency presentations on a patient with subacute obstruction in relation to the indication for operation. Our rule is that within a year one admission is a warning, two is an indication and three admissions an indictment.

In many of the patients there is an element of inflammatory oedema that precipitates the attack and such oedema may respond, particularly to steroids. Many patients presenting in the manner described will still be on low-dose steroids and some will have had a relapse of the symptoms once their steroids were decreased.

We have another working rule that no patient should remain on steroids for subacute intestinal obstruction for longer than three months without serious consideration being given to the alternative of surgical intervention and stopping the steroids. We believe that the risks of strictureplasty are less than those of continued steroid medication.

The majority of patients who respond to conservative management usually have liquid feeding restarted when the gut is shown to be transmitting its content satisfactorily, which is usually when the patient is passing large quantities of gas or stool. Depending on progress, the patients are gradually promoted through a liquid only to a blended diet. In my experience it is rarely necessary to have to institute parenteral feeding or even prolonged fluid enteral feeding, such as an elemental diet. However, in some patients in whom there are frequent attacks of food bolus colic that recur as soon as a semi-solid diet is restarted, a prolonged course of liquid nutrition is often tried with surgical re-intervention always considered as the ultimate sanction. It is the practice on our unit to consider the option of surgical intervention in all patients who require emergency admission more than twice in six months. A few of these patients choose to remain on a liquid or totally blended diet. However, most of those who have already experienced the safety and lack of trauma associated with non-invasive surgical procedures such as strictureplasty usually volunteer for further strictureplasties.

Chronic blood loss

Persistent moderate anaemia with a haemoglobin between 9 and 11 g/l is common in Crohn's disease but a serious degree of anaemia is rare: it appears to be commoner with colonic than with small bowel Crohn's disease. The repeated necessity for blood transfusion to "top-up" the haemoglobin in a patient with known colonic Crohn's disease is a relative indication for surgical intervention. A running flow chart, completed at each review and showing a haemoglobin and haematocrit levels will provide a graphic indication of the need for transfusion. Furthermore the size of the ulcerated area of bowel responsible for the blood loss can be determined either by contrast radiology or endoscopy. I feel that, in the large bowel, endoscopy provides the clearest indication of area involved in ulceration and predicts the extent of any bleeding. If transfusion is needed more than twice in six months, I usually advise surgical resection. I have employed anastomotic strictureplasty without resection in some patients in whom the bleeding apparently came from a post-operative anastomotic stenosis.

Fistula

In our series a fistula is the second commonest indication for elective surgical intervention in small bowel Crohn's disease.

We classify fistulas into post-operative or spontaneous. Post-operative fistulas are those occurring within 60 days of operative intervention, associated with an obvious or suspected anastomotic leakage or abscess. Such anastomotic complications in the absence of distal obstructing disease often heal spontaneously without surgical reintervention.

A spontaneous fistula occurs as the result of the rupturing of a abscess, almost inevitably secondary to a penetrating ulcer in an area of stenosis. In such patients the stenosis and penetrating ulcer are persisting factors preventing the healing of the fistula and, almost inevitably, they require surgical intervention. The subject of intestinal fistula is dealt with in greater detail in a subsequent section.

Chronic ill-health

Patients who have an intra-abdominal abscess secondary to stenosis in small bowel Crohn's disease are often acutely ill and patients with fistulas are often chronically ill. However, in the absence of such obvious complications, chronic ill-health in Crohn's disease is most commonly associated with extensive colonic ulceration.

The chronically ill patient with Crohn's disease tends to have a continued fever and malnutrition. They are usually unable to work or study and lose weight. Such a state of chronic ill-health should always evoke the question "Can surgical intervention help?". In former years when the consequence of all surgical intervention in Crohn's disease was loss of functioning gut and when surgical intervention was often followed by continued morbidity, there was a natural reluctance to operate simply for chronic ill-health; most patients were encouraged to accept it. However, since the adoption of strictureplasty for stenosis and the application of the principle of temporary exteriorisation of the gut to overcome the consequences of abscess or fistula, surgery should be associated with very little morbidity. Safe surgery is an attractive alternative to chronic ill-health.

Urgency and incontinence

Urgency and incontinence are symptoms which often go together and are associated particularly with distal large bowel and perianal Crohn's disease. A patient with unremitting urgency with up to ten stools by day and two or three by night is likely to be much happier and able to achieve more goals if she or he has a well-managed ileostomy. Those sensitive patients to whom the thought of faecal material discharging from their abdomen is an anathema inevitably find that a well-managed ileostomy is preferable to constant anal incontinence. If the faecal incontinence is slight or intermittent or if it is simply purulent, many patients are prepared to put up with it rather than having an ileostomy. For such patients it is often helpful to offer them a temporary loop ileostomy with the promise of restoring continuity if they find it less convenient and more distasteful than their present complaint. I have employed this strategy frequently and find that once they have had a well-managed stoma about 60% of patients willingly opt to retain it. If they decide to have a permanent stoma then they must realize that the defunctioned rectum and any remaining large bowel will have to be removed because of the long-term risk of the development of cancer.

Anal pain is a common indication for minor surgical intervention because it usually signifies pus under tension that needs draining. This subject is dealt with in detail under perianal Crohn's disease (Chapter 18).

8 Reducing the Risks of Operation

J. Alexander-Williams

Principles

As patients with Crohn's disease are likely to need many operations during the course of their life, it is important that the surgeon should make surgery as safe as possible. Our goal is that no patient should die as the result of an operation for Crohn's disease. This ideal depends, partly, on the patients being referred for surgery before they become too ill and partly on the acceptance that surgeons should tailor their operative intervention to the fitness of the patient presented to them. They should always try to operate with the patient in optimum condition and, when they do operate, they should try to consider and avoid all possible complications.

The principles behind minimising operative risk including minimising the blood shed during the operation, preventing damage to adjacent tissues and recognising any damage that might occur, minimising infection, avoiding unnecessary sacrifice of gut and ensuring that anastomosis do not leak.

Minimise blood loss

The principles that should be adopted to achieve minimal blood loss are good technique to ensure that the minimum number of small vessels are divided, that large blood vessels are securely ligated and that the normal physiological mechanisms that prevent bleeding are compromised as little as possible by, for example, anticoagulants or other drugs that interfere with clotting mechanisms.

Haemostatic technique

Principles

There is no point in dividing by sharp dissection, tissues that do not need to be divided. Those tissues containing arteries and veins should be carefully secured, which may be difficult when operating on oedematous tissues with fatty infiltration and large lymph nodes. Ligatures placed around clamps that have picked up a large mass of oedematous tissue may easily slip and let the blood vessel retract into the pedicle and form a mesenteric haematoma or continue to bleed. The technique is illustrated for doubly ligated large oedematous pedicles to ensure complete, safe haemostasis (Fig. 8.1).

It is not possible to achieve total instant haemostasis of all tissues that are divided when operating on inflamed, hyperaemic tissues as in Crohn's disease. The surgeon has to be aware of the amount and type of bleeding that will stop if it is simply left or pressed on with an operating gauze swab. I find it useful to have very fine tissue forceps (Adson, Fig. 8.2), as used in plastic surgery, to enable me to coagulate with diathermy fine bleeding points. However, I leave most raw hyperaemic divided tissues that are not bleeding from any obvious point, in the knowledge that the

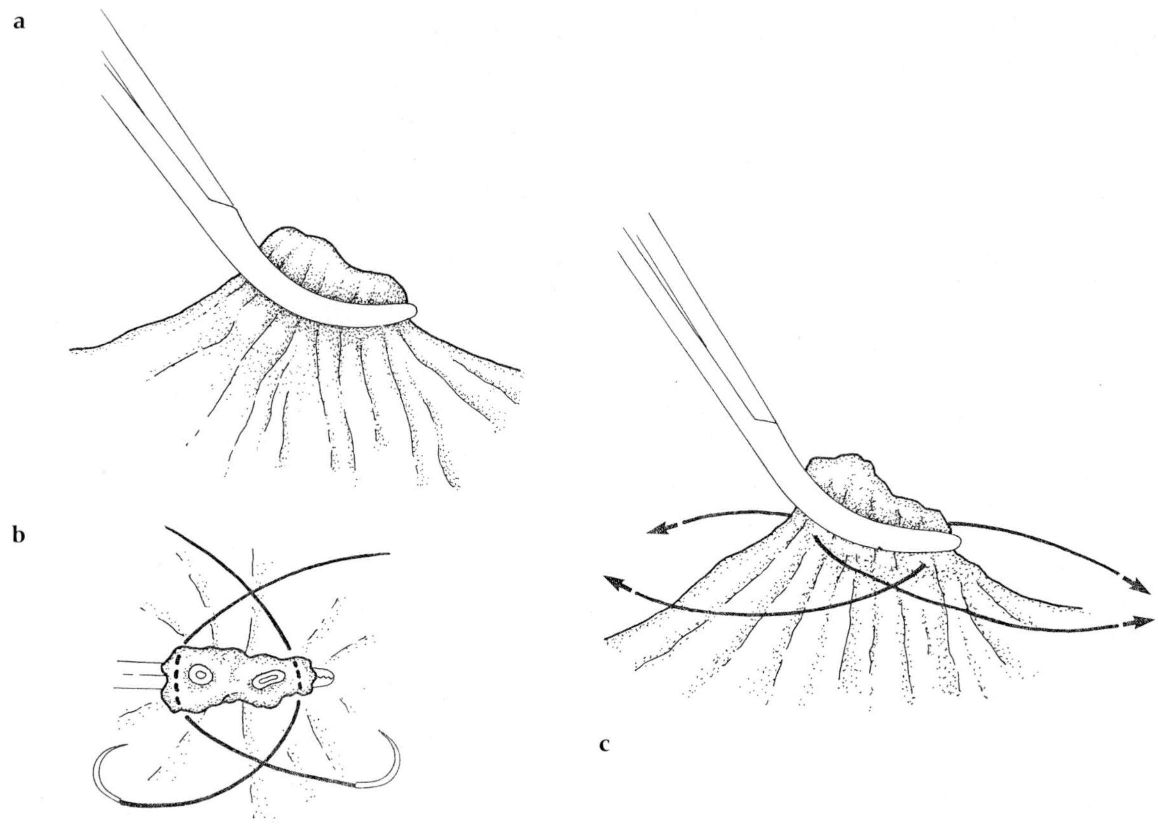

Fig. 8.1. Double-interlocking ligation sutures to control thick vascular pedicles.

bleeding will satisfactorily arrest in a short time. There is usually such a lot of surgical intervention to perform that it is counter-productive to attempt to achieve total haemostasis in each operative move. The advantage that we have in operating on patients with Crohn's disease is that they are mostly young and that the natural factors that control haemorrhage are surprisingly effective.

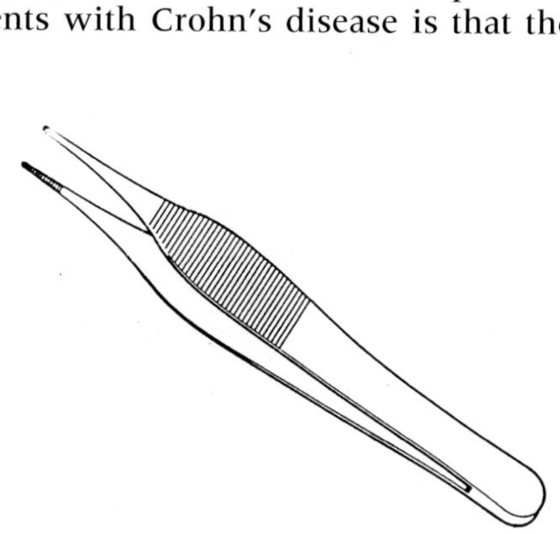

Fig. 8.2. Adson fine dissecting forceps.

Avoid anticoagulants

When operating on patients with Crohn's disease I always tend to try to avoid systemic anticoagulants. Although I use prophylactic subcutaneous heparin widely in the management of patients with malignant bowel disease, I tend to avoid heparin in patients with Crohn's disease unless there are very strong factors favouring phlebo-thrombosis such as a past history of phlebo-thrombosis and embolus. My early experience of serious bleeding during and after pelvic operations for rectal Crohn's disease in patients receiving prophylactic heparinisation was so worrying that I made a decision, about 20 years ago, to avoid heparinisation. I also avoid other systemic anticoagulants such a Dextran. I rely for thrombo-phlebotic prophylaxis on graduated compression stockings (Fig. 8.3) and pneumatic leggings during the operation (Fig. 8.4).

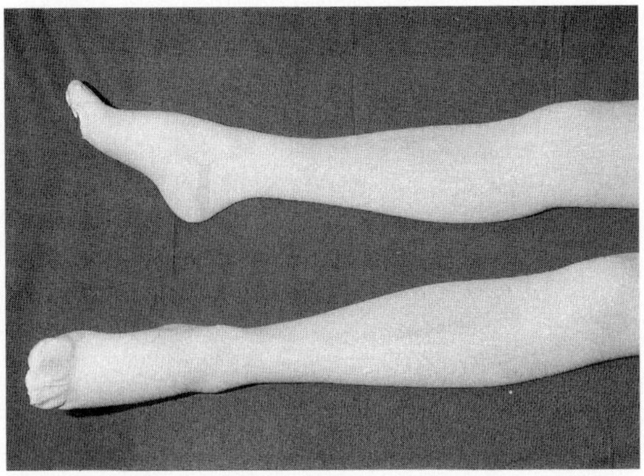

Fig. 8.3. Graduated compression stockings worn before and after operation.

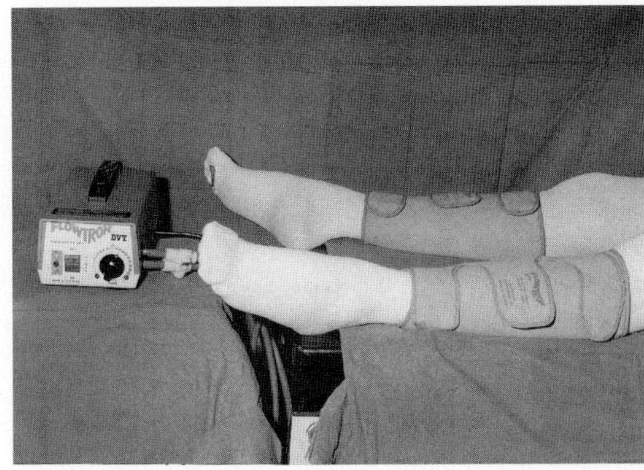

Fig. 8.4. Pneumatic leg bags to provide intermittent pressure.

Although in our earlier analysis of the causes of death in patients with Crohn's disease we had a number of patients who had fatal pulmonary emboli, in the past 20 years we have not had any fatality from pulmonary embolus, although we have had a few patients survive a pulmonary embolus. Some of the most serious postoperative bleeding complications that I have ever experienced were during the time that we were conducting clinical trials with an antibiotic (Meslacillin) which appeared to destabilise the patients' clotting mechanism.

Preventing damage to adjacent tissues and organs

The gut

The structures that are at greatest danger of inadvertent damage during operation for Crohn's disease are adjacent loops of gut that may have become secondarily adherent to a primary inflammatory mass. Some of the well-known danger areas include adherence between the hepatic flexure of the colon and duodenum and between the terminal ileum and sigmoid colon. However any loop of gut proximal or distal to the principal lesion in Crohn's disease can become secondarily adherent to the inflammatory mass and the separation of these secondarily adherent loops of gut may be damaged. The serosa and muscle layers are frequently damaged but the only damage of great significance is that of mucosa. I will be describing later methods that minimise this risk of damage but equally important is the instant recognition of such damage should it occur. Some of the worst catastrophes that I have experienced after operating on Crohn's disease have followed undetected operative damage to loops of bowel that are stuck firmly to the major lesion for which the operation was undertaken. Particularly dangerous adhesion involvement is between the third part of the duodenum and the hepatic flexure of the colon or between the terminal ileum and sigmoid colon. Under these circumstances is it quite easy to breach the mucosa of gut that is not primarily involved in active Crohn's disease. This breach of the mucosa is serious enough in itself but if it is undetected and therefore unsutured it can be disasterous.

The next most important structure that might be damaged during operative dissection is the urinary system. The bladder is particularly at risk when inflammatory masses of the terminal ileum or the sigmoid colon or both are stuck on to the fundus of the bladder and sometime lesions of the terminal ileum or of the sigmoid colon are involved in inflammatory masses that are closely related to the ureter.

Planes of cleavage

One of the first happy realisations of the surgeon encountering complex problems from Crohn's disease is that it has some inherent advantages over the sort of operative problems encountered with other advanced conditions in the abdomen such as malignancy and diverticular disease. The first surgical happiness in the management of Crohn's disease is the privilege of operating on young tissues, the second privilege is that the nature of the adhesion of one structure to another in Crohn's disease seems to be quite different from that in other conditions, in that it seems to be much easier in Crohn's disease to find a plane of cleavage between the involved gut and adjacent structures. This plane of cleavage that occurs when the inflamed serosa of gut sticks to an adjacent area of serosa can usually be separated by gentle finger pressing or pinching. One of the delightful experiences of a surgeon managing Crohn's disease is how easily apparently densely adherent organs separate one from another once the correct plane of cleavage has been entered. The plane of cleavage is usually easy to establish unless there has been some secondary complication such as abscess or an infected operation. In the absence of such complications, simple finger pressure or pinching between the forefinger and thumb is enough to establish and enlarge on the plane of cleavage. There are times during the dissection in which the easy plane of cleavage is held up by a firmer fibrous adhesion that cannot be easily broken down. Therefore from time to time it is necessary to undertake some sharp dissection either with scissors or, as I prefer when possible, diathermy dissection. Sometimes it is possible to use the closed blades of dissecting forceps to continue the plane of cleavage when simple finger dissection is not possible. I refer to this manoeuvre as a "tyre lever manoeuvre" (Fig. 8.5).

The separation of planes of cleavage between loops of gut is further aided by distending the adjacent loops by CO_2 insufflation. By this method two loops of gut that appear firmly stuck to each other show a line of separation which can be developed as before with finger tip or closed dissecting scissors once they are tightly distended with CO_2. I find that with the gut distended with gas it is much easier to avoid finding a false plane such as that between the mucosa and the muscle.

The CO_2 insufflation to distend the gut can be achieved by blowing CO_2 through a nasogastric tube into the stomach and then propelling the gut onwards by manually compressing the stomach and pushing the gas through the pylorus. Another option is to introduce the gas into the lumen of the gut through a fine bore needle passed obliquely through the gut wall into the lumen. Once the gut has been opened because there is either a stricture or an abscess or some lesion that is going to need to be resected, the opened gut

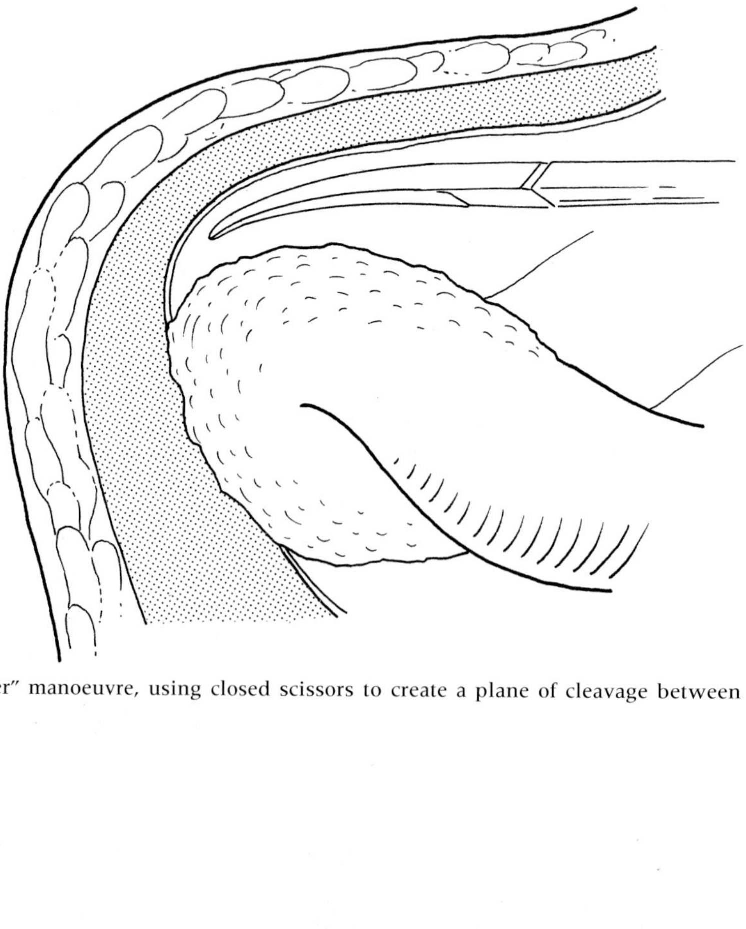

Fig. 8.5. "Tyre lever" manoeuvre, using closed scissors to create a plane of cleavage between oedematous gut and abdominal wall.

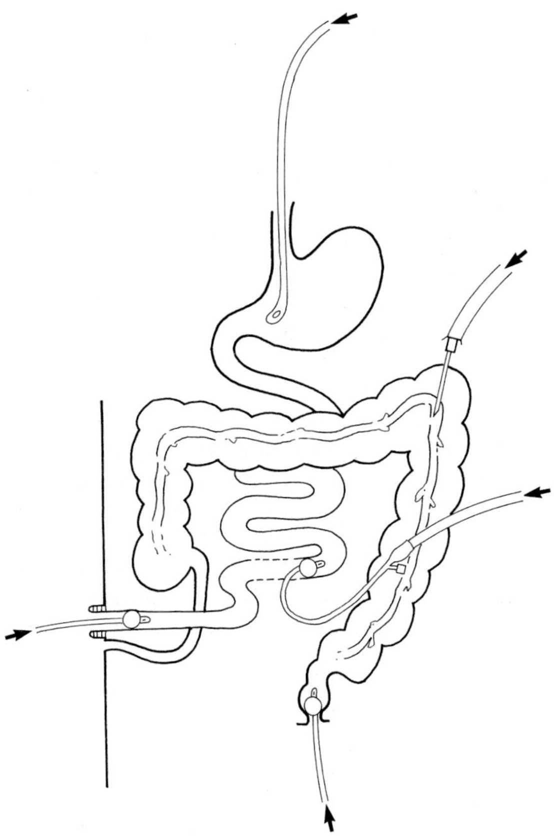

Fig. 8.6. Diagram of potential sites for CO_2 insufflation of the gut.

can then be used as a port to insufflate with CO_2. I use a transparent sterile suction tubing to distend the gut with CO_2 from the laparoscopy inflation apparatus (Fig. 8.6).

Urinary system

The urinary system is also in danger during dissection of oedematous inflamed loops of gut. There tends to be a particular danger to the ureter at the pelvic brim. The possibility of ureteric obstruction can often be predicted clinically and investigated pre-operatively by ultrasound; it is rarely necessary to have further confirmation from excretion urography. Whatever method is used to warn of the possibility of ureteric involvement should prompt the surgeon to identify the ureter proximal to the Crohn's disease inflammatory mass and trace it downwards towards the pelvis and to the bladder. Once the ureter has been identified proximally it is relatively easy to find the plane of cleavage between the ureter and the gut mass or phlegmon. The separation of this plane of cleavage is rarely difficult and using this method I have never caused injury to the ureter or failed to be able to separate it from the mass. This experience is in contrast to that of comparable inflammatory masses produced by carcinoma or diverticular disease. In both of these diseases I have found ureter damage difficult to avoid.

Adherence of the inflammatory mass to the bladder can usually be resolved by dissecting, by finger pinching, the "tyre lever" manoeuvre or occasionally sharp dissection with knife, scissors or diathermy. When it is difficult to find a good plane of cleavage between the gut and the bladder I inflate both organs with CO_2. Then, when both are distended, it is usually possible to cut between them with a cutting diathermy without entering either organ, unless there is a fistula. This will, of necessity, involve making a small hole in the bladder. This hole is usually dealt with simply by suturing the bladder wall and continuing bladder catheter drainage for about a week.

In general damage to the urinary system during operations for Crohn's disease is easy to avoid. Damage to adjacent loops of gut is less easy to avoid but, once detected, is simple to correct by transverse suturing and rechecking with CO_2 inflation.

Minimise infection

Principles

The partially obstructed gut in Crohn's disease is always heavily colonised with anaerobic and aerobic microbacteria and therefore all operations are invariably heavily contaminated. It is not possible to sterilise the gut or gut contents before operation. Bowel preparation for the small gut is both impractical and ineffective. Surgeons have to accept that this type of operation is contaminated.

The next principle is that the peritoneal cavity is resistant to microbacterial contamination. Small quantities of microbacteria are readily dealt with by the body's defence system and overwhelming peritoneal infection is virtually unknown following operations for Crohn's disease, unless there is anastomotic leakage and continued contamination.

Other tissue spaces apart from the peritoneal cavity are much more susceptible to infection, particularly the fat of the abdominal wall and the extra peritoneal tissues of the pelvis after excision of the rectum. It follows that it is unnecessary to drain the peritoneal cavity. However, some form of drainage or antibacterial irrigation might minimise the risk of extra-peritoneal infection.

Plastic wound guards

I always use plastic wound guards in an attempt to minimise the quantity of bacterial contamination of the fat of the abdominal wall. I also thoroughly irrigate the abdominal wall with an antiseptic (chlorhexidine) solution before skin closure. If contamination is heavy I leave the skin wound partially open to drain.

In the extra-peritoneal tissues I always drain with a vacuum drain. In the pelvis after proctectomy, I either close the extra-peritoneal space with a vacuum drain or I leave the pelvic wound open to be managed by irrigation, awaiting healing by second intention.

Minimising spillage of gut contents

In an attempt to minimise or prevent contamination with small bowel contents I used to use a soft intestinal clamp. However, in Crohn's disease it is so difficult to achieve that I have abandoned the attempt. It is impossible to achieve in those cases having strictureplasties or having the small bowel luminal diameter investigated by balloon pull-through. Under these circumstances contamination is inevitable and accepted. If the small bowel is obviously distended with fluid, I will suck this out with a sump suction drain. When there is food bolus impaction proximal to an obstructing lesion, I remove this with a small teaspoon. If there is much faecal fluid in the lumen of the gut proximal or distal to an anastomosis or strictureplasty I will often tamponade the lumen of the gut with a small gauze swab soaked in an antiseptic solution such as colloidal iodine. These swabs are inserted before the anastomosis is begun and both are removed before the final few sutures are placed in the anterior layer.

After the completion of anastomosis or strictureplasty, I wash out the abdominal cavity with more than 2 litres of saline. This lavage helps to remove small particles of fatty tissue or intestinal contents or phlegmonous exudate that otherwise would have imposed a burden on the body's defence mechanism. At one time I used an antimicrobial agent in the washout fluid but no longer do so since I have found that after such contaminated operations for Crohn's disease intra-abdominal abscess or peritonitis is virtually unknown. I have decided that intra-peritoneal antibiotics are not necessary and regard them as an unjustifiable expense.

Prophylactic antibiotics

Prophylactic antibiotics are given as with all intestinal operations. Fashion in the use of antimicrobial agents changes and whatever I am using now is likely to be superseded by some newer, more effective and, possibly, even cheaper preparation. For many years it has been our practice to use a single dose of intravenous metronidazole and a cephelosporin intra-operatively and once post-operatively. Those preferring a single antimicrobial preparation currently find Augmentin both convenient and economical.

Avoid unnecessary sacrifice of gut

The gut, particularly the small bowel is a vital organ which is essential for adequate nutrition. At present there is no known cure for Crohn's disease and so sufferers are likely to need repeated operations. There is the theoretical possibility of repeated resections reducing available small gut to a critical level and in the past many cases were recognised with the so-called "short gut syndrome". In some centres permanent home parenteral nutrition is required for such patients. Therefore, it is a reasonable principle to try to avoid resection or to resect as little as possible when managing the complications of Crohn's disease. This is particularly so in young patients and in those who have already had a number of operations for recrudescence. Although it is difficult to give relative physiological values for different parts of the small bowel, it is generally considered that the duodenum is the most important part of the small bowel both for digestion and absorption, the jejunum is also vital. The ileum is considered to be a little less vital apart from its role in the reabsorp-

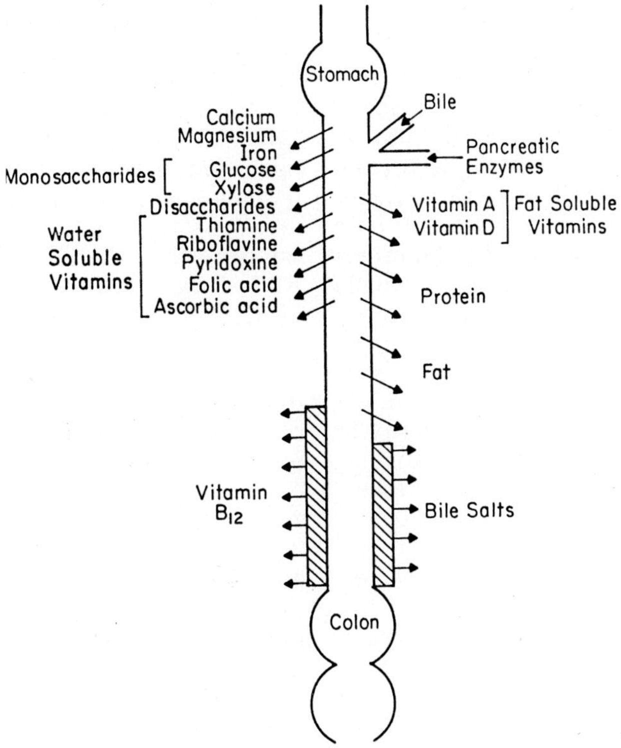

Fig. 8.7. Sites of absorption in the small intestine.

tion of bile acids and some nutrients such as Vitamin B_{12} (Fig. 8.7). The large bowel is relatively unimportant from the point of view of absorption of nutrients, as is shown by the perfect health of most patients who have had a panproctocolectomy and permanent ileostomy for ulcerative colitis, familial polyposis or Crohn's colitis. The only part of the large bowel that has a vital physiological function is the rectum; it has storage and water absorption properties vital for normal continence. It is always my policy to attempt to preserve the rectum in patients with Crohn's disease. A healthy rectum is important in the preservation of continence and avoidance of frequent watery stools. Apart from the rectum there seems to be little physiological advantage in sacrifice of all of the colon or in the sacrifice of 60 cm of the terminal ileum. Nevertheless the principle of maximum gut conservation is one that I feel should be applied throughout the whole of the alimentary tract. We must remember that we are only operating for the complications of Crohn's disease, we are not having to eradicate every vestige of Crohn's disease from the patient.

To avoid unnecessary sacrifice of gut

In reoperations for Crohn's disease I believe that it is important to always dissect out the whole of the residual bowel and to free all kinks and adhesions. This enables the surgeon to make an accurate assessment of the amount of remaining small bowel. It also enables the particular lesion or lesions for which the operation is being performed to be mobilised and brought out on to the surface of the abdomen. The exceptions to the this rule are the duodenum and rectum; the rest of the gut can usually be brought up to the surface. The point of bringing the gut to the surface of the abdomen is to be able to unravel the various loops of gut and to sort out any possible dense adhesions and enteroenteric fistulae. Enteroenteric fistulas are often unnoticed unless this is done. The principal importance in their detection is to avoid the en bloc excision of matted loops of small gut. This was a policy that I used to employ before being converted to the cult of gut conservation.

The advantage of bringing the affected part of the gut to the surface is that it is possible to be more precise about what part is affected by Crohn's disease and what part is simply oedematous and adherent to the inflammatory process or an abscess. I find that what at first appears to be a mass of several matted loops of gut can be slowly and carefully sorted out by freeing the adherent loops; usually with the aid of CO_2 inflation. A number of these oedematous adherent areas can be shown not to be affected by Crohn's disease in their luminal aspect and not associated with any stenosis when examined by an intraluminal balloon. In the early days of our experience with the management of Crohn's disease, such masses of matted gut were often resected as a single mass of inflamed and adherent tissue only to find, on subsequent dissection, that a relatively small area was involved in active ulcerated Crohn's disease and narrowed by a fibrous stenosis.

The process of total dissection of inflamed masses of gut brought to the surface of the abdomen is referred to on our unit as a "bench-job". This is a term borrowed from the automobile repair trade when the affected engine or gear box is lifted out from the automobile to be repaired more carefully and precisely on the work bench. I feel that by using this technique I have been successful in preserving many tens of centimetres of gut that might otherwise have been resected. Many patients in whom gut was so preserved have inevitably returned for further stenotic problems in succeeding years. At the next operation it is a common observation that gut that was matted together and freed at the last operation now appears normal; it is another part of the gut that is the subject of the stenosis that is the indication for the latest operation. This anecdotal evidence has no scientific basis but is presented only as an explanation for the philosophy of trying to retain as much gut as possible in Crohn's disease.

Avoiding anastomotic leakage

Principles

The best conditions for satisfactory complete healing of gut that is sutured together, either as an anastomosis or strictureplasty, is that the ends to be sutured should be healthy with a good blood supply. The patient should be in optimum condition with optimum nutrition and the ability to mount the appropriate inflammatory response to activate the normal repair mechanism. The patient should not be under the influence of any drugs that might impair healing.

It is rarely possible to achieve all these optimum conditions when operating on a patient who is ill with Crohn's disease, therefore it is important to try to give a relative importance value to each of these desiderata. As will be referred to later under the section of the results of strictureplasty, we have attempted a retrospective analysis of those patients who experienced leakage of strictureplasty suture lines in an attempt to find which of the factors are important in predisposing to poor healing. The personal views now to be expressed have been acquired by such retrospective studies of patients who have experienced anastomotic complications; although it is recognised that few if any of them have been submitted to strict scientific prospective trial analysis. All of us working in this field will realise how difficult it would be to mount reliable prospective trials to test most of these hypotheses.

The patient's fitness and the inflammatory response

I always prefer to make an anastomosis in a patient who had a normal haemoglobin, a normal serum albumin, normal lean muscle mass and grip strength and who is not receiving any form of immunosuppression. At a time when we are considering carefully the cost and possible disadvantages of blood transfusion, we no longer tend to replace blood until the patient has a normal level of haemoglobin before operation. The combined team of physician, surgeon and anaesthetist usually agree that a haemoglobin of above 11 grams per cent is desirable and patients below this level usually have a transfusion to achieve this. We would like patients to be well nourished but usually the indications for operation include the patient's failure to maintain adequate oral nutrition. The question therefore is: how much does nutritional "supercharging" benefit the patient and decrease the risk of anastomotic leakage? My own instinctive feeling used to be that we should attempt to achieve an optimal nutritional status by giving high-calorie, high-nitrogen liquid feeding and if this was not possible by giving total parenteral nutrition.

However, I have slowly modified these ideals on realising that an impractical amount of time and resource was involved in achieving significant changes in serum albumin levels and lean body mass and in improving the patient's ability to mount an inflammatory response as judged by skin testing for evidence of anergy. Our retrospective analysis of those patients who came to operation still severely malnourished has not shown any clear evidence of the adverse factors predisposing to leakage. The same lack of statistical evidence has led us to believe that the presence of steroid therapy in standard doses does not significantly affect healing. However, I am still wary of operating on patients receiving active immunosuppression with, for instance, azothiaprine.

A good blood supply

Nothing prejudices good anastomotic healing more than an inadequate blood supply. Poor blood supply is a factor that is considered to prejudice the healing of colonic anastomosis in malignancies, particularly in the elderly and to compromise anastomoses when gut is being resected for irradiation damage. Some have thought that a poor blood supply may be a factor compromising anastomoses in Crohn's disease. This hypothesis does not fit with my experience when dividing the gut at the level of an anastomosis in Crohn's disease. I tend to divide the bowel with cutting diathermy without the use of occlusion clamps. Using this method it is inevitable that there is vigorous bleeding from multiple sites at the cut edge of the gut, indicating an excessive rather than impoverished blood supply.

Avoid factors that may impair healing

It is obviously unwise to perform an anastomosis or make a suture line in the presence of distal obstruction; yet in Crohn's disease it is often difficult to detect an obstruction distal to a line of resection simply on external appearances or past radiological findings. It is usually possible to have detected the presence of large bowel Crohn's disease before an operation. Furthermore, any Crohn's disease of the large bowel sufficiently severe to cause obstruction is usually obvious at laparotomy. However, the danger is that fibrous strictures of the terminal ileum can be missed when making, for example, an anastomosis after resection in the mid-ileum. For this reason I advocate checking by the passage of a 25 mm balloon through the lumen from any proximal gut anastomosis as far as large bowel. Any distal stenosis is dealt with by strictureplasty (see strictureplasty, Chapter 13).

I believe that the presence of drainage tubes down to, or across anastomoses may impair healing. There is good experimental evidence that intra-abdominal intestinal anastomoses are more likely to break down in the presence of an impervious drain in their immediate vicinity. Although there is no scientifically acceptable trial evidence in man, I still believe that there is no evidence that an intra-peritoneal drain carries any advantage in Crohn's disease and therefore I never use them and advise against their use.

The presence of intra-abdominal abscess, particularly any residual abscess cavity or granulation tissue, seems to be a major factor in predisposing to anastomotic breakdown. The evidence in favour of this hypothesis is presented below under strictureplasty (Chapter 13). The exact mechanism of impairment of anastomoses is not known, it may simply be that patients with intra-abdominal sepsis are generally sicker than those without. Nevertheless, I am always apprehensive about the integrity of an anastomosis or a suture line in the gut in someone who is known to have, or is found to have, an intra-abdominal abscess. Although on occasions I will make an anastomosis knowing this risk, it strongly influences me towards creating a stoma for proximal diversion. I do this with a view to re-establishing intestinal continuity when the sepsis has resolved and the patient is fitter, usually after 12 weeks.

Surgical technique

There are many variable factors in the anastomotic technique that may influence healing. The surgeon has to consider the number of layers, whether the suture is continuous or interrupted, how close together are the sutures, the type of suture material and how tight to pull the knots or the continuous suture. It is not my intention to review the pros and cons of the different forms of anastomotic technique, I intend simply to tell you of what I have chosen and why. The principle behind the selection is that I always choose the simplest and quickest technique, unless I find evidence or experience that suggests that a more complex technique has advantages. I use as fine as practical a continuous absorbable seromuscular suture, pulling the seromuscular edges to be sutured into gentle apposition. At present I use 3/0 continuous Polyglactin using between two and four additional stay sutures simply to hold up the bowel during the suturing to make it easier and also to allow occasional knotting of the continuous suture to prevent a "purse-string" tightening effect. The distance between the sutures depends on the thickness of the bowel to be sutured. The thicker the bowel the further apart are the sutures. I tend to err on the side of taking larger rather than smaller bites; knowing that after completing the suture line I am going to test it by gas distension. At any point where the continuous suture is not quite tight enough, a gas leak will be detected that can then be reinforced by an extra suture. Experience has taught me that I need to put in an extra, reinforcing, airtight suture to supplement a suture line in about every four or five suture lines. I argue that if my suture lines never leaked gas on distension, I am probably pulling most of them rather too tight. On healthy small gut I find that the stitches are usually 5–7 mm apart and in most instances I am able to avoid picking up the mucosa with the seromuscular stitch (Fig. 8.8).

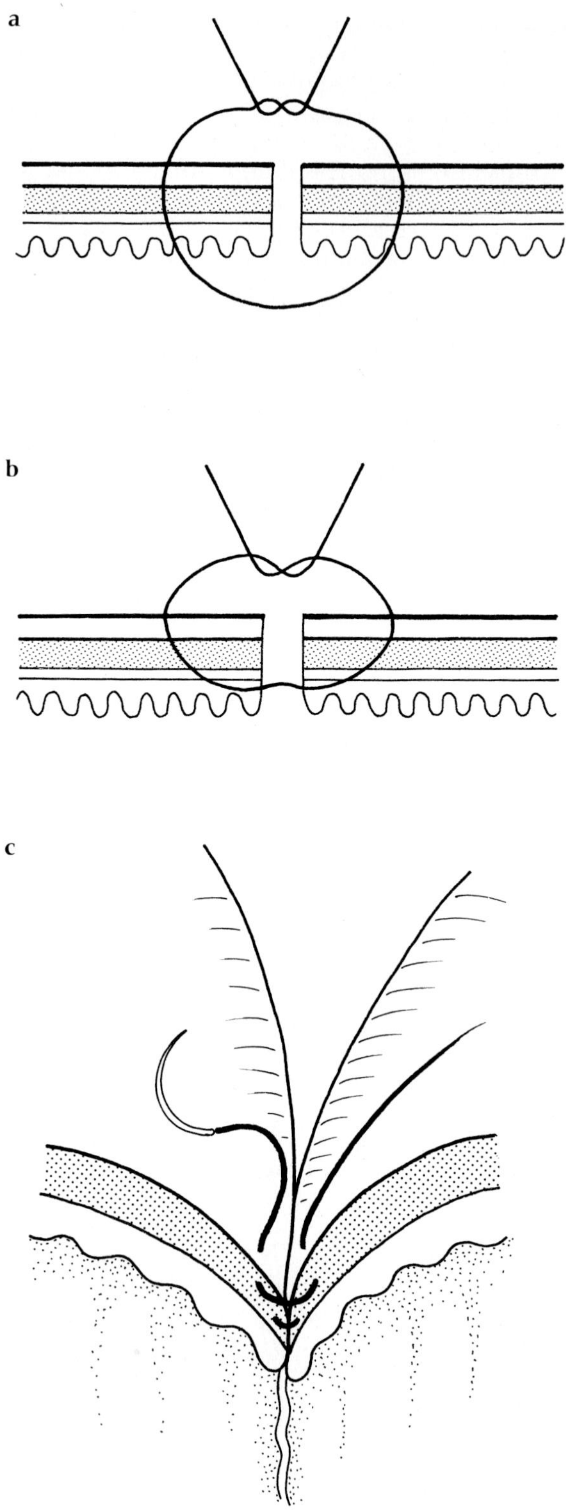

Fig. 8.8. **a** Diagram of full thickness all layer suture. **b** Seromuscular sutures missing the mucosa. **c** seromuscular suture seen from within the lumen: the mucosa is approximated.

Testing and reinforcing

I always test anastomoses to see if they are gas-tight by gently compressing the gas within the lumen of the bowel and putting the anastomosis under gentle distension pressure. Obviously with very high gas pressure any anastomosis will leak gas. The pressure within the lumen during testing is not monitored so that the testing process that I use is wholly empirical. Nevertheless, experience soon gives the operator the feeling of how much pressure is necessary. I put the sutured bowel under gentle distension resembling that experienced when operating on a patient with intestinal obstruction.

The leakage of gas that occurs when the sutures are not sufficiently tight or sufficiently close together is easily recognisable. At one time I tested the distended gut under fluid but, even without immersion, it is easy to detect a gas leak. Sometimes the gas leak only occurs as the tension is taken up on a running suture so that it is worthwhile repeating the pressure once before resorting to suture reinforcement. I usually use a single horizontal

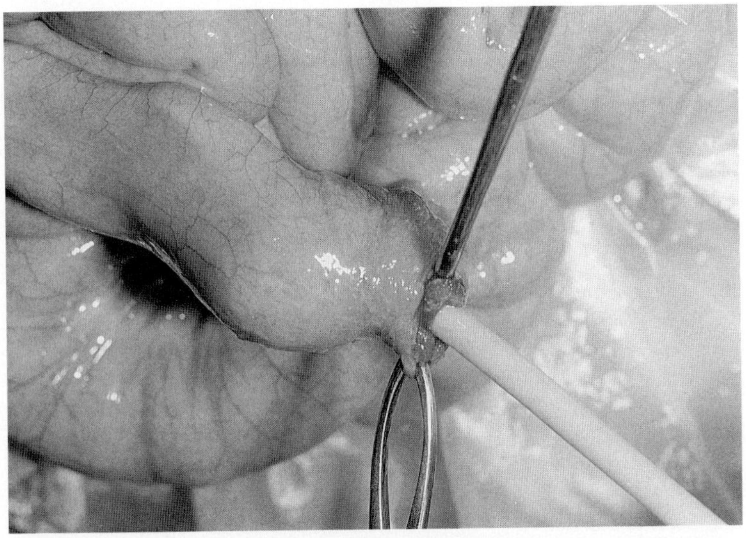

d

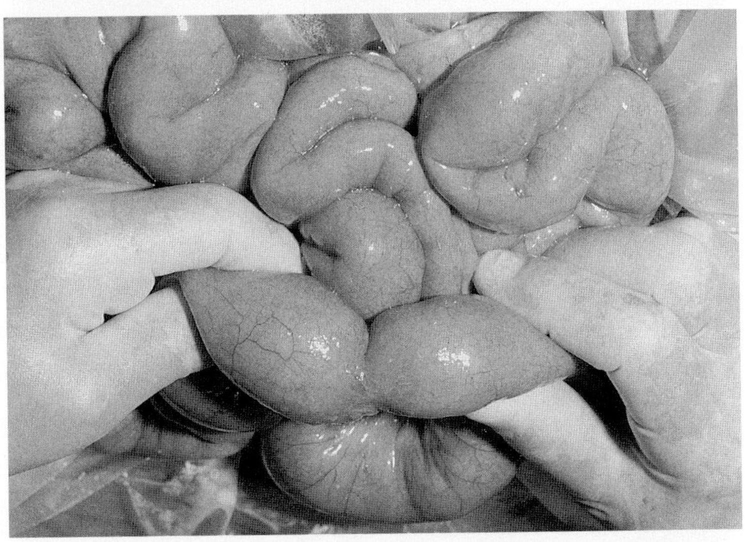

e

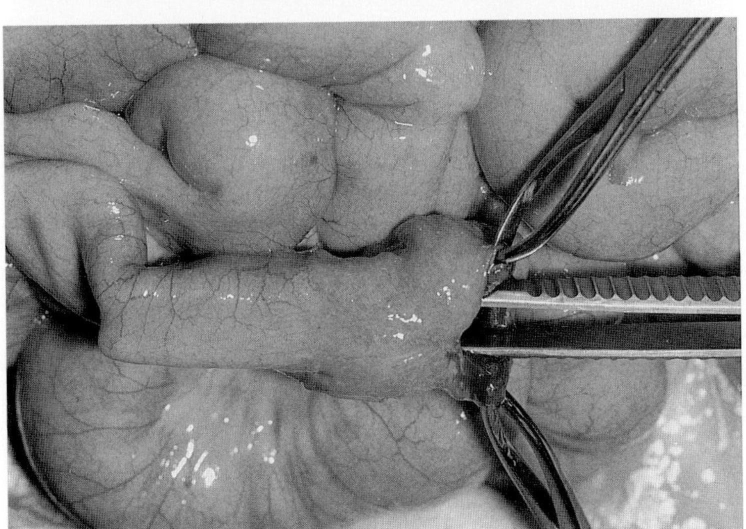

f

Fig. 8.8. d–f Stricture detection and strictureplasty: **d** balloon catheter inserted into gut; **e** stricture detected by inflated balloon; **f** incision just beyond stricture and dissecting forceps inserted and allowed to spring apart.

g

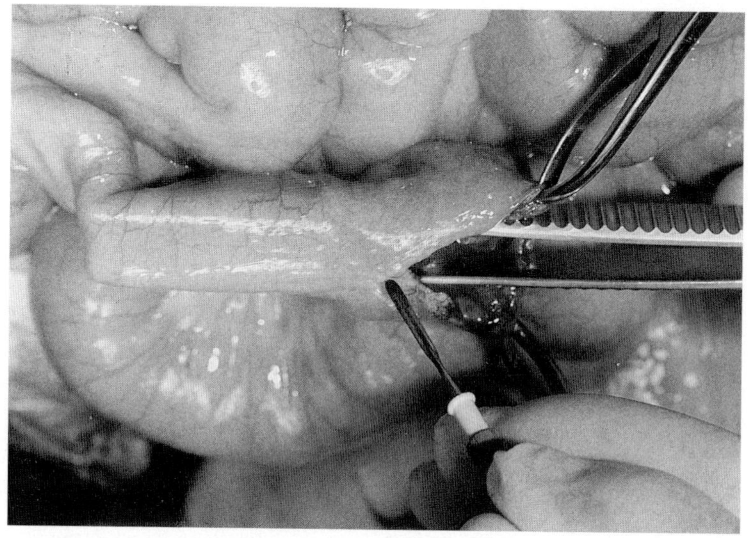

h

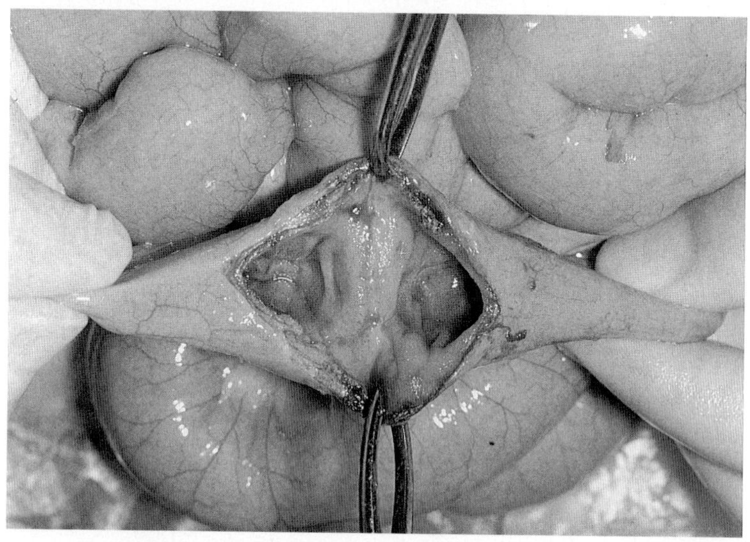

i

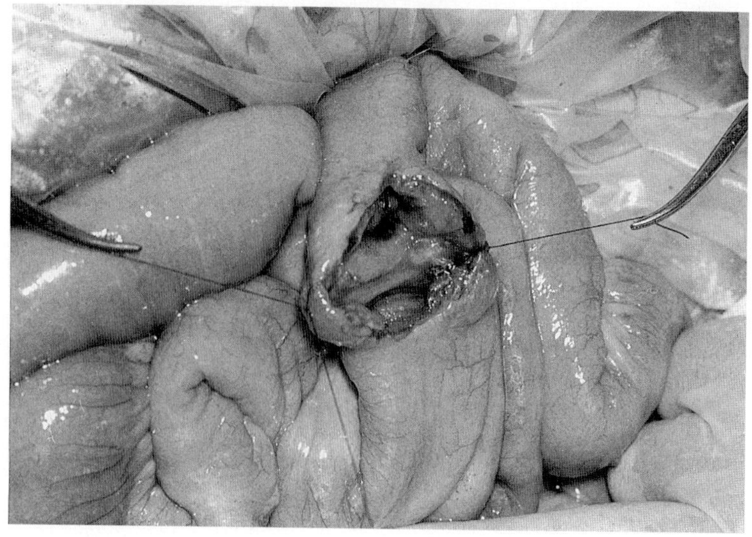

Fig. 8.8. **g** Cutting through stricture with diathermy. **h** Stricture displayed after longitudinal incision. **i** Gut lumen pulled transversely with stay sutures.

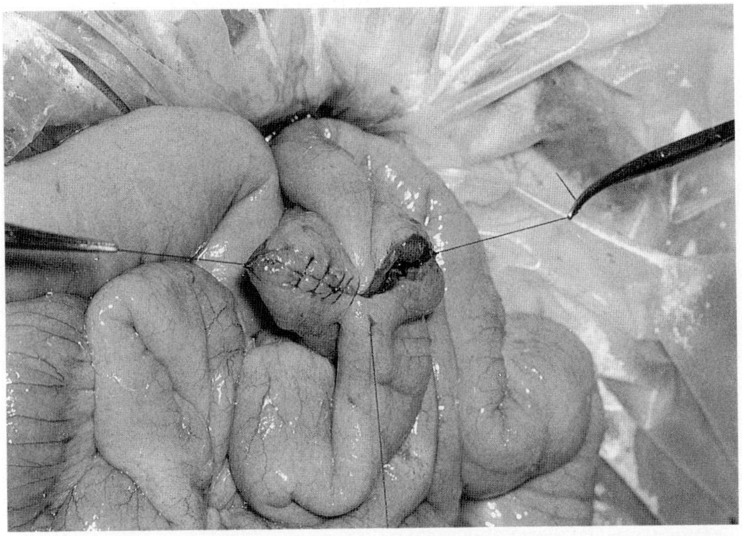

j

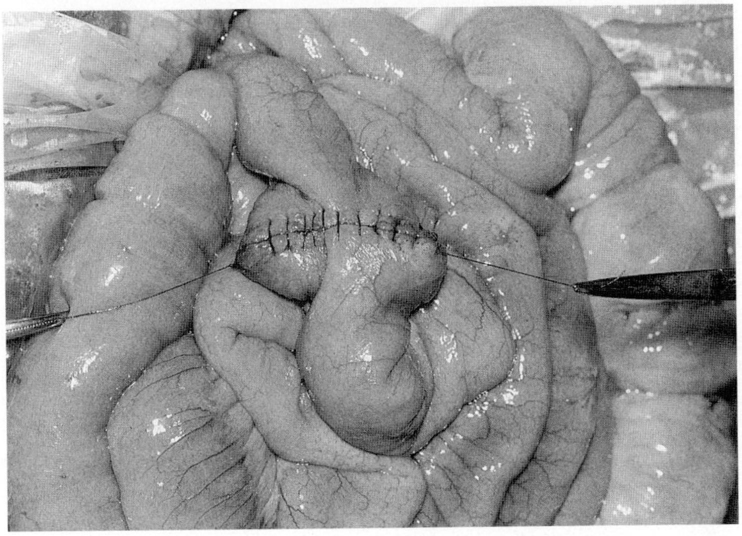

k

Fig. 8.8. j Half the row of continuous seromuscular sutures. k Completed transverse suture.

mattress, 3:0 Polyglactin, seromuscular suture at the site of the leak and then retest. I rarely find it necessary to put more than two reinforcing sutures in an end-to-end anastomosis or in a long strictureplasty.

Risk of recrudescence and how to minimise it

Principles

I reiterate, at the risk of inducing boredom, the axiom that surgical excision does not cure Crohn's disease, which has a multi-focal, pan-intestinal potential. Surgery merely overcomes the effects of the complications of longstanding chronic inflammation and ulceration. If surgery does not significantly alter the natural history of the disease, the disease is most likely to manifest itself again in the course of the patient's life. When this recrudescence occurs after an operation it is regarded as a recurrence and some regard it as a measure of failure of surgical management. Furthermore, there is a predilection for recrudescence at, or close to a suture line and so the concept of post-surgical recurrence has a lot to support it; particularly in the mind of a conservative gastroenterologist.

Because the subsequent clinical manifestation of Crohn's disease after resection is so likely to occur at the suture line, surgeons tend to become obsessed and to consider what possible actions they might have to take at operation to minimise this risk of recrudescence. It is routinely observed, and frequently reported, that endoscopic, intraluminal surveillance of patients after resection for Crohn's disease indicates that, soon after operation, a high proportion of patients can be observed to have mucosal lesions at or around the anastomosis. These are usually superficial ulcers resembling aphthous ulcers in the mouth. They are almost invariably asymptomatic, they heal, reappear and sometime coalesce (Rutgeerts et al. 1984, Tytgat et al. 1988).

It is this observation that prompts the question as to whether medical therapy, soon after resection, might reduce the risk of clinical or symptomatic recurrence. The fact that these lesions occur around the anastomosis prompts the question: is it the relative narrowing of the lumen or slowing of the intestinal content at the anastomosis that is the particular factor predisposing to new complications at that site? It also prompts the question: was the pre-anastomotic recrudescence determined before the resection and had more been resected could the recrudescence have been avoided? The answer to these questions is the observation that there appears to be no significant difference in the reoperation rate in patients who have had resections up to the point of histological normality and in those in whom the suture line has been microscopically abnormal (Pennington et al. 1980).

Attempting to eradicate the disease

Excising the primary lesion

A surgeon, faced with the need for surgical intervention in a patient with small bowel Crohn's disease because of an acute inflammatory recrudescence causing severe symptoms, may feel that it would be advisable to remove all macroscopically diseased bowel because of the fear that leaving some of the disease behind would invite early post-operative recrudescence. The wish to remove all obvious disease is understandable; although it must be said that it may not be necessary. I have adopted the policy of total excision of all macroscopic disease at the first operation, which is most commonly for the ileo-caecal complications of Crohn's disease. Under these circumstances I resect the ileum and caecum from the point in the terminal ileum where the bowel appears normal to that part of the ascending colon that seems to be uninvolved in the disease process. The segment and its draining lymph nodes are removed and end-to-end anastomosis performed between macroscopically normal bowel. The justification for this policy is the extremely low complication rate of the primary operation and the recently published figures from our unit showing that the large majority of patients so treated were, more than five years later, enjoying good health and not requiring drug therapy (Andrews et al. 1991).

For the surgeon brought up on the management of neoplastic disease of the bowel the presence of grossly enlarged lymph nodes immediately evokes an excisional response. The lymph nodes must be bad and their removal must benefit the patient. This "knee-jerk" reaction seems reasonable, providing that the removal of the lymph nodes does not mean that more gut has to be resected than would have been if the nodes had been left behind. The advantage of a wide excision at the first operation is that there has been no previous sacrifice of gut, that healthy tissues are anastomosed and the specimen produces adequate material for careful histological diagnosis and for the exclusion of such other diseases as tuberculosis.

Skip lesions

A problem arises if, at the time of primary ileo-caecal resection, there are skip lesions detected with isolated, thickened areas of partial luminal obstruction, proximal to the major lesion requiring surgical intervention. What should be done about these skip lesions? Should they be noted but not treated in the expectation that most of the inflammatory reaction in Crohn's disease is intermittent and may well resolve or should they be either resected or enlarged by strictureplasty? There is no one correct answer to these questions and the decision in each individual must be made on its merits. If there are one or two skip lesions situated within 20 cm immediately proximal to the main area that is to be resected and providing that excising these two also does not involve more than a 60 cm resection, I usually excise the skip lesions. If there are more of them, if they are more proximal or if their excision would mean excising more than 60 cm, I try to avoid resection either by leaving them alone or performing strictureplasty.

As will be discussed in more detail under strictureplasty (Chapter 13), my empirical rule is that if the stricture determined by intraluminal balloon measurement is 20 mm or less then I will enlarge the stricture by strictureplasty.

A wide anastomosis

As most recrudescence tends to occur at or near to an anastomosis it can be speculated that it is the hold-up of intestinal contents at the anastomosis and the possible narrowing of the lumen consequent upon the anastomosis itself that is a major factor disposing to recrudescence of that site. Therefore, many surgeons believe that it is as well to make the anastomosis as wide as possible. For this reason I always avoid a two-layer anastomosis that may invert gut wall and so narrow the lumen (Fig. 8.9). I prefer to cut the gut wall obliquely, with the longer end on the mesenteric side to preserve the blood supply. I then rotate the one loop of gut through 180° and make a single layer continuous anastomosis as described (Fig. 8.10). I have experimented with side-to-side stapled anastomoses, believing that this would give a wider lumen but I have now abandoned the practice (Fig. 8.11). It seems unnecessarily expensive and takes me rather longer to perform than a simple handsewn anastomosis. I also believe that an oblique end-to-end anastomosis gives less potential disruption to the normal flow of intestinal contents.

Continued drug therapy

As anti-inflammatory drugs are used in the treatment of exacerbation of Crohn's disease it is not surprising that there are some who have advocated continued prophylactic therapy after resection in the hope of minimising recrudescence. There are those who have advocated sulphasalazine because it is relatively inexpensive or 5-aminosalicylic acid (5-ASA) compounds because they are less likely to induce sensitivity reactions. There are some who have advocated low doses of systemic steroids. In my opinion there has as yet been no convincing evidence that any of these regimens decreases the risk of the patient with Crohn's disease needing reoperation. Furthermore, there is no evidence that these drugs provide prophylaxis and decrease the risk of exacerbation as they have been shown to do in ulcerative colitis. There are serious side effects of long-term steroid therapy such as osteoporosis and in the male sulphasalazine causes reversible azoospermia. At the time of writing there is interest in the effects of poorly absorbed steroids which appear to have a topical rather than a systemic effect on inflammatory diseases of the gut. These have been shown to be effective in the large bowel when administered as enemas and we await

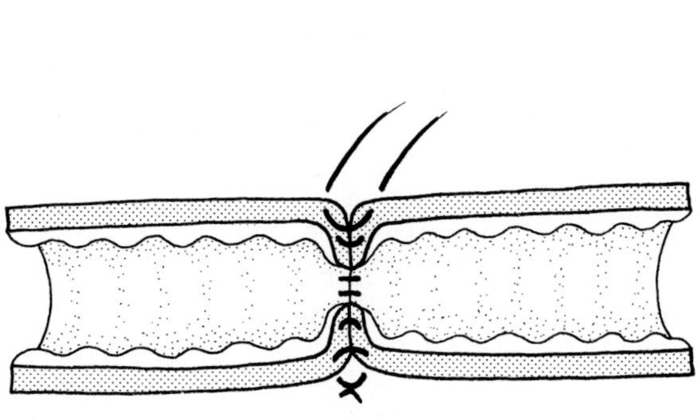

Fig. 8.9. Double-layer inverting sutures narrow the lumen.

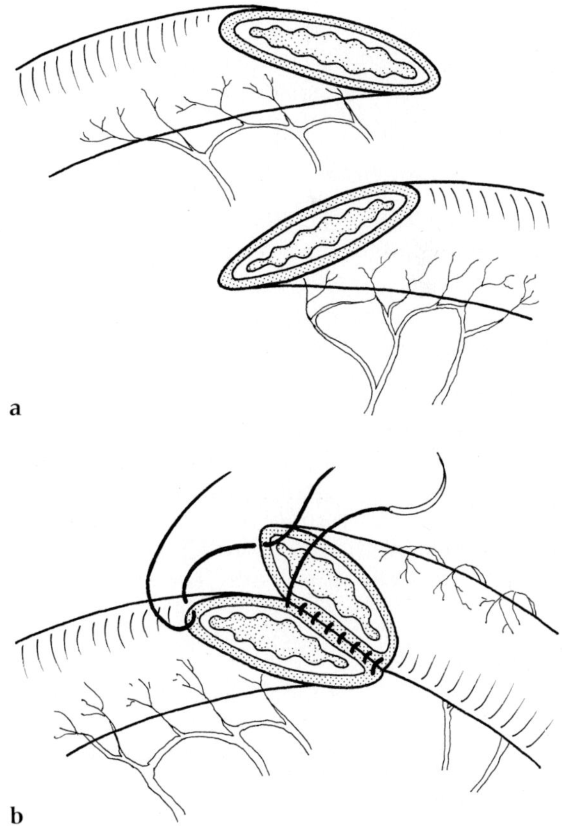

Fig. 8.10. a Small gut cut obliquely. **b** Rotated through 180° and sutured with a single layer continuous suture.

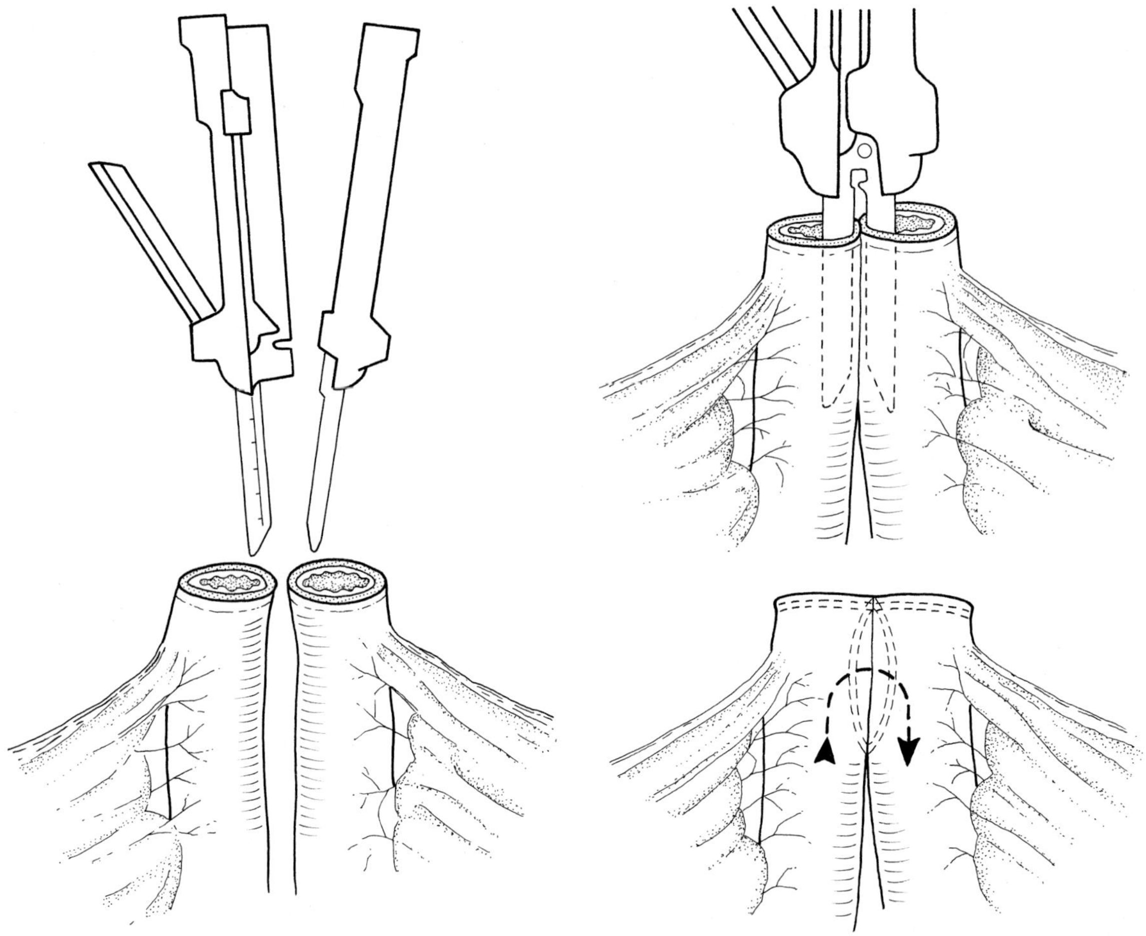

Fig. 8.11. a–c. Side-to-side stapled anastomosis using the GIA stapler. **a** Step 1: introduce stapler, close limbs and fire. **b** Side-to-side stapled small bowel anastomosis. **c** Step 2: cut ends closed with staples. Luminal flow shown with arrow.

evidence of their efficacy when administered orally (Olaison et al. 1990).

The ideal trial to assess the value of prophylactic therapy on preventing recrudescence in Crohn's disease would be to take patients who have had a primary excision of all macroscopically involved bowel and then performed surveillence endoscopy of the anastomosis and adjacent ileum. The trial would compare prospectively the prophylactic effects of topically active steroids with 5-ASA compounds and a control placebo. This important trial would be difficult to set up, would require large numbers and would have to be multi-centre. At the time of writing an attempt is being made to run a two-arm trial, simply comparing the topically active steroids with a placebo.

References

Andrews HA, Keighley MRB, Alexander-Williams J, Allan RN (1991) Strategy for management of distal ileal Crohn's disease. Br J Surg 78:679–682

Olaison G, Sjodahl R, Tagesson C (1990) Glucocollicoid treatment of ileal Crohn's disease: relief of symptoms but not of endoscopically viewed inflammation. Gut 31:325–328

Pennington L, Hamilton SR, Bayliss TM, Camera JL. (1980) Surgical Management of Crohn's disease: influence of disease on margin of resection. Ann Surg 192:311–318

Rutgeerts P, Geloes K, Van Trappen G. Kewemans R. Coenegrachts J, Coremans G (1984) Natural history of recurrent Crohn's disease at the ileocolonic anastomosis after curative surgery. Gut 25:665–672

Tytgat GNJ, Mielder GJJ, Blummelkamp WH (1988) Endoscopic lesions in Crohn's disease early after ileocaecal resection. Endoscopy 20:260–262

9 Assessment and Preparation

J. Alexander-Williams

Principles

Pre-operative preparation is to make sure that the patient is in the best attainable health with as good as possible nutrition. The patient should have the local conditions in the most favourable state and be able to mount an inflammatory response. It is obviously desirable not to have the bowel distended or full of indigestible material or faeces. The application of these principles has been discussed already in Chapter 8.

General and nutrition

Anaesthetists prefer to have the patient with a haemoglobin of above 11 g/dl and often wish to have the patient transfused to achieve this. I like the patient to have good grip strength, which I judge manually. I prefer to have the patient's serum albumin level above 24 g/l. However, I often operate on patients with low albumin levels because it is deemed impractical to devote resources to prolonged nutritional supplements when a relatively simple operation will soon allow the patient to take oral food. For further details see Chapter 3.

Psychological preparation

The reader is referred to Chapter 4 for an account of our philosphy of counselling. Here I am referring to the specific pre-operative preparation and the patient's attitude to the forthcoming operation. It is best if the patient is positively welcoming the thought of the operation. Many patients who are severely symptomatic and have previously experienced the benefit of surgical relief for recrudescence in Crohn's disease, positively look forward to an operation. I have many patients who make their own decision that the time has come for them to have further correction of stenotic complications. If, once again, I may draw a picturesque analogy from the automobile service industry, I have many patients present to the surgical clinic saying that they feel that the time has come for them to have another "10 000 mile service".

Not all patients are so psychologically motivated; particularly those who have not had operative intervention before. I find that the most important factors in psychological preparation are to provide the patient with an optimistic explanation of the disease and its natural history and try to convince them that the large majority of patients with Crohn's disease work normally and live to a ripe old age. However, I am careful to explain to them that the operation is only going to take care of a specific complication of the disease not eradicate the disease completely.

I believe that it is important to try to determine what it is that the patient fears most about the forthcoming operation. I question them as to whether they fear pain, disfigurement, death or even simple discomfort from a nasogastric tube. Many of the fears of a patient coming to reoperation are due to the memory of the unpleasant incidents of the last operation, particularly any of the complications that might have occurred. The anaesthetist explains to the patient about post-operative pain relief which is now very effective; particularly with "on demand" patient – control analgesia. I explain to the patient how we will take steps to minimise disfigurement. Although I rarely use nasogastric suction after operations on the alimentary tract I am particularly keen to avoid them in patients who have found this distasteful before. For example, I often place a gastrostomy drainage tube in a patient with a particularly high-risk operation on Crohn's disease of the stomach or duodenum if I think there is a risk of prolonged ileus.

Bowel preparation

It is impossible to sterilise the bowel. The most that intraluminal antimicrobial agents can do is to decrease temporarily the concentration of microbacteria in the lumen. Colonisation of the lumen is heavy if there is any degree of obstruction in the small bowel, as in the "blind loop syndrome". In such patients the reduction of microflora by even the most rigorous antimicrobial agents is unlikely to produce changes that would materially decrease the risk of post-operative wound infection. As we are usually operating on patients with Crohn's disease who have some degree of obstruction, we have to accept that it is always a contaminated operation. We attempt to minimise the degree of contamination and to give appropriate antimicrobial prophylaxis. In patients who have been operated on for subacute food bolus obstruction there are often quantities of partly digested fibrous food particles in the obstructed gut (Fig. 9.1). In theory it would seem advisable not to have these in the lumen of the gut but I do not think that they can be avoided by taking a "liquid only" diet for two or three days before operation. From questioning patients carefully about the identification of material retrieved at operation I am sure that such particles may remain undigested for many weeks. Therefore it seems impractical to have any prolonged period of food restriction pre-operatively, apart from that normally required to ensure that there is an empty stomach. We do not normally request more than six hours starvation.

Many patients with small bowel Crohn's disease have some degree of faecal loading in the large bowel and sometimes patients with

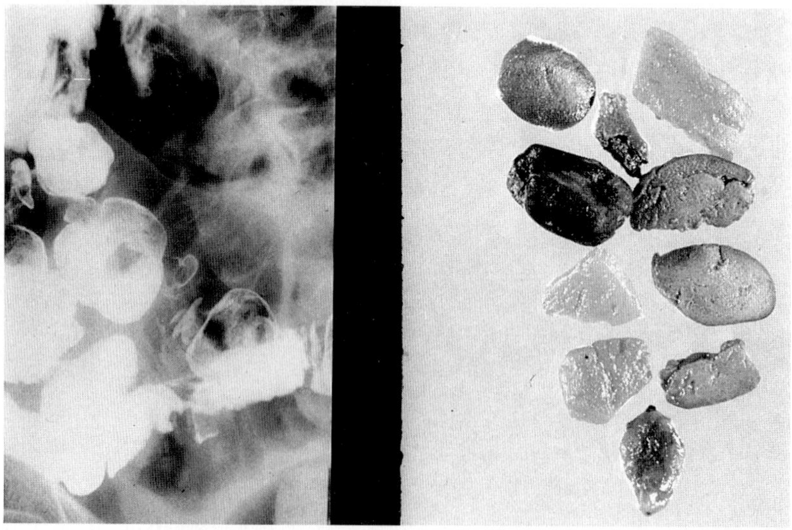

a b

Fig. 9.1. **a** Detail of barium contrast showing defects in lumen between strictures. **b** Undigested particles of food removed from between strictures at operation. Some were identified as being consumed more than two weeks before.

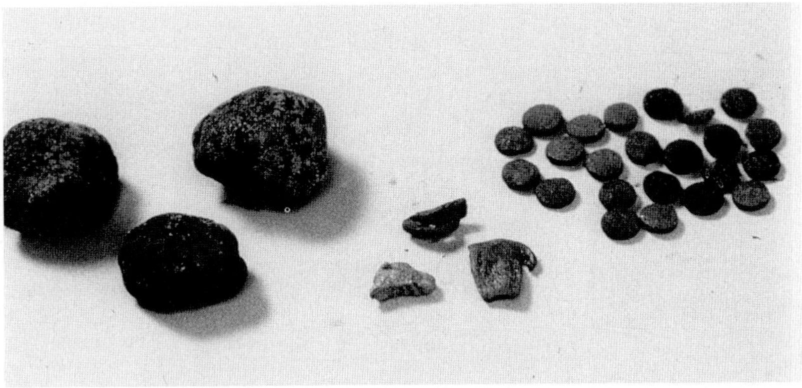

Fig. 9.1. c Debris recovered from lumen of gut between multiple ileal strictures. Distally were 3 enteroliths (diameter 1.7–2.2 cm), next were slices of button mushrooms and proximally were 22 tablets of sulphasalazine (500 mg). The patient complained of colic and borborygmi but no vomiting.

left-sided colitis have right-sided constipation. Therefore it is difficult to give precise rules about the pre-operative preparation of the large bowel. I always consider carefully how much bowel preparation might inconvenience or distress the patient and consider in each operation whether it is important to have an empty gut.

If the operation is to be a simple ileo-caecal resection with a primary anastomosis, then it is sensible to ensure that the distal large bowel is not loaded with hard faeces and so an enema is given. If the patient is suffering from diarrhoea and there is no evidence of faecal impaction on physical examination, or on the last plain radiograph of the abdomen, we do not consider it necessary to give a cathartic or an enema. Patients with stenotic lesions of the terminal ileum are often distressed by saline or high volume cathartics and those with perianal Crohn's disease often have difficulties with enemas. Our rule is not to employ bowel preparation routinely but only if there is clinical or radiological evidence of constipation or the particular operation necessitates an empty bowel. For example, a patient having a left hemicolectomy for a phlegmonous lesion of the descending and sigmoid colon, who had faecal loading in the right colon would have a saline cathartic preparation with sodium picosulphate and a 36-hour fluid only dietary restriction. Whereas a patient who is to have an ileostomy rarely needs to have bowel preparation before the operation.

Some anal operations, particularly those involving sphincter repair, are better performed with the large bowel empty. Some operations involving severe stenosis of the left colon such as a combination of diverticular disease and Crohn's disease in the elderly may be totally resistant to attempts at emptying the right colon. Some of these patients will not need to have the right colon emptying because they have a total colectomy and ileostomy. However, we often employ on-table colonic lavage in those in whom an anastomosis to a relatively unaffected rectum is being considered. The technique of on-table lavage is exactly the same as that used for emergency operations for large bowel obstruction by carcinoma or diverticular disease. A wide bore tube is inserted and tied into the distal lumen at the site of resection; it drains by gravity into a closed receiver. The large bowel is irrigated usually with four or more litres of normal saline at 37 °C via a balloon catheter inserted into the appendix stump after appendicectomy.

There are many who recommend oral prophylactic antibiotics such as streptomycin and erythromycin (Nichols et al. 1972). However, we do not believe that this regime is likely to make any significant difference to the gut flora and for the reasons outlined above, we do not use it. We rely entirely on a five-day course on systemic prophylaxis as will be described in the chapter on post-operative management.

Reference

Nichols RH, Condon RE, Gorbach SL, Nyhus L (1972) Efficacy of preoperative antimicrobial preparation of the bowel. Ann Surg 172: 227–232

10 Resection of the Ileum or Ileocaecum

J. Alexander-Williams

Operative position

The patient is operated on in the prone position. The bladder is drained with a (16F) catheter and a large balloon catheter (24F) is placed in the rectum and connected by drainage tubing so that the sigmoid colon can be inflated with carbon dioxide if necessary. An adhesive unipolar diathermy pad is fixed to a shaved patch on the thigh. The right-handed surgeon usually stands on the patient's left. The most difficult access usually involves the freeing of the gut from the right side of the abdomen and pelvis as the ileocaecal junction is mobilised and delivered into the wound. The assistant and the scrub nurse stand on the opposite side of the table. Only one assistant is usually required.

Skin preparation and draping

Minimal abdominal shaving is performed. I prefer the shaving to be performed after the patient is anaesthetised as I think this is better psychologically and there are likely to be fewer micro-organisms or infected follicles on the skin than if shaving is performed on the previous day. I do not shave young patients or patients who are not particularly hairy and in women I often only shave the upper centimetre or two of the public hairs. The previously marked potential stoma sites are shaved if they are hairy, even though it is most unlikely a stoma will have to be performed. The skin is prepared with a spirit-based antiseptic such as a povidone-iodine or chlorhexidine. Care has to be taken that any spirit-based preparation is completely removed particularly as cutting diathermy is used on the skin.

If there is a fistula or there has been a previous defunctioning stoma these are included in the prepared area and the drapes are placed around them so that the stoma or fistula is exposed. I find it impractical to cover fistula sites or stomas with transparent adhesive drapes to occlude them; there is inevitably a need to have access to them during the course of the operation and it is impossible to prevent infected material escaping from them. I feel it is better to have them under view so that they can be sucked or swabbed as necessary. I have observed some surgeons injecting antiseptic agents down fistula tracks but I do not consider it worth the time or expense.

The incision

Principles

There are some special factors in patients with Crohn's disease that influence the choice of incisions.

1. Many operations may be required in the course of the patient's life-time
2. The patients are often young and may be psychologically disturbed by unsightly incisions

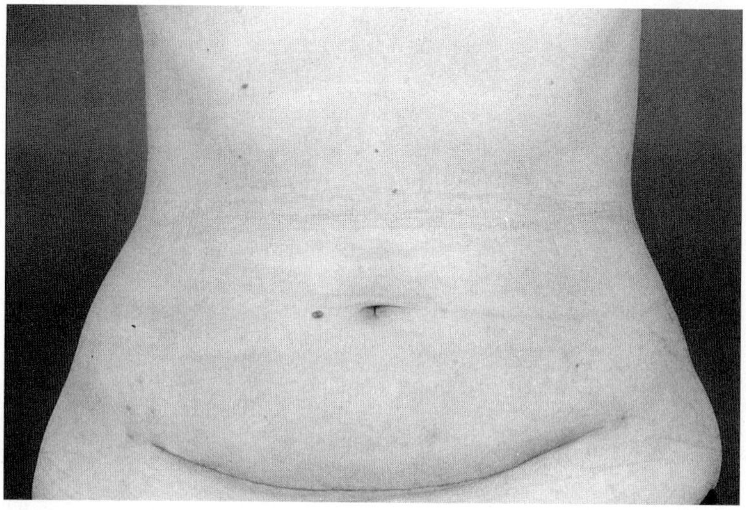

Fig. 10.1. A sub-total colectomy and ileo-sigmoid anastomosis was achieved safely through this low transverse incision. The stoma sites are available and unscarred should severe rectal recurrence necessitate an ileostomy.

3. Wound infection is commoner in Crohn's disease then in many abdominal operations that have less microbacterial contamination and infected wounds tend to leave unsightly scars
4. Already there may be unsightly scars that may need to be excised (Fig. 10.1).

The choice

The optimum sites for incision in patients with Crohn's disease are shown in the diagram (Fig. 10.2). The midline incision gives the quickest access to the whole of alimentary tract, it is suitable for reoperation and in Crohn's disease it is extremely uncommon for an incisional hernia to develop. The reason for this relative rarity of incisional hernia is difficult to document or to explain. While I have experienced many problems with incisional hernia after operation in patients with conditions such as diverticular disease or carcinoma particularly after operations that have become infected, I have rarely ever found the same problem following many hundreds of abdominal operations for Crohn's disease. Therefore one of the main theoretical objections to a midline incision does not appear to be valid. I use a infra-umbilical midline incision as my standard approach to ileo-caecal Crohn's disease. I avoid the supra-umbilical incision wherever possible because young patients find upper abdominal scars more difficult to conceal than lower.

For what appears likely to be a straightforward ileo-caecal resection in a young girl who is fearful of the consequences of an unsightly abdominal scar I try to avoid a vertical incision. I frequently explore the abdomen through a skin crease supra-pubic incision usually sited just below the level of sun-tanned skin. This is well away from any stoma site, the ileo-caecal region even in a

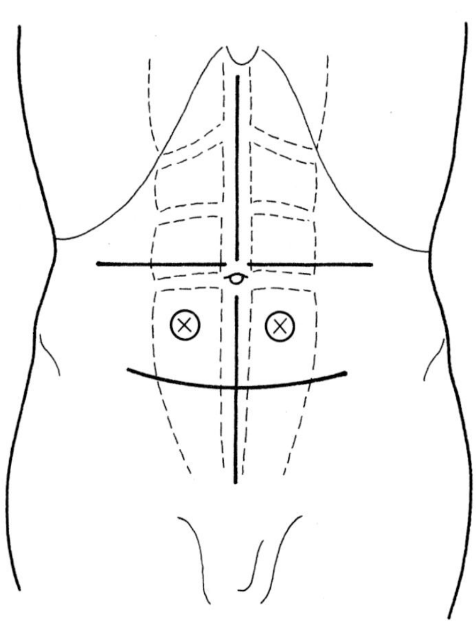

See also Fig. 7.2.

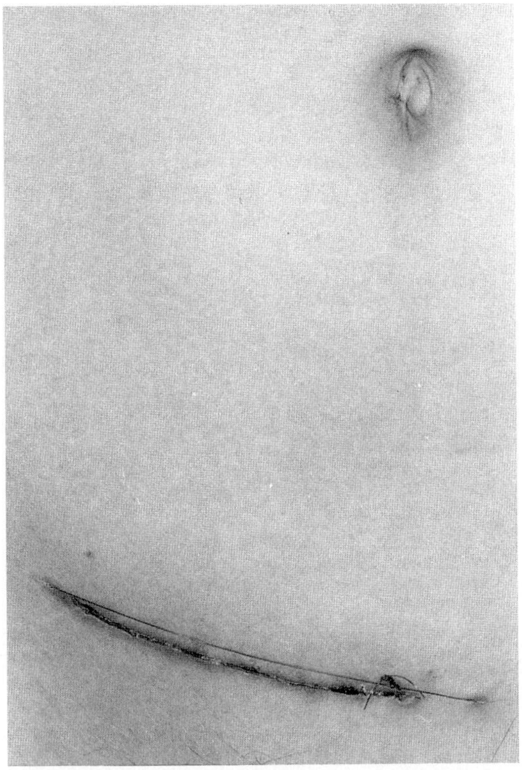

Fig. 10.3. An ileo-caecal resection for primary Crohn's disease was performed through this low right iliac fossa incision in the "bikini line" in an 18-year-old girl. Photograph of the wound, with subcutaneous Prolene stitch, on the sixth post-operative day.

grossly diseased state can be brought up into this wound without difficulty and patients are appreciative of a good cosmetic result (Fig. 10.3). A paramedian incision should never be used as there seems to be no justification for the extra time it takes and it is likely to encroach on potential stoma sites.

Cutting the skin and abdominal wall

When opening on the abdomen, my personal preference is to incise skin with a unipolar diathermy point. I do so because diathermy causes less bleeding than scalpel incision and because many of the operations for inflammatory bowel disease are reoperations and diathermy produces a less vascular field of access. Also the delicate control of the diathermy point allows one to incise accurately around the edges of complex scars from previous operations. Diathermy skin incision also allows a neat and accurate trephining of a stoma site. To those of you who are horrified at the thought of using diathermy to cut the skin, I recommend a personal randomised trial comparing the efficacy of healing and the cosmetic assessment of the result of the scar. We performed such a study on my unit, comparing the cosmetic results of scalpel and diathermy incisions, for both vertical and transverse scars (Sharif et al. 1992). At one month after operation we were unable to detect any difference between the scars of the two different methods of incision.

The linea alba and the parietal peritoneum are also incised with diathermy as two separate layers.

When there has been a previous scar, particularly one that has been infected and had healed an ugly cicatrix, I normally excise the whole of the cicatrix to the edges of healthy skin. Using diathermy to incise through the centre of an old scar results in there being one fibrous edge to the wound, without the normal separation of layers that occurs even with a primary midline incision. Thereafter, before the closure of the wound, I undercut the skin for about 1 cm along the edge with diathermy (see below) to facilitate a neat skin closure.

Peritoneal access

In primary operations I incise down to the linea alba, which I pick up with tissue forceps at the level of the umbilicus. I then incise a little at a time with the tip of the diathermy point. In primary operations it is almost unknown for the gut to be adherent to the umbilicus at this level. By cutting slowly with the fine diathermy tip there is no bleeding and so it is immediately evident when there is a change from the white tissue of the fascia to the browner tissue of adherent gut muscle. It should always be possible to avoid entering gut even in secondary operations when the gut is stuck to the back of the previous incision.

When adherence of the gut to the parietes is expected, I aim to enter first into an unexplored part of the abdomen. When reoperating on patients who have previously had operations for Crohn's disease I often extend the vertical incision a centimetre or two above the previous incision and aim to enter the peritoneal cavity just above the old scar. I do this because any adherence of gut is almost always immediately behind the scar; particularly behind any point where there has been sepsis and a broad, hard scar. Often the omentum is adherent behind the midline and, once the intra-abdominal fat is recognised, it is easy to push it away with the finger tip. In this manner it is possible to gain access to the abdomen, even when there has been extensive obliteration of the peritoneal cavity from preceding sepsis. The gentle finger separation of omentum from the parietal peritoneum of the anterior abdominal wall gradually enlarges a space. The successive sweeps of the finger will eventually separate enough of the omentum and whatever is left of the free peritoneal cavity can be entered; once this is achieved the dissection becomes easier and successive sweeps of the exploring finger, combined with retraction on the abdominal wall, by the assistant holding it up with tissue forceps, enables the plane of separation between the omentum or the gut and the parietal peritoneum of the anterior abdominal wall to be seen clearly. Usually it will separate well with gentle finger or scissor dissection.

The easier parts of the separation of the abdominal cavity are undertaken first. Whenever resistance due to apparent firm adherence is encountered, I stop and move to another part of the abdominal cavity where separation is easier. Eventually I find that I am left with one or two areas where the gut is fixed to the parietes. Then, by working all around these points as far as possible, I come to the dangerous areas where there is firm adherence of inflamed gut to the abdominal wall. If there is an abscess or a fistula then it is inevitable that the granulation tissue space will have to be entered before the gut is freed enough for it to be able to be delivered into the wound. I consider it to be an unnecessary hazard to enter the lumen of the gut where there is not already an abscess or a fistula. Therefore, dissection of adherent gut from the abdominal wall is best done by keeping well on the abdominal wall side of any adherence. I always do this with cutting, unipolar diathermy because I am happy with the precision of this method and it reduces bleeding to the minimum. Others, including some of those who have been trained by me, are less happy with this method and prefer to use sharp dissection with scissors.

Whenever the adhesion of the gut to the abdominal wall is very hard and difficult to separate, I take away a small portion of the parietal peritoneum with the gut, leaving exposed muscle on the abdominal wall side. This manoeuvre, which we call "postage-stamping" (described and illustrated below, see Fig. 10.5), ensures safety of the underlying gut and will allow the inflamed mass of gut to be freed and brought up to the abdominal wall. The "postage stamp" can later be removed if necessary but there is no harm in leaving a thick plaque of mesoderm tissue attached to the gut.

If the gut if firmly adherent to the posterior abdominal wall there are further dangers in store. In what I term "neglected disease" that has been treated for too long medically and when abscesses have been allowed to develop, there are dangers to the ureter and the gonadal vessels on the posterior abdominal wall. Any involvement of the urinary system should have been suspected from the findings on preoperative ultrasound assessment. However, whenever a mass of gut appears to be stuck to the posterior abdominal wall, it must be considered as a potential hazard, particularly to the ureter.

Division of the gonadal vessels is apparently innocuous and they may be ligated with impunity; although, if seen, they are better spared. The ureter is at particular hazard and always remember that there may be two ureters. In such a case it is best to start to explore the retroperitoneal space just below the kidney and then work downwards in the line of the ureter. With primary resection, it is a posterior abscess or adherent mass, usually the ileo-caecal region, that is having to be mobilised towards the midline. Mobilisation of the ascending colon and hepatic flexure soon exposes a bloodless tissue plane where the ureter can be identified. It is then immediately obvious whether or not the ureter is obstructed. Furthermore, whenever there is duplication two ureters should be seen easily. The ureter is then traced downwards towards the adherent mass. It is usually possible to lift the inflammatory mass forward with finger dissection without difficulty, while displacing the ureter posteriorly. In operating on a large number of such patients I have never encountered any difficulty with the ureter or damage to it. For this reason I never feel that

a b

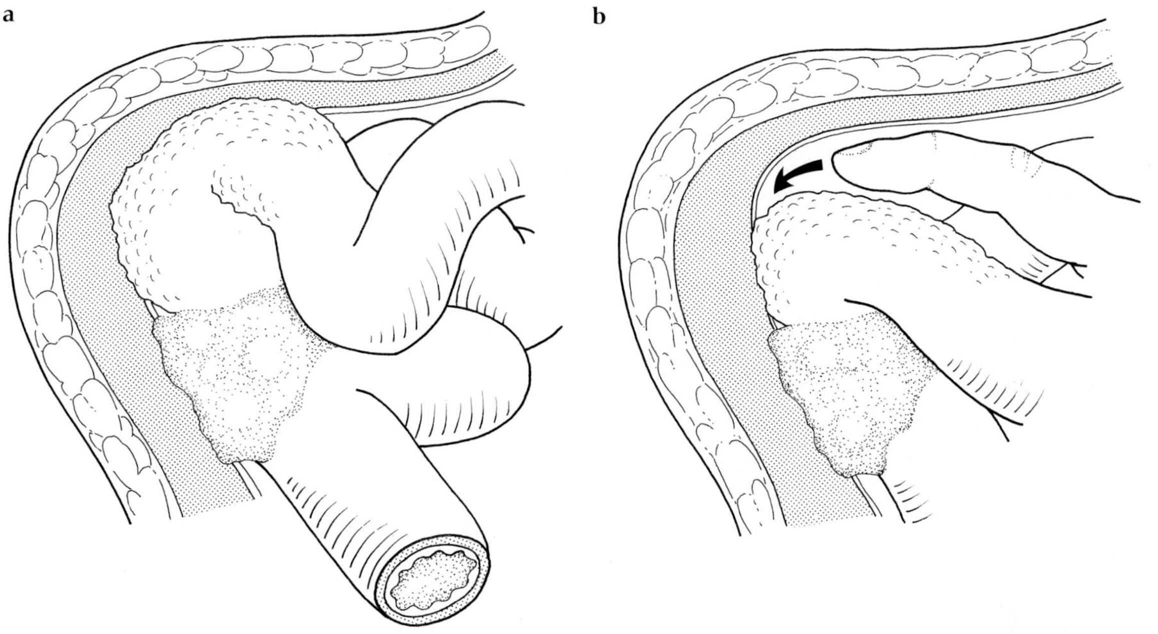

Fig. 10.4.a Diagram of oedematous gut and adjacent abscess stuck to abdominal wall. **b** Simple finger separation "scratching".

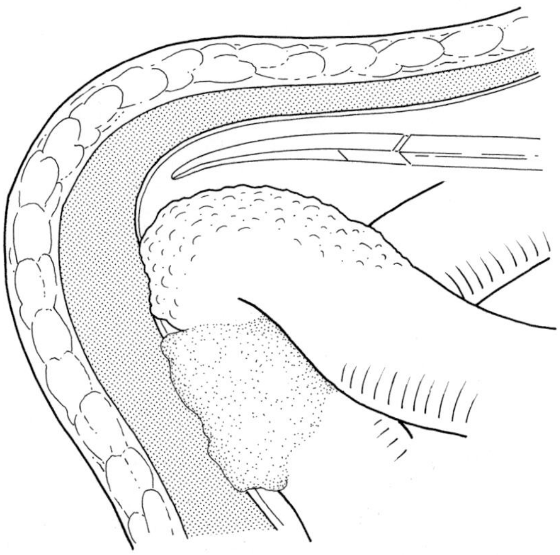

Fig. 10.5. For more resistant adhesion the tips of the closed scissors performs the "tyre-lever" manoeuvre. (See also Fig. 8.5.)

it is necessary to place a stent in the ureter before operation, although I know that this technique is recommended by others.

Technique of dissection

These are illustrated in diagramatic form in figures. The simplest method is finger separation of adherent omentum or gut. There is usually an odematous tissue plane in which this separation can be performed quite easily by "scratching" with the finger tip (Fig. 10.4). When separation becomes more difficult but the line of cleavage can still be seen dissection with the tip of closed scissors is helpful (Fig. 10.5). This I refer to as the "tyre lever" manoeuvre, although I recognise that there are now many surgeons who have never had to fit a tyre even to a bicycle wheel. I suppose that the next generation will have to invent a new contemporary descriptive term.

As dissection becomes more difficult and the gut densely adherent the "postage stamp" manoeuvre is performed as described above (Fig. 10.6). As dissection through all the easy planes of cleavage is performed this usually leaves an area of dense adhesion where granulation tissue may be entered. This is found whenever there is a fistula. Under these circumstances the quickest and most effective way of separating the gut from the parietes is to encircle the adherent area in a pincher

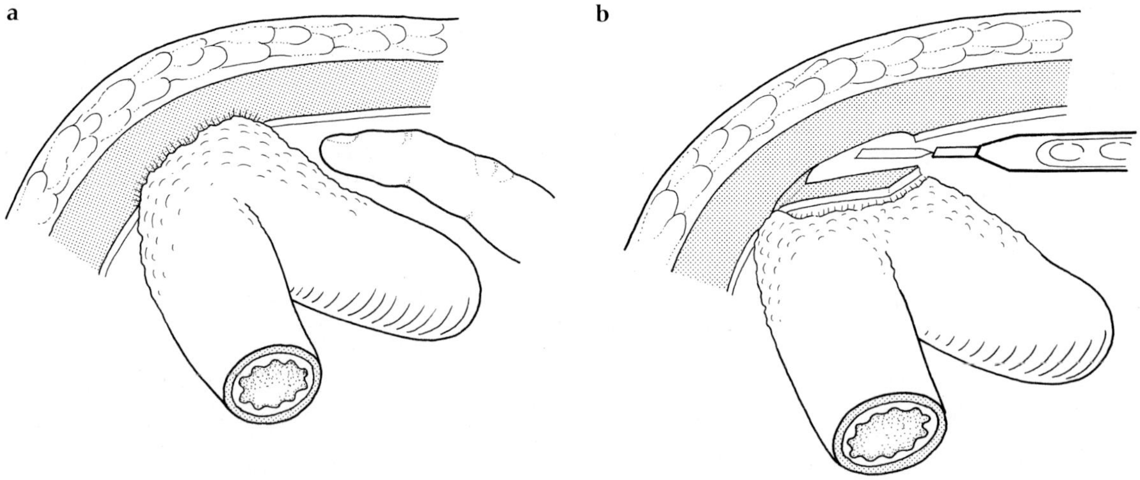

Fig. 10.6.a When the gut is so densely adherent that it may be damaged if it is levered off the parietes. **b** A portion of the attached parietes is cut off with diathermy: the "postage-stamp" manoeuvre.

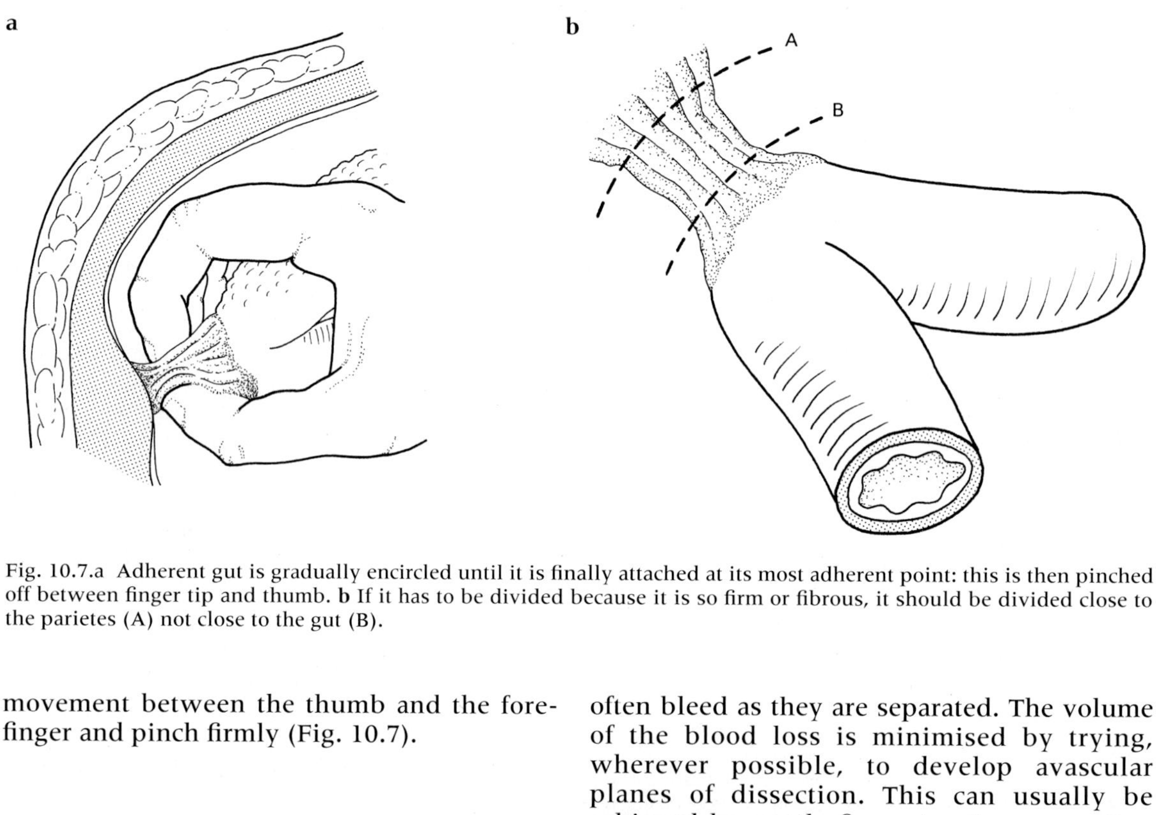

Fig. 10.7.a Adherent gut is gradually encircled until it is finally attached at its most adherent point: this is then pinched off between finger tip and thumb. **b** If it has to be divided because it is so firm or fibrous, it should be divided close to the parietes (A) not close to the gut (B).

movement between the thumb and the forefinger and pinch firmly (Fig. 10.7).

Haemostasis

The hyperaemic, inflamed gut often bleeds as it is separated from the parietal peritoneum and the omentum or adjacent loops of gut often bleed as they are separated. The volume of the blood loss is minimised by trying, wherever possible, to develop avascular planes of dissection. This can usually be achieved by gentle finger traction separating loops of gut, as described above. Because of my preference for diathermy dissection and for carbon dioxide gut insufflation, I believe that I can perform rapid and relatively bloodless separation of loops of gut in Crohn's disease. The diathermy dissection is particularly valuable and time-saving when operating on complex recurrences, particularly when there have been previous septic complications. When there are abscesses, the residual granulation tissue always bleeds when it is separated.

Most of the bleeding that occurs from the dissected gut wall is relatively minor and will stop spontaneously. It may be aided by gently wrapping the gut in moist towels or swabs. Any recognisable bleeding point, from which blood can be seen to be flowing, is controlled by a fine pair of (plastic surgery) dissecting forceps (Adson). I rarely use the "spray" diathermy facility as most of this type of bleeding stops spontaneously.

Major bleeding occurring during this preliminary dissection of the adherent gut usually comes from omental vessels, the poorly supported veins and arteries of the omentum that are a major source of bleeding and are never adequately controlled by diathermy. I always pick them up with artery forceps and ligate them.

The greatest danger of major bleeding comes from the division of the thickened mesentery during the resection of gut. In a primary ileocaecal resection the mesentery is usually infiltrated with fat, grossly thickened with oedema and contains many enlarged nodes. Almost invariably it is impossible to identify the major vessels visually and attempting to dissect through the thickened inflamed tissue can lead to uncontrolled bleeding. The technique that I employ relies on gentle pinching of the thickened mesentery, which pushes away oedema and fat; the pinching pressure must not be so hard that it can damage veins. Once a thin window has been pinched it is inspected carefully with counter pressure from the forefinger on the far side of the mesentery. Gentle scissor dissection is used to confirm that there is no major vessel being pushed forward by the finger and the scissors then complete the window. If a vein is divided inadvertently during the formation of the window the bleeding can be immediately controlled by the finger and thumb and a fine artery forceps applied.

One or two major windows are created in the mesentery and the vessels between them clamped with heavy duty, curved (cholecystectomy) artery forceps. The tissue between the clamps is divided with scissors and the clamp on the gut side is tied with a simple ligature. The clamp that is to be left behind has to be secured particularly firmly because it is easy for the ends of the vessels to retract into the large oedematous pedicle. If this occurs a mesenteric haematoma develops and is difficult to control. If the tissues are not particularly thick and there is obviously a simple pedicle, containing obvious large vessels, I

Table 10.1 Summary of measures to prevent or treat bleeding during operations

Site	Prevention	Management
Vascular adhesions	Coagulation diathermy division	Hot wet pack
Adherent bowel wall	Postage stamp manoeuvre (see Fig. 10.6)	(1) Fine point diathermy coagulation (2) Hot wet pack (3) Stitch if torn
Omentum	Clamp fine vessels divide and ligate	Always occlude with haemostat and tie
Root of mesentery	Finger pinching Clamp and lock stitch (see Figs 8.1 and 10.8)	– of haematoma. Squeeze between finger and thumb for 2–3 minutes – a deep lock-stitch as last resort
Cut edge of gut when resecting or making strictureplasty	Divide with diathermy	They usually stop Fine point diathermy coagulation They all stop when anastomosis completed

will usually tie this with a simple, strong surgeon's knot, using 2:0 Polyglactin or an equivalent. If, however, the pedicle is grossly thickened and the vessels are not obvious, which is usually the finding in primary operations for Crohn's disease, a more secure form of pedicle ligation is needed. A transfixion ligation is more secure than simply just tying a ligature round the forceps. For large pedicles I prefer a double interlocking ligation as shown (see Fig. 8.1). Two sutures of 2:0 Polyglactin or equivalent are placed through the pedicle, taking care to avoid major vessels if these can be identified. The two interlocking sutures are then tightened simultaneously by the surgeon and the assistant while the clamp is removed either by a second assistant or the scrub nurse.

Another good method of controlling a less oedematous mesentery is to first divide the gut and then place parallel straight toothed forceps towards the root of the mesentery step by step, securing each bit with a single or double interlocking suture (Fig. 10.8).

The next step is to remove the gut to be resected. The selection of the particular length to be removed will be discussed below. Once it is determined where the level of division of the gut is to occur, haemostasis has to be secured in the mesentery. The periphery of the mesentery near the gut contains only relatively small vessels and these are usually simply diathermied or clamped and divided under direct vision. This is not difficult as in a primary resection the limits of resection are into macroscopically normal bowel with macroscopically normal mesentery.

There are two types of haemostasis that I strongly condemn in operations for Crohn's disease. The first is the use of staples and the second the use of non-absorbable ligatures. The main reason for condemning stapling is that all the difficult aspects of haemostasis in Crohn's disease already described are unsuitable for stapling while the peripheral minor vessels that are easy to staple are also easy to clamp and ligate. Therefore I believe that the expense of stapling cannot be justified for what is a small part of the operation.

My condemnation of non-absorbable suture material, particularly for ligated major pedicles, is based on my experience in earlier decades of reoperating on patients who had their primary operations for Crohn's disease elsewhere. I often found multiple intra-abdominal abscesses. These were associated with non-absorbable sutures, placed around major vessel pedicles, that continued as the foci of minor or even major suppuration.

a b c

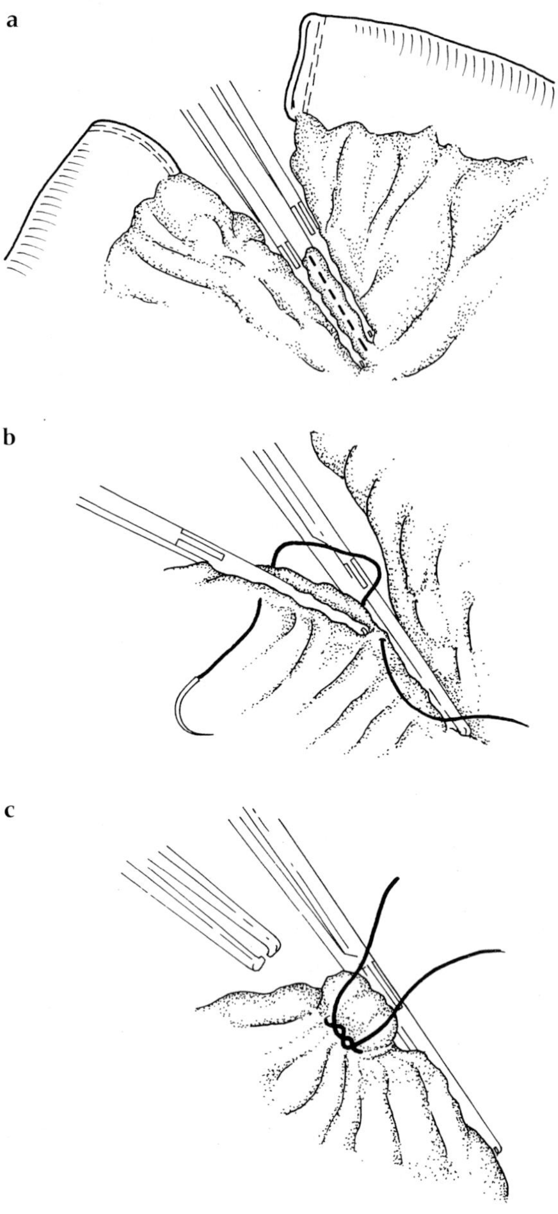

Fig. 10.8. **a** Parallel straight toothed clamps placed down towards the root of the mesentery. **b** Each bite is secured by a suture ligature. **c** Which is secured and tied step by step.

First operation

In a primary operation, which is usually for ileo-caecal Crohn's disease, the policy that I adopt is of maximum excision. If there are no proximal skip lesions, I excise the whole of the macroscopic disease, including the lymph nodes. I then anastomose apparently normal ileum to apparently normal colon. Usually I excise all the enlarged lymph nodes, unless their removal necessitates excision of much normal gut.

This philosophy may seem to be at variance with the later philosophy of maximum conservation. However, the reasons for this dichotomy of approach are based on our experience of the favourable long-term follow-up of patients with primary presentation of ileo-caecal disease, treated by our unit by the technique of maximal excision that I have described. There is, of course, the inevitable 3% per year recrudescence reoperation but even that means that at the end of 10 years, there is still 60%–70% of patients who have not had further trouble. The majority of those who have recurred we have been able to deal with in a simple manner, usually with minimal excision of gut or strictureplasty. The other advantage of the wide primary excision is that it gives a good opportunity for complete histological examination and is acceptable for such other diagnoses as tuberculosis or lymphoma.

Reoperations

The philosophy adopted at any subsequent operations is one of maximal conservation. The histological diagnosis is already known without doubt from the primary operation and, from now on, the objective is to sacrifice as little as possible of the remaining functioning bowel. It is for recurrent operations that I particularly favour the use of strictureplasty (see Chapter 13).

The question of which skip lesions to resect with the primary excision and which to leave alone have already been described.

The methods for detection of occult proximal strictures are discussed in further detail under Chapter 13 (Strictureplasty).

Extent of excision

I have two distinct philosophies governing the choice of the extent of excision, depending whether it is the first or a subsequent operation; radical for first operations and conservative for subsequent ones.

Opening and occluding the gut

A general principle of gut surgery is that no intestinal contents should spill during anastomosis. This ideal has to be modified in Crohn's disease for a number of reasons. The sizing of the luminal diameter of the proximal and distal gut is best achieved with the bowel not occluded. Therefore, some slight contamination is inevitable, although the escape of intestinal contents are usually easily controlled by suction. Furthermore the occlusion with soft intestinal clamps proximally and distally may interfere with the ease of end-to-end anastomosis; the two ends usually are of different size and the walls of different thickness.

To minimise contamination I advocate a combination of a number of manoeuvres, depending on local conditions. If the small bowel is empty, as is usual, I apply a soft clamp (Doyen, Fig. 10.9) to the gut only, about 10 cm proximal to the line of division. I then

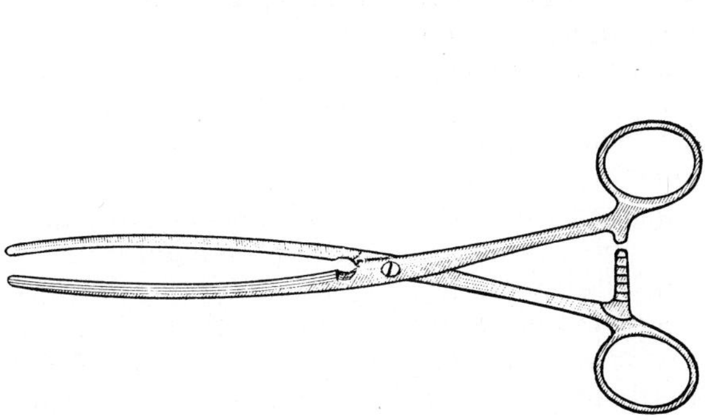

Fig. 10.9. The Doyen soft intestinal clamp.

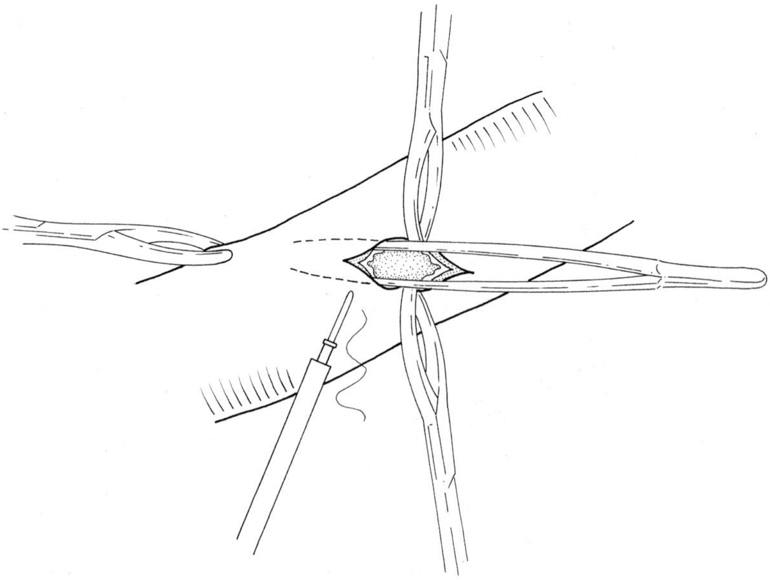

Fig. 10.10. Cutting with diathermy with the aid of long dissecting forceps in the lumen. (See also Fig. 8.8g.)

cut the wall of the gut obliquely with diathermy, aiming to create an opening of approximately the same size as the transverse incision in the ascending colon to which it will be anastomosed. The first cut is on the anterior wall of the gut. As soon as the lumen is opened the gut wall is held up with two tissue forceps while the third holds up the serosal aspect of the gut at the apex of the incision on the antimesenteric border. (Fig. 10.10). This enables gentle tension to be put on the bowel wall and acts as a guide to the subsequent diathermy incision. Any liquid intestinal content is removed with a sucker and the mucosal aspect of the gut is wiped with a povidone-iodine swab. Haematosis from the cut edge of the gut is secured by diathermy; fine arterial bleeding points are picked up by small dissecting forceps (Adson) and cauterised. I then remove the proximal soft occluding clamp and place a small povidone-iodine soaked tampon into the lumen of the proximal bowel. It is best that this is attached to a linen tape to make sure it does not migrate proximally and become left behind inadvertently after the anastomosis.

It is likely that the descending colonic end of the resection will have some faecal contents in the lumen and so it is advisable to gently milk these onwards towards the hepatic flexure with gentle finger pressure and then to apply a soft non-crushing (Doyen) clamp to occlude the lumen of the gut but not the mesentery.

I open the colon directly at 90° to the line of the gut, using a similar manoeuvre to that employed in cutting the small bowel. The ascending colon up to the occluding clamp is carefully sucked out and, once again a povidone-iodine soaked occluding tampon with a tape is placed distally. If the colon contains only little faecal material I will then often remove the occluding clamp from the colon also as this gives greater freedom of mobility for the subsequent anastomosis.

Suturing

The gut ends to be anastomosed are aligned correctly so that the mesenteric sides of the ileum and the colon are together.

If the excision is of a length of terminal ileum or jejunum only the two ends of small gut to be anastomosed are rotated through 180° so that the mesenteric edges are not in opposition (Fig. 10.11).

With an ileo-caecal anastomosis I start by placing one seromuscular stay suture on the mesenteric borders. On the antimesenteric border the cut ends of the gut are held with tissue forceps to provide the right amount of tension. This manoeuvre shows whether the edges of the gut lie easily together without gross size discrepancy. If the ileal end is smaller by more than a centimetre, I make a further antimesenteric cut into the ileum (Fig. 10.12).

Once the two luminal cut edges are of equal size, I place and tie the suture at the antimesenteric end and hold it with an artery forceps to provide the appropriate tension. I then usually insert a second stay suture in the centre of the posterior wall to help provide the correct tension and apposition of cut edges that are now about to be sewn. If there is much size or thickness discrepancy I may use two more stay sutures in the centre of each half (Fig. 10.13).

The assistant holds the end of the running suture and the stay suture at such an angle that the gut to be sutured is approximately 45° from the line across the surgeon's shoulders. This enables the suturing to be performed comfortably with a simple pronation movement of the forearm holding the needle holder. It is the assistant's task also to keep the edges of the gut under gentle tension and gently lifted up towards the surgeon.

For anastomosis I use a single layer of 3:0 Polyglactin on a 30 ml needle, picking up only the submucosa, muscle and serosa and sparing the mucosa. With the appropriate traction on the stay sutures it is usually possible to define these layers easily. If they are not seen easily it is better to perform an all layer running suture, taking up only the minimum amount of mucosa. I used to employ interrupted sutures but I find that a running suture is more likely to give a gas tight anastomosis (see below). This is because the suture line is "taken up" satisfactorily when the gut is distended with gas at the end of the anastomosis. The presence of three stay sutures along the continuous line of the anastomosis, which are tied to the running suture as it passes, prevents there being a "purse-string" effect. When the running suture reaches the end of the posterior row it is tied to the first stay suture after the needle has come out of the serosal surface. Another stay suture is then placed in the middle of the anterior row. The tampons are removed from the proximal and distal lumen before the central stay suture is tied. The assistant once again puts the edges of the gut on the correct tension and the correct 45° angulation

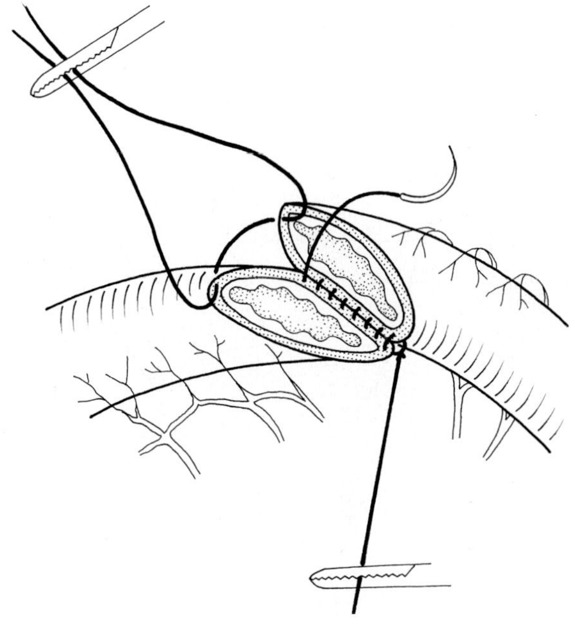

Fig. 10.11. Small bowel to small bowel anastomoses are performed by rotating the obliquely cut gut end through 180°. (See also Fig. 8.10b.)

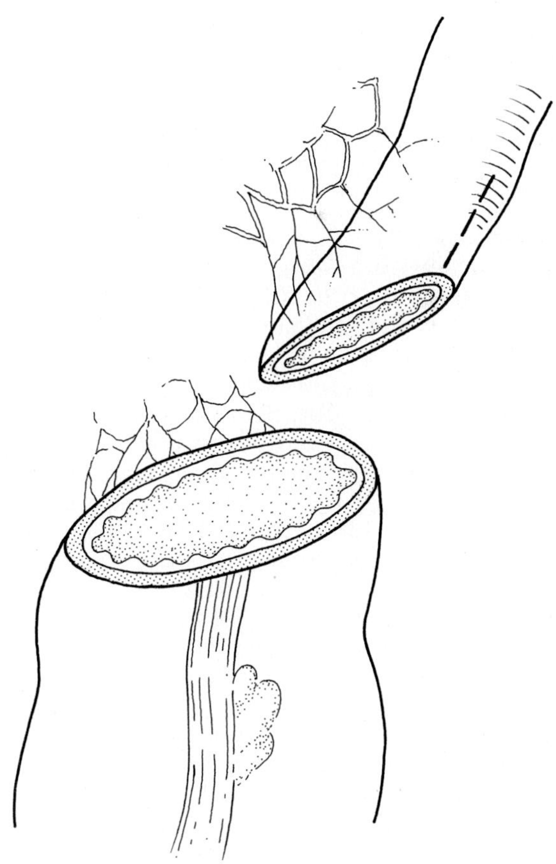

Fig. 10.12. If there is still a size discrepancy between ileum and colon, a further antimesenteric incision is made.

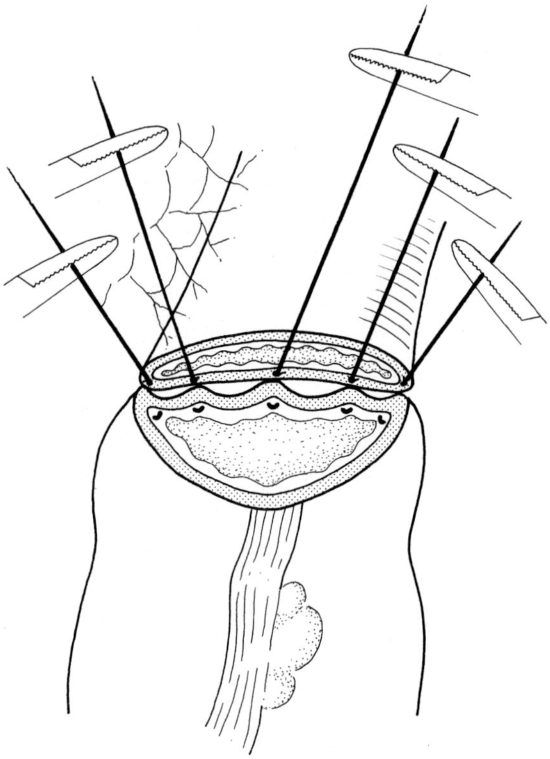

Fig. 10.13. The end and centre stay sutures are supplemented by quarter stay sutures to facilitate accurate end-to-end anastomosis.

to the surgeon. The anterior row is then continued with a mucosal sparing, seromuscular suture. After the anastomosis is complete it is tested with CO_2 distension to "take up" the running suture and reveal any gas leak.

If more gas is required in the lumen to achieve adequate distension of the anastomosis, the end of tubing that is attached to the CO_2 laparoscopy insufflating machine is placed into the proximal lumen of the gut just before the final sutures are placed in the anterior row. The proximal gut is then inflated with about 500 ml of CO_2 and the anastomosis completed rapidly. When the starting point of continuous suture is reached it is knotted and all sutures are cut. The insufflated CO_2 is then milked back to the anastomosis and gentle intraluminal gas distension is performed, controlling the lumen of the gut above and below the anastomosis with gentle finger pressure. I employ about as much distension of the lumen as I am accustomed to see when operating on patients with intestinal obstruction. It would obviously be possible to apply enough intraluminal pressure to leak through any recently sutured line. However, it is not difficult, with experience, to judge the right amount of pressure to put the suture line under reasonable tension. Gas leaks are quite obvious: some of them stop spontaneously as the running suture is "taken up"; those that do not are secured by a single stitch, usually a horizontal mattress suture. The anastomosis is then re-checked and, once it is satisfactorily gas tight, the gap in the mesentery is sutured with the same suture material, taking great care not to transfix any vessels in the mesentery. Then I usually place the greater omentum over the anastomosis and may suture it in place.

As is usual in primary ileo-caecal resections there is minimal or no contamination and, if so, I do not irrigate the peritoneal cavity. In complex operations, particularly reoperations, where there is contamination or has been bleeding from separated tissues, I complete the operation by peritoneal lavage; usually with two litres of normal saline at 37 °C. I do not use antibiotics in the peritoneal lavage.

When to avoid anastomosis

Distal obstruction

In a primary ileo-caecal resection it is usually simple to exclude the presence of distal obstruction. The pre-operative "work up" should always include a flexible sigmoidoscopy, although not necessarily a barium enema or colonoscopy. However, it is easy to assess the absence of gross colonic disease by palpation and observation, even when access is limited by a low transverse laparotomy incision. Therefore there should be no problem in exclusing distal large bowel obstruction in the simple primary operation. It is vitally important to ensure there is no distal obstruction when the operation is for more proximal disease or particularly when it is a reoperation. Obstruction should easily be detected and readily corrected, usually by strictureplasty.

The compromised patient

The patient's power of healing may be compromised by drugs, anergy from chronic illness and possibly also by malnutrition. In my opinion it is compromised by immunosuppressive drugs that present a significant problem in patients with Crohn's disease. If a patient has to undergo resection for Crohn's disease while still on immunosuppressive drugs I always try to perform a proximal stoma with the aim of later re-anastomosis once the patient has recovered and the drugs withdrawn. We have to operate on many patients with Crohn's disease who are on corticosteroid therapy and this has not appeared to be a significant risk factor in anastomotic failure in our series (see also Chapter 8, Avoiding anastomotic leakage).

Intra-abdominal sepsis

I always try to avoid performing a primary anastomosis when Crohn's disease is associated with an intra-abdominal abscess. Nevertheless, exceptions can be made and an anastomosis performed in an otherwise healthy patient providing the site of the anastomosis lies well away from the septic focus (see also Chapter 8, A good blood supply).

Creation of a stoma

The technique of the creation of an end or a loop stoma will be described under proctocolectomy and also in the section on ulcerative colitis.

I think that it is rarely ever necessary to perform a proximal defunctioning ileostomy to protect an anastomosis in Crohn's disease. If it is considered necessary to perform a proximal defunctioning stoma then it would have been better to bring out the ends as a definitive stoma and mucus fistula for later reconstruction when the patient is fit.

An exception to the "do not protect an anastomosis" rule is when there is a sigmoid or upper rectal disease that has to be resected so leaving a short rectal stump. The options then are to close the rectal stump or anastomose to it with or without a protecting stoma. I feel that it is often safer to anastomose to the cut end of the rectum than to try to close a thickened rectal wall.

Abdominal wall closure

As stated above (Cutting the skin and abdominal wall) a reopened abdominal incision often does not have distinct layers as the incision is through scar tissue. When this occurs I undercut the skin until a healthy fat layer is entered and I prepare at least a centimetre of abdominal wall on each side to take the mass closure sutures. If the incision was through only thin skin scar tissue I excise this also until the edge of the rectus muscle can be identified. Although incisional hernias are uncommon in patient's with Crohn's disease I still think it is preferable to ensure that the mass closure suture is through both anterior and posterior layers of the rectus sheath. When the edges of the abdominal wall have been prepared and haemostasis secured with diathermy the abdominal wall is then sutured with monofilament, slowly absorbed, suture material. I use a delayed-absorption (PDS) loop suture of zero gauge on a 50 ml taper cut needle. All layers are sutured and the bites are approximately 1 cm apart and 1 cm from the edge of the abdominal wall. The suture is followed by the assistant and pulled only sufficiently tight to approximate the edges. The assistant must be restrained from pulling the suture too tight. As the suture progresses the gentle apposition of the edges of the abdominal wall can be checked as the suture progresses by palpation inside the recently placed sutures. At the proximal end of the wound the one end of the loop is divided close to the needle and one extra bite placed at the apex of the suture line and knotted securely with a surgeon's knot, followed by a reef knot. The subcutaneous fat plane is then washed with an aqueous chlorhexidine solution and, providing there has been minimal contamination and factors are favourable for primary healing, I approximate the wound edges with a fine subcuticular, monofilament, non-absorbable suture. I never drain the peritoneal cavity after operations for Crohn's disease. Although, as will be discussed later under protectomy (Chapter 16), there is occasionally an indication to drain the extraperitoneal space in the pelvis, I believe there is no justification for an intra-peritoneal drain and is some evidence to suggest that drains may compromise the healing of anastomoses.

If there is a fistula track extending to the skin, well away from the main wound, I enlarge the skin opening of the fistula somewhat by trephining the skin with diathermy to ensure that it does not heal over before the track has healed. Often, but not invariably, I curette out the contents of a complex track to remove any foreign material from the gut that has become lodged there.

Management of contaminated wounds

If the wound is contaminated, particularly if there has been an abscess or fistula in the wound, I close the abdominal wall with a mass suture as described but I do not perform a primary closure of the skin wound. I try to take sufficiently wide a bite with the abdominal wall suture so that the edges of the skin are brought into close proximation. When the skin edge is reasonably close together I do not do anything to the skin but, if there is a gap of 7 mm or more I close it with a few non-absorbable skin stitches. In the length of a full length midline wound I may place four sutures to avoid a large gap for rapid healing by granulation but sufficiently loose to allow blood or serum to escape (Fig. 10.14).

Until recently I used to lightly pack between these widely spaced skin sutures with a little ribbon gauge soaked in an aqueous chlorhexidine solution and remove it after 24 hours. However, in recent years I have omitted packing; this seems to result in less discomfort for the patient and I have detected no disadvantage. I now simply apply an absorbant dressing over the skin wound.

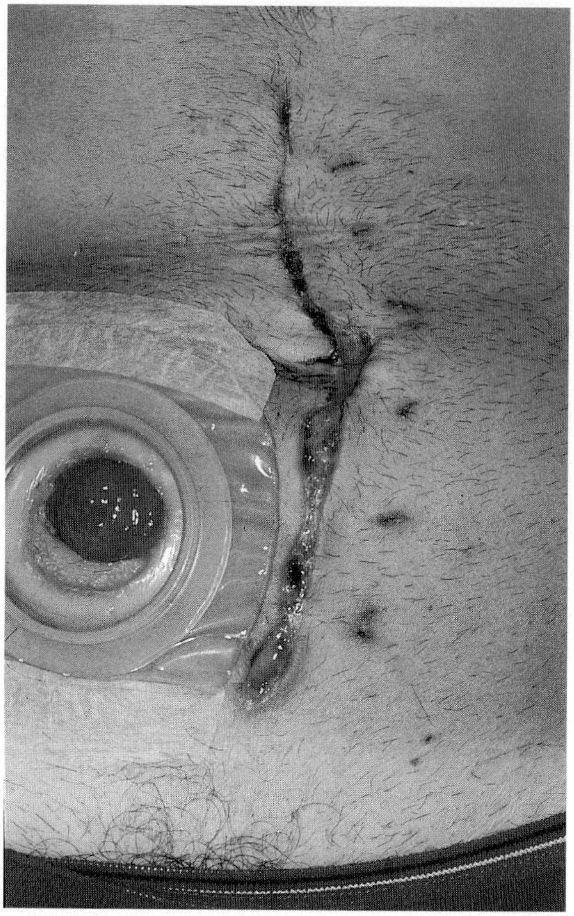

Fig. 10.14. A contaminated reoperation involving refashioning the ileostomy. The wound was partially closed with six loosely placed sutures, allowing it to drain between. The sutures have just been removed on the seventh post-operative day just before the patient left hospital.

11 Bypass, Diversion and Dilatation

J. Alexander-Williams

Bypass overcomes obstruction and may allow inflammatory oedema to settle. The traumatic aspect of the disease process that is being provoked by intestinal contents being forced under pressure through the stitches is relieved if the narrow area is bypassed. The effect of the bypass on the local disease is similar to that produced by total parenteral nutrition, when there is little apart from intestinal secretion passing through the area. However, bypass does not cure the disease or necessarily overcome the complication of stenosis.

Indications and principles of bypass

In the early years of surgical intervention in Crohn's disease surgeons considered that a complicated adherent mass in the ileo-caecal area was an indication for a bypass; either in continuity or exclusion. There is no indication today for the anastomosis of the ileum proximal to the obstructing disease to the transverse colon. Some suggest that inexperienced surgeons encountering a fixed mass of inflamed tissue in the right iliac fossa should simply bypass the mass and close the abdomen when the diagnosis is not clear or they do not consider themselves competent to remove it. I believe that such a situation should not occur if pre-operative assessment is adequate and, if ever it does occur, the surgeon should summon experienced help.

Others think that bypass can be used in an operation on a sick patient when it is impossible to improve the patient's health before operation such as in a patient who is septic with a psoas abscess that does not respond to percutaneous drainage. Under these circumstances the mass of gut and the abscess could be put "out of circuit" by bypass. I think that this is best done by a proximal ileostomy and mucous fistula. This is an external bypass rather than an internal bypass using a ileo-transverse anastomosis. However, I always try to remove the affected gut from which an abscess is arising. Some decades ago when we employed such diversion without excision we encountered continued complications from the abscess and gut left behind.

Multiple short strictures, particularly with active disease have been treated by short side-to-side bypass. This can be performed quite rapidly by a side-to-side staple apparatus (GIA) as described by Keighley (1991) but in my opinion it has no advantages over a strictureplasty, it takes longer to perform and is much more expensive.

Ileo-transverse and entero-enteric bypass

In my opinion the ileo-transverse anastomosis as a means of treating an ileo-caecal mass no longer has any place (see above). The obstructed area of the gut can be bypassed by a side-to-side anastomosis of small bowel to small bowel using an entero-anastomosis. If the bypass is for a very short inactive stricture it can be performed by side-to-side stapled entero-anastomosis (GIA) (Keighley 1991).

External bypass

External bypass can be achieved by a loop ileostomy which will be described below or by an end ileostomy with the distal end brought out as a mucous fistula either in a separate stoma site or at the lower end of the wound (Truelove et al. 1965; Lee 1976; Harper et al. 1983). The latter is the so-called "split ileostomy" popularised by the Oxford school. I do not use the procedure of end ileostomy with closure of the distal segment. The dangers of this procedure are similar to the dangers of the exclusion bypass popularised in Mount Sinai Hospital, New York which in our experience led to continued sepsis in the bypassed segment and, in one patient, to a sudden rupture of the closed stump.

Closure or reversal of bypass

The Oxford group (Lee 1976) reported a few cases in which bypassed disease settled to such an extent that, without resection it was able to be put back into continuity. This has not been our experience and we have always had to perform some sort of excision before continuity was restored. It is for this reason that, wherever possible, I excise the main obstructing lesion at the first operation and exteriorise the end of healthy bowel as a mucous fistula. Therefore this does not really fall into the category of bypass.

In my opinion the closure of either a loop ileostomy or a mucous fistula be performed only if it can be demonstrated that there is no hold-up distal to the stoma. It is difficult to assess this radiologically and also difficult and impractical to instil ileostomy effluent into the distal lumen, as has been recommended by some. I believed that the only way to restore continuity in a patient who has had a bypass is for the original obstructing lesion either to be resected or the strictures treated by strictureplasty. This would necessitate a full laparotomy, separation of all the adherent loops of bowel and checking by intraluminal balloon exploration to be sure there were no hidden strictures. The reconstruction operation should always be undertaken by a specialist unit if the original bypass had been performed as an emergency by inexperienced staff.

Dilatation with balloon or dilator

The reason for attempting to dilate an intestinal stricture is obvious and the procedure should be straightforward. It is similar in principle to the well-established practice of oesophageal dilatation for peptic oesophageal strictures or even malignant oesophageal strictures (Atkinson et al. 1978). The same principle is applied to the dilatation of atheromatous arterial strictures.

Oesophageal dilatation for peptic stricture is invariably accompanied by appropriate medical therapy and is usually successful in controlling the disease. No such therapeutic option is available in Crohn's disease and therefore dilated strictures are likely to recur; in our experience most do.

Indications

Dilatation is indicated particularly for short strictures in quiescent disease. It is, of course, essential that the strictures are accessible. Balloon dilatation is contraindicated in long strictures in active disease and impractical if there are multiple strictures. It is possible that improvement in technology and expertise will widen the present indications for dilatation but I do not see a great future for it.

Technique

The stricture is approached by direct vision through an end viewing endoscope; duodenal strictures via the stomach and ileo-colonic anastomotic strictures via the rectum. It is usually helpful to have some clear radiological picture of the stricture, particularly to determine its length and to ensure that there is not another stricture immediately adjacent. I would also advise that this should be done under mild sedation and not under general anaesthesia. It is vital to be able to assess the patient's response to the dilatation; pain is a danger signal. Once the stricture is clearly visualised the deflated balloon is passed through it. This is done either under direct vision or, if this is not possible, over a guide wire in the same manner as is practised in the dilatation of oesophageal strictures. Usually X-ray screening control is not required. When the balloon is in position it is inflated with saline under controlled pressure monitored by a pressure gauge. The pressure is maintained for a minute or two and then repeated on two or three occasions (Williams and Palmer 1991).

Complications and precautions

The most important complication of dilatation is tearing or disruption of the gut as it is stretched. This can occur even in the absence of any immediate painful response. If there is a rupture of the bowel, gas will escape into the peritoneal cavity and cause pain. If rupture is suspected, a plain radiograph of the abdomen may show free gas or gas may be seen in tissues. If there is any doubt about the diagnosis, an immediate water-soluble contrast examination should be performed. We have had one patient who had an ileo-colonic anastomosis dilated followed by mild pain and a small pneumoperitoneum. The patient was treated conservatively with antibiotics and rest, she was unwell for some days and then recovered. She returned to have a strictureplasty six months later after which there was a rapid, uncomplicated recovery.

Bleeding is a theoretical complication if the bowel wall is torn. The risk is probably small but it would be as well to take care in patients receiving anticoagulants.

Infection of the tissues following splitting the wall of the bowel by dilatation is a theoretical danger and for that reason the same antimicrobial prophylaxis should be given as for an operation.

Results

Balloon dilatation of upper gastrointestinal strictures of the upper gastrointestinal track is now widely accepted (Lindner et al. 1985; Hogstrom and Haglund 1985). Endoscopic balloon dilatation of Crohn's disease strictures under intravenous sedation in seven patients was reported by Williams and Palmer (1991). Five were at an ileo-transverse anastomosis, two of which were technical failures and two were successful after two dilatations each. They took four attempts to achieve temporary improvement in the nutritional intake of one patient with a duodenal stricture and two attempts before relieving the pain of a patient with a colonic stricture. Our own experience (Alexander-Williams et al. 1986) was in 12 patients. We achieved short-term success in three patients with duodenal or pyloric strictures (Fig. 11.1) but had less success with rectal

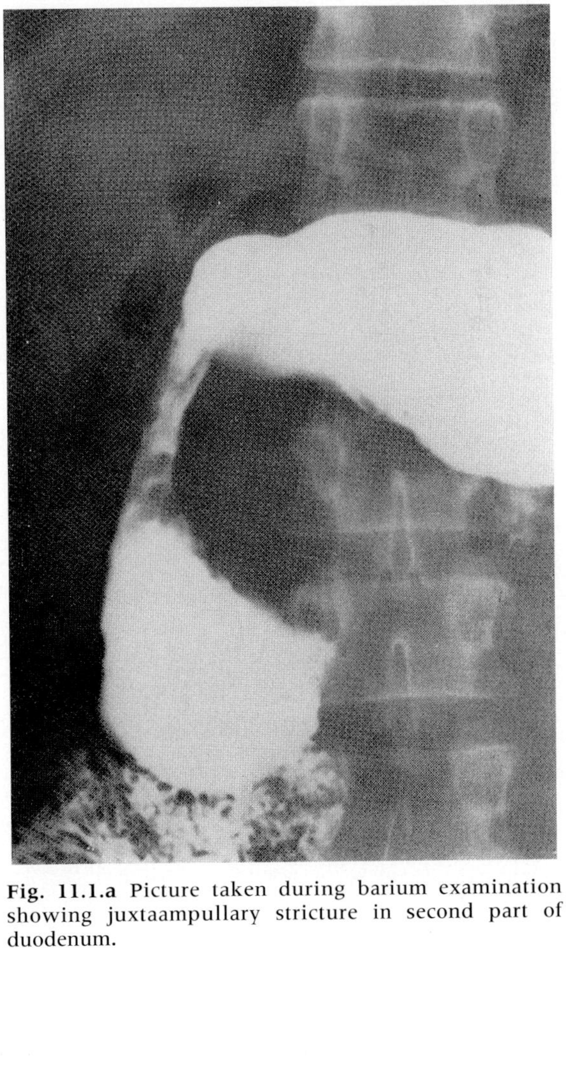

Fig. 11.1.a Picture taken during barium examination showing juxtaampullary stricture in second part of duodenum.

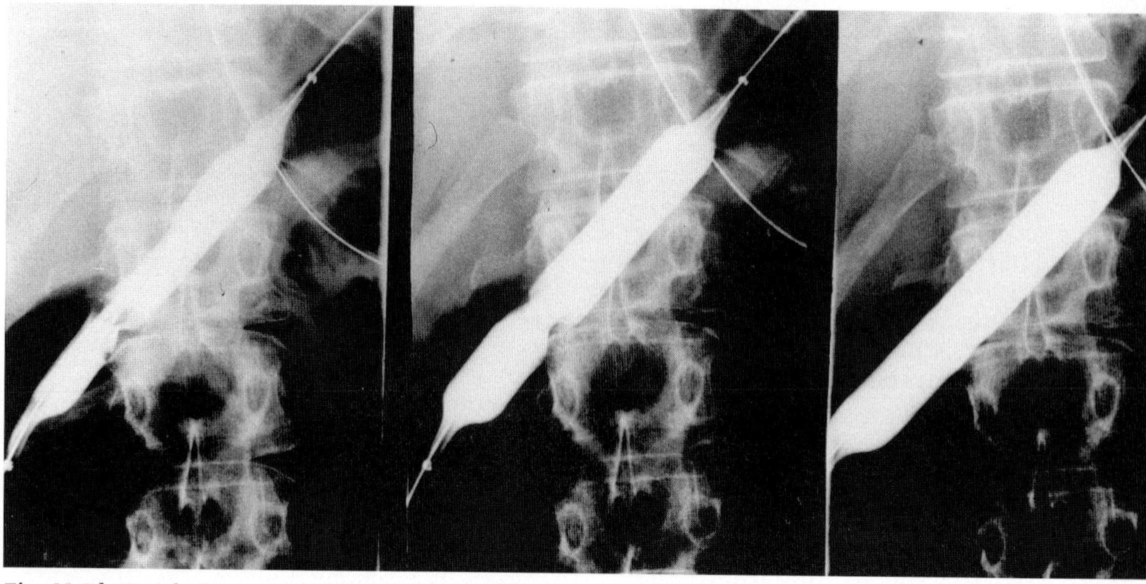

Fig. 11.1.b Serial pictures taken during balloon dilatation of stricture with 20 mm oesophageal dilatation balloon introduced via an endoscope.

or anastomotic strictures in one of which we caused a perforation that settled on conservative treatment but later needed a resection.

Although we were enthusiastic about the future of this method of stricture management we have rarely been successful in any patient since 1986. We now prefer strictureplasty for ileo-colonic anastomotic strictures, we reported 24 of these (Sharif and Alexander-Williams 1991) and have performed three more since without complication. In 1986 we concluded that the technique of balloon dilatation for enteric strictures due to Crohn's disease is a relatively safe procedure. Its value in comparison to strictureplasty is not proven but it may fulfil a similar role for a shorter duration.

Some strictures may be more amenable to dilatation than others and less mature strictures may be dilated more readily than fibrotic ones. However, our series includes one rectal stricture that has been present for five years. Whether or not disease activity at the time of dilatation will have a significant effect on stricture re-stenosis remains to be assessed. Further studies must seek to identify which stricture can be dilated with safety and which may be expected to re-stenose soon.

In the last six years our enthusiasm for balloon dilatation has waned despite two or three attempts each year. We have usually found as did Williams and Palmer (1991) that technical failure was due to a long tortuous stricture or to an acute kink in the bowel being mistaken for a stricture on endoscopy.

References

Alexander-Williams J. Allan A, Morel P, Hawker PC, Dykes PW, O'Connor, H (1986) The therapeutic dilatation of enteric strictures due to Crohn's disease. Ann R Coll Surg Eng 68:95–97

Atkinson M. Ferguson R and Parker GC (1978) Tube introducer and modified Celestin tube for use in palliative intubation of oesophageal neoplasms at fibreoptic endoscopu. Gut 19:669–671

Harper PH, Truelove SC, Lee ECG. Kettlewell MGW, Jewewll DP (1983) Split ileostomy and ileocolectomy for Crohn's disease of the colon: a 20-year survey. Gut 24:106–113

Hogstrom M, Haglund U (1985) A technique for endoscopic balloon dilatation of pyloric stenosis. Endoscopy 17:224–225

Keighley MRB (1991) Stapled strictureplasty for Crohn's disease. Dis Colon Rectum 34:945–947

Lee ECG (1976) Results of split ileostomy in Crohn's colitis: In: Weterman IT, Pena AS, Booth CC (eds) The management of Crohn's disease. Excerpta Medica, Amsterdam, pp 220–223

Lindner KD, Ott BJ, Hughes RW (1985) Balloon dilatation of upper digestive tract stricture. Gastroenterology 89:545–548

Sharif H, Alexander-Williams J (1991) Strictureplasty for ileo-colic anastomotic strictures in Crohn's disease. Int J Colorectal Dis 6:214–216

Truelove SC, Ellis H, Webster CU (1965) Place of a double-barrelled ileostomy in ulcerative colitis and Crohn's disease of the colon: a preliminary report. Br Med J i:150–152

Williams AJK, Palmer KR (1991) Endoscopic balloon dilatation as a therapeutic option in the management of intestinal strictures resulting from Crohn's disease. Br J Surg 78:453–454

12 Strictureplasty

J. Alexander-Williams

In animal experiments we have shown that there is a critical narrowing beyond which the pressure required to transmit low viscosity (saline) or high viscosity (motor oil) rises rapidly (Morel et al. 1990; Linares et al. 1992). We have postulated that the high pressure of perfusion could cause mocosal damage at the maximal part of narrowing.

Why strictures cause problems

Intestinal strictures result from the maturation and shrinking of the granulation tissue that is the basis of healing of ulceration (see Chapter 16). They cause problems when they are so tight that they impede the passage of intestinal contents. If the contents are solid, as in the distal large bowel, a stricture can cause distal obstruction when it is 20 mm or less in diameter; whereas in the upper jejunum strictures as narrow as 10 mm can usually be passed by the thin, low viscosity fluid. These narrow areas of gut usually need widening because they cause obstructive symptoms or because the force needed to push through the gut contents is high enough to cause pressure necrosis (stercoral ulceration). The strictures can be dilated (Alexander-Williams et al. 1986; Williams and Palmer 1991), resected, bypassed or widened by strictureplasty (Alexander-Williams 1986).

Towards conservative operations

Early attempts at surgical management of stenotic areas of Crohn's disease in the 1930s and 1940s involved bypass procedures which were marred with serious complications of sepsis, development of cancer and increased rate of recurrence (see Chapter 1). By the 1950s resection became the preferred operation but there soon arose a controversy about the amount of bowel that should be removed. There were some who advocated radical excision; removing all diseased bowel with a large margin of apparently normal tissue on each side of the resection. Others found less radical resection safer as it preserved gut and also had no apparent effect on the rate of recrudescence of the disease. Although this argument continued, the balance gradually shifted towards less radical surgery. Perhaps the ultimate in surgical conservatism is the concept of managing strictures by widening the bowel rather than resecting it.

The concept of strictureplasty

The concept of strictureplasty came initially from the Indian subcontinent in the management of strictures complicating quiescent intestinal tuberculosis. Katariya et al. (1977)

reported that tuberculous enteric strictures were treated more safely and effectively by strictureplasty than by excision.

In 1982 Lee and Papaionnou in Oxford reported their experience with a group of patients who underwent what they described as "minimal surgery". Most patients had strictureplasty constructed through inactive disease. The procedure was reported as being safe and effective in relieving symptoms and improving health. Although strictureplasty was performed in our unit as early as 1957, it was not until 1981 that it was adopted as a serious option in treatment for obstructing Crohn's disease (Alexander-Williams and Fornaro 1982).

The principles guiding our surgical intervention have been that surgical treatment for Crohn's disease should be for complications only, it should be safe and it should preserve as much gut as possible. Furthermore, if most of the complications of small bowel Crohn's disease are stenotic, then only the stenosis needs to be treated. We have gradually adopted a conservative approach to the surgical treatment because Crohn's disease is multifocal, recurrent and cannot be cured by resection.

Multifocal disease

Many reports have shown Crohn's disease to have a multifocal potential. Histological abnormalities have been demonstrated on routine rectal biopsies of apparently normal rectum from patients with small bowel disease (Kovelitz and Summers 1977). In our centre and elsewhere, histological and cellular changes were found in biopsies of the mucosa of the intestine well away from overt disease (Dunn et al. 1977; Goodman 1980). Furthermore, random biopsies taken during upper gastrointestinal endoscopic examinations have shown inflammatory cellular infiltration and even granuloma in macroscopically normal mucosa (Hamilton et al. 1981).

Resection of all the disease is neither necessary nor feasible

The incidence of anastomotic leakage and recurrence have been shown to be independent of the presence or absence of disease at the suture line (Lee and Papaioannou 1980; Heuman et al. 1983; Williams et al. 1991). More than 20 years ago it was our policy to perform ileo-caecal resections in patients who had diffuse large bowel disease and anastomosed ileum to abnormal, but not stenosed, large bowel. We found no higher incidence of anastomotic leakage than we experienced with anastomosis when bowel ends were macroscopically normal (Alexander-Williams and Haynes 1985).

Frequent recrudescence means many operations

Almost all who suffer from Crohn's disease eventually require surgical intervention and some require multiple bowel resections (Greenstein et al. 1975; Mekhjian et al. 1979). Data of our unit (Andrews et al. 1991) have shown that, in a mean follow-up of 10 years, 30% of patients with distal ileal disease needed more than one resection. More than three resections were needed in 5%; had these all been extensive resections there would be the potential for the development of the short gut syndrome and its metabolic consequences (Andrews et al. 1991). Hellers (1979) reported a 1.5% incidence of the short gut syndrome in his series of Crohn's disease patients in Stockholm County.

Indications

When Crohn's disease first presents, usually in the terminal ileum, it is our policy to perform simple resection of the abnormal segment of bowel with end-to-end anastomosis of macroscopically normal gut. We also resect segments containing multiple adjacent strictures, provided it is not necessary to remove more than 50 cm of gut. The results of this policy have been reviewed (Andrews et al. 1991) and referred to in Chapter 11.

It is now our policy to use strictureplasty for the following indications:

1. For recurrence after initial resection when there are single or multiple short fibrous strictures of the small bowel
2. Strictures in skip lesions well proximal to the resection margin in patients undergoing local resection
3. Ileo-colonic or ileo-rectal anastomotic strictures that do not respond easily to balloon dilatation (see Chapter 11)
4. For duodenal strictures (since it is not feasible to resect the duodenum, bypass, in the

form of gastrojejunostomy, has usually been the recommended treatment (Murray et al. 1984). Vagotomy has also been recommended to reduce the risk of stomal ulceration but this may lead to exacerbation of troublesome diarrhoea after operation. We now prefer duodenal strictureplasty to gastrojejunostomy whenever possible

5. Patients who already have a serious shortage of gut as a result of previous resections.

Technique

Preparation

To reduce the risk of infection, all patients receive prophylactic antibiotics; usually a five-day course of cephalosporin and metronidazole as described in Chapter 9. Our routine anti-embolic measures consist of stockings and compression leggings during the operation. Routine prophylactic heparinisation is not used.

I usually employ a midline incision although in patients who had previous operations we incise through the old scar. We recommend not to use a paramedian incision, as most patients with Crohn's disease have the potential for temporary or permanent ileostomy so stoma sites should be left free from scars.

All adhesions are freed so that all viscera and the whole gut can be inspected. This allows unexpected strictures to be identified and associated conditions such as gallstones to be treated. Freeing of the entire small bowel may involve a tedious and difficult dissection but can be facilitated by CO_2 insufflation through a nasogastric tube or via a fine needle introduced obliquely into the lumen through the muscle wall of the gut (Cabrol et al. 1991). The entire bowel is displayed to avoid missing distal strictures with potential disastrous consequences for a proximal anastomosis or suture line.

Detection of strictures

1. Strictures may have been demonstrated on contrast radiographic studies but it is often difficult to determine the luminal diameter or to differentiate fibrous strictures from spasm. Endoscopy may have demonstrated an obvious stricture but often they are inaccessible; multiple strictures usually defy intubation.
2. The best demonstration of strictures is at laparotomy. The appearances of the serosal aspect of the gut is typical in active Crohn's disease (Fig. 12.1) but in quiescent disease with submucosal fibrous strictures (Fig. 12.2). It may be difficult to detect them from outside the gut.

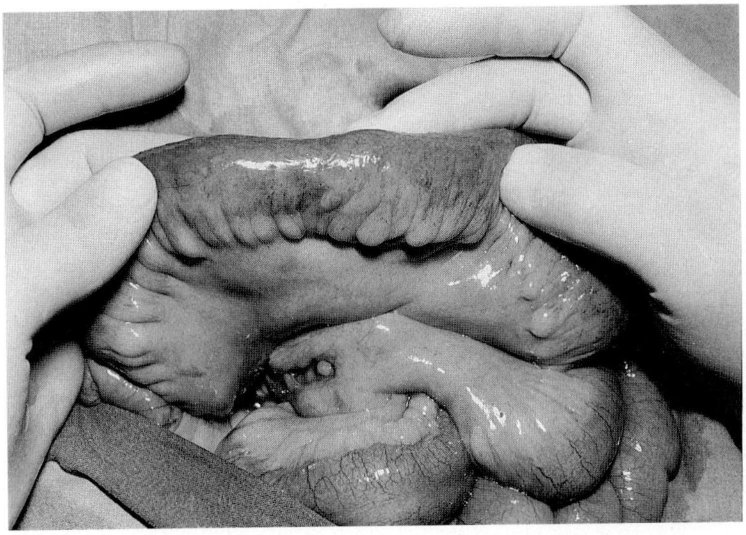

Fig. 12.1.a Active skip lesions and strictures are usually identified easily by inspection and palpation.

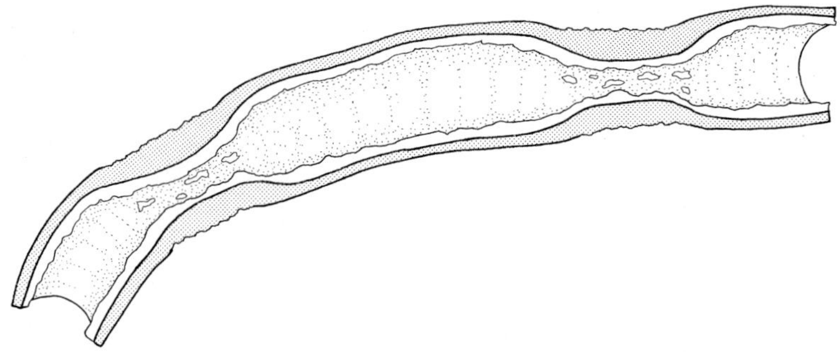

Fig. 12.1.b The thick-walled gut of skip lesions invariably indicates luminal ulceration.

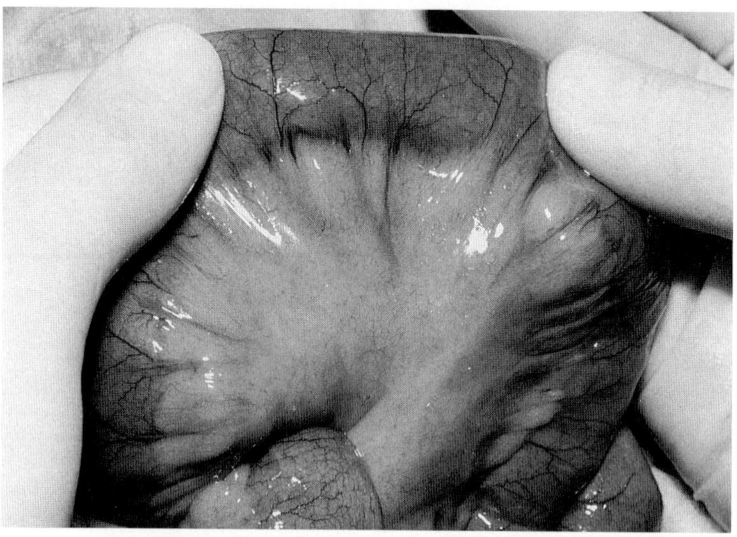

a

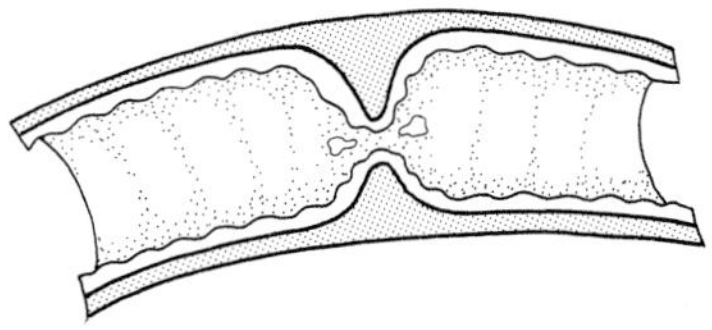

b

Fig. 12.2.a Quiescent fibrous strictures may not be obvious from external inspection but may be detected when the gut is distended by CO_2 or when an intraluminal balloon is held up. **b** Diagram of mucosal stricture.

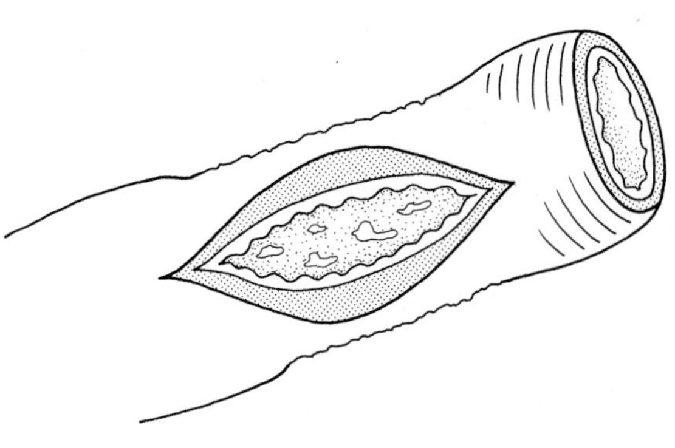

Fig. 12.3. Mucosal ulcers are present at site of stricture.

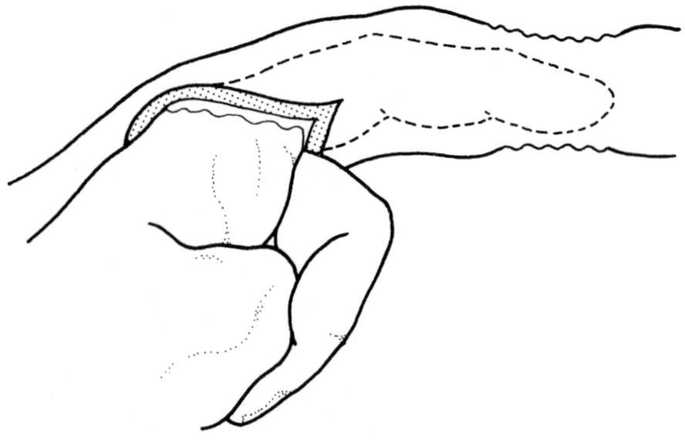

Fig. 12.4. Index finger explores lumen to detect next stricture.

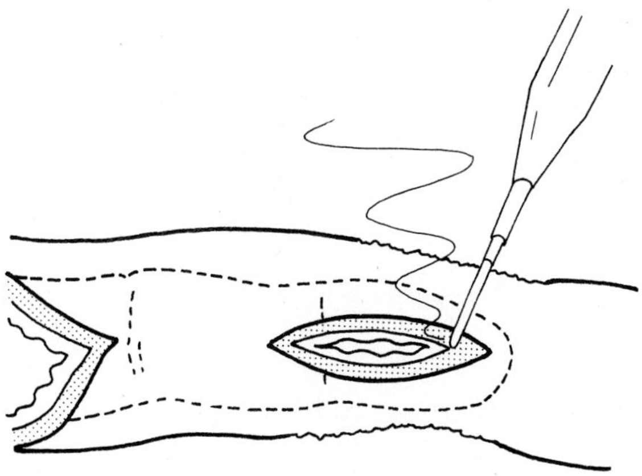

Fig. 12.5. Diathermy incision whenever there is a stricture too tight to admit interphalangeanl joint.

3. Usually at least one stricture site is obvious and this is first opened by a longitudinal diathermy incision, aided if necessary by dissecting forceps springing apart in the lumen. On the mesenteric side of the lumen there is usually an ulcer at the site of the stricture (Fig. 12.3).
4. The index finger is then introduced into the lumen and the gut concertinaed on to it to search for other strictures within the adjacent 10 cm on either side (Figs. 12.4, 12.5). If another stricture is located that is too tight to pass the finger, the gut is incised over it with diathermy. Be sure you have no hole in your glove or you may experience a diathermy burn!
5. To detect more distant strictures a balloon "pull through" technique is used. A standard 18f balloon catheter on an introducer is threaded along the bowel. Most of the small bowel can be concertinaed over one introducer but sometimes a second enterotomy is needed. If another stricture is detected and is incised, this becomes a new point of entry for the catheter. Once the catheter is passed up to the duodenum or down through the ileo-caecal junction, the balloon is inflated with 8 ml of water to give a balloon diameter of 25 mm. The balloon is then withdrawn and is held up wherever the lumen is less than 25 mm. If necessary the lumen can be sized by serial deflation (8 ml = 25 mm, 6 ml = 20 mm, 4 ml = 10 mm) (Fig. 12.6). Most 25 mm and all 20 mm or less strictures are incised longitudinally with diathermy. It is convenient to cut down on to the latex catheter but not onto the balloon, which may be ruptured by the diathermy incision.

Longitudinal incision

The method of longitudinal diathermy incision cutting down on to the left index finger in the lumen of the gut or on to the catheter has been described. Usually I cut at least 1 cm proximal and 1 cm distal to the stenosis. I always then check by inserting the index finger into lumen of the gut and increasing the length of longitudinal incision until the finger passes into the lumen without difficulty.

Haemostasis is secured along the cut wall of the gut using very fine dissecting forceps (Adson) and coagulating diathermy.

Methods of closure

Three methods of closure are employed depending on the length of the incision and the amount of thickening and oedema of the gut wall.

The simplest method used for short quiescent strictures is shown in Fig. 12.7. The index finger can be inserted through the incised stricture from an adjacent opened stricture. The presence of the finger stents the anastomosis and helps the cut edges to be everted (Fig. 12.7). A 3:0 Polyglactin suture is used starting furthest away and working towards the operator. Seromuscular sutures are used, sparing the mucosa wherever possible (Fig. 12.8). The distance between the bites of the continuous sutures depends on the thickness of the gut wall; it is always thinnest in the centre of the suture line where there is also the most tension. I usually place the bites between 5 and 8 mm apart; preferring to err on the side of too large a gap which can always be reinforced with a single stitch or two if the suture is not gas-tight when tested later. This simple method of suture only takes a minute or two for each strictureplasty; time economy is important if there are many strictures.

For the longer stricture or if the gut wall is thickened and there is some tension at the centre of the suture line, a central mattress stay suture is used (Fig. 12.9). When this is tied it indicates how much tension there is at the centre of the suture line and helps to hold the edges together while the seromuscular continuous sutures are used as before (Fig. 12.10).

a

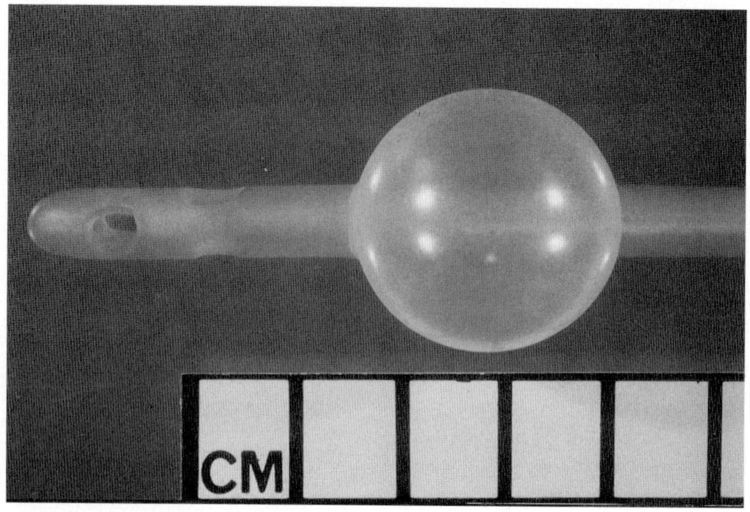

b

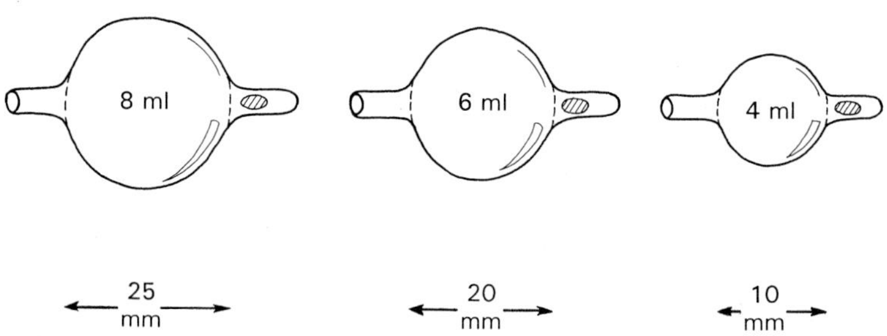

c

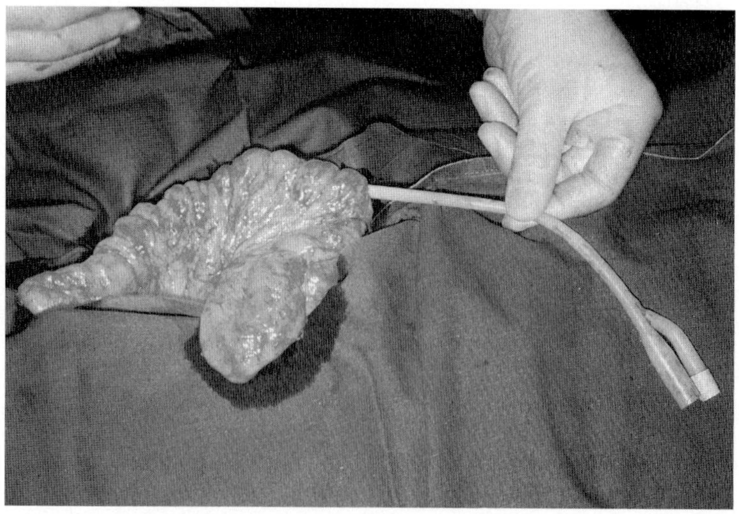

Fig. 12.6.a No. 18f balloon catheter containing 8 ml of H_2O. **b** Serial balloon distention with H_2O produces incremental enlarge
Balloon diameters with 8, 6 and 4 ml shown. **c** Balloon catheter inflated in lumen of gut.

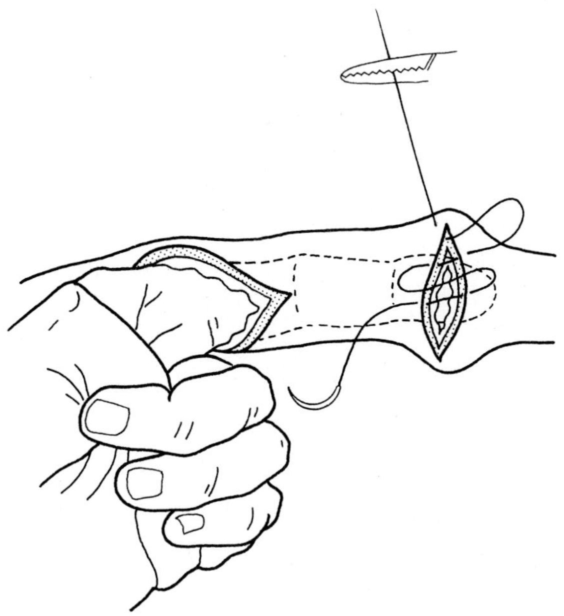

Fig. 12.7. The tip of the left index finger stents the incision and everts the mucosa for ease of transverse suturing.

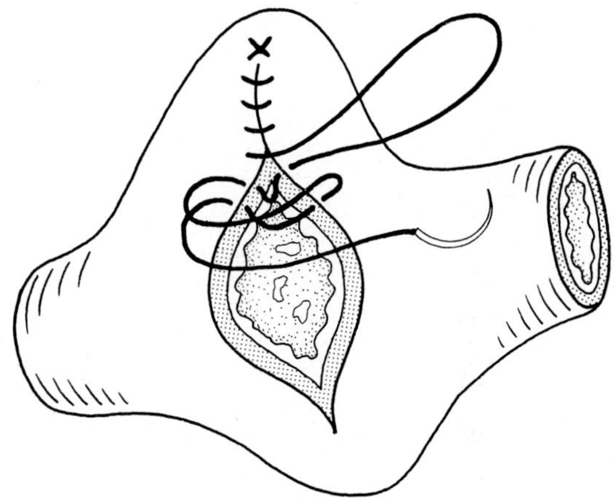

Fig. 12.8. Simple strictureplasty transverse suture when there is no tension. No stent is being used. Note seromuscular only sutures.

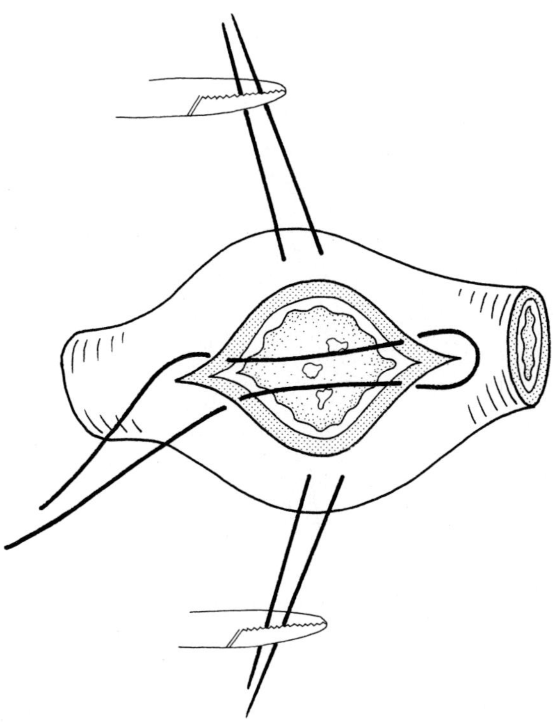

Fig. 12.9. Central stay sutures are used if gut thickening or a long incision make it difficult to approximate the ends of the incision to the centre of the transverse suture line.

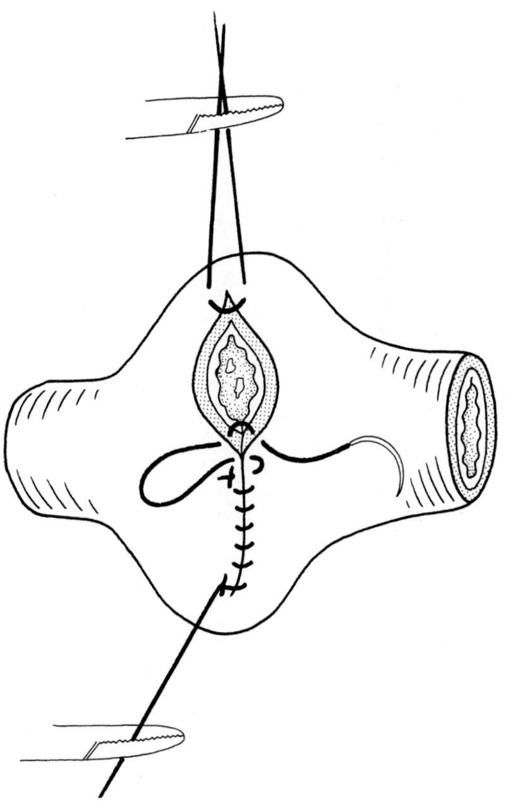

Fig. 12.10. After the central stay suture is tied a simple running seromuscular suture is used; knotting it to the stay suture as it passes.

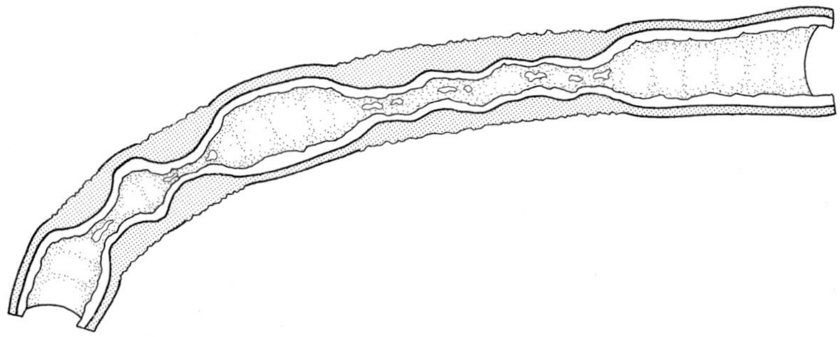

Fig. 12.11. Multiple adjacent or confluence strictures are all opened longitudinally from normal gut proximally to normal gut distally.

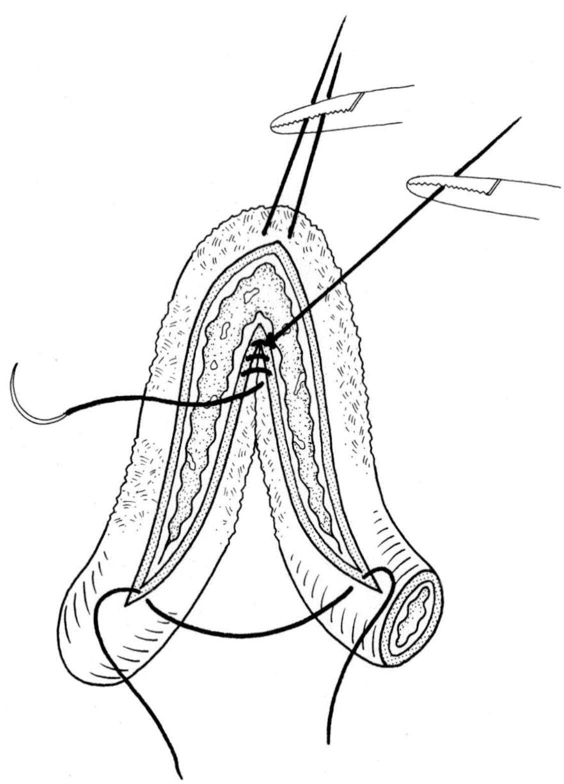

Fig. 12.12. The incised gut is bent over in a loop and the posterior wall is sutured with a continuous seromuscular stitch. A stay suture approximates the apices of the long incision.

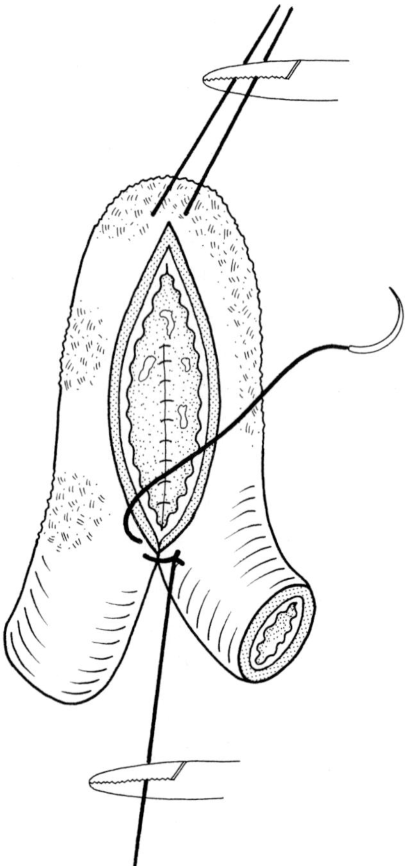

Fig. 12.13. When the posterior suture meets the apical stay suture they are knotted and the seromuscular continuous stitch is continued up the anterior wall.

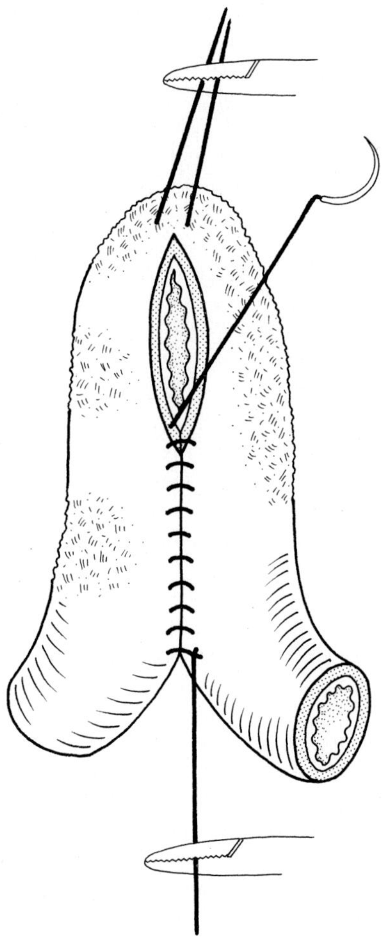

Fig. 12.14. A nearly completed "Finney" type strictureplasty.

For long or multiple confluent strictures a technique is used that resembles the "Finney" side-to-side pyloroplasty used for long or immobile peptic strictures of the duodenum.

The gut containing the stricture is cut longitudinally, often guided by the index finger in the lumen until normal diameter soft gut is entered (Fig. 12.11). If the length incised is such that it cannot easily be brought together in the centre by stay sutures, as in the method for longer strictures above, then the length of incised gut is bent over like a loop or a pouch and the posterior wall is sutured as in Fig. 12.12. The posterior wall is sutured until the central stay suture is reached (Fig. 12.13) and knotted to the running 3/0 Polyglactin suture. The anterior row is then completed (Fig. 12.14). All sutures lines are tested by CO_2 inflation to ensure that they are gas tight.

Results

The series to date

Over a period of 10 years, 80 patients underwent 309 strictureplasties at 97 operations. The principal indication for surgery at each operation was recurrent intestinal obstruction in 87, enterocutaneous fistula in nine and recurrent ileostomy bleeding in one. Bowel resection was undertaken in addition to strictureplasty in seven operations. We performed strictureplasties in the following sites: duodenum 9, jejunum 126, ileum 128, and ileocolic anastomosis 28.

Mortality and morbidity

There was no post-operative mortality. Three patients have since died, of carcinoma of lung, uterus and small bowel respectively. During follow-up 26 patients (42.6%) have required reoperation. All but four of the previous strictureplasties were unstrictured at reoperation.

Fourteen major complications developed in ten patients: eight enterocutaneous fistulas, two pulmonary emboli, two abdominal sepsis and one drug-induced haemoperitoneum. These are discussed in detail below.

Symptoms and weight gain

At a six-month review we reported a mean weight gain of 3.4 kg which was maintained on subsequent follow-up (Alexander-Williams and Haynes 1985). Over the mean follow-up of 72 months 70 of 77 survivors (91%) have complete symptomatic relief and satisfactory nutritional state. The remaining seven patients have recurrent symptoms because of underlying diffuse small bowel disease.

Other centres have reported good quality of life after strictureplasty and attested to the safety of the procedure (Dehn et al. 1989; Fazio et al. 1989; Kendall et al. 1986; Silverman et al. 1989).

Complications

Major leakage

Initially we feared that a strictureplasty, constructed through grossly diseased bowel, would lead to a high rate of anastomotic leakage and enterocutaneous fistula. However, experience with strictureplasty has shown that bowel affected by Crohn's disease has a good blood supply and strong fibrous tissue to take sutures; it appears to heal well. There seems to be little evidence that the presence of active Crohn's disease hinders healing of anastomoses or suture lines.

Of the 97 operations with 309 strictureplasties in our series, eight were followed by enterocutaneous fistulae. This is no greater than we have found after resection for complicated Crohn's disease in ill patients.

Fazio et al. reported that three (6%) out of their 50 patients who underwent 225 strictureplasties (Fazio et al. 1989), developed enterocutaneous fistulae, whereas Dehn et al. (1989) who reported 86 strictureplasties performed in 24 patients in Oxford had no anastomotic leakage or fistulae (Dehn et al. 1989). One explanation for the high incidence of post-operative enterocutaneous fistulae in our series is that we performed strictureplasty in patients even in the presence of severe intra-abdominal sepsis. On 14 occasions we found gross intra-abdominal sepsis (peri-intestinal abscess, entero-enteric enterocutaneous fistula related sepsis and psoas abscess), seven (50%) were followed by an enterocutaneous fistula. The remaining seven healed without complications. Nutritional factors did not seem to influence post-operative recovery; eight patients in the series had serum albumin levels between 16 and 23 g/dl. Only one developed anastomotic leak and enterocutaneous fistula.

Minor leakage

After 12 of the 97 operations there have been episodes of abdominal pain, fever and transient ileus that resolved slowly, many with continuation of the perioperative antibiotic therapy. We have presumed that these represented minor suture line leakages that resolved. One of these patients was unwell for six months before an abscess pointed and a fistula supervened.

Restenosis after strictureplasty

Strictureplasty tends to be used for patients with multifocal Crohn's disease and is often used after multiple previous resections. A higher incidence of recrudescence might therefore be expected than after a simple resection, in which a single site of Crohn's disease is resected with an end-to-end anastomosis.

An appropriate randomised prospective comparative trial of strictureplasty and resection does not seem to be feasible, but we have calculated the risk of recurrence at individual sites of stenosis that have been treated either by resection or strictureplasty (Sayfan et al. 1989). We compared 41 patients, treated by resection only, in whom 93 separate resections had been performed with 41 other patients whose treatment had included strictureplasty and in whom 129 separate strictureplasty sites could be analysed. The number of sites treated by either strictureplasty or resection that had required a further operation in the months and years following the first definitive operation were analysed statistically. There appeared to be no significantly greater risk of recrudescence at an individual site where the lesion had been treated by resection or by strictureplasty. It was concluded that strictureplasty was a reasonable alternative to multiple resections for multifocal stenotic small bowel disease.

Evidence from some of the patients who required another operation months or years later for further stenotic complications suggests that the active disease process may become quiescent at the site of strictureplasty. It is not known whether there is a significant long-term risk of the development of small bowel carcinoma at the strictureplasty site, but the risk of carcinoma developing in such an area appears to be no greater than that in residual areas of Crohn's disease in which there was no specific indication for surgical operation.

Strictureplasty now and in the future

Strictureplasty is not the surgical answer to all the problems of Crohn's disease. At present it is a safe technique when used in the correct circumstances for quiescent, multifocal, stenotic disease. In less favourable circumstances, in the presence of fistulas or sepsis, it may still be the best of a number of poor options. However, it is always worth

a

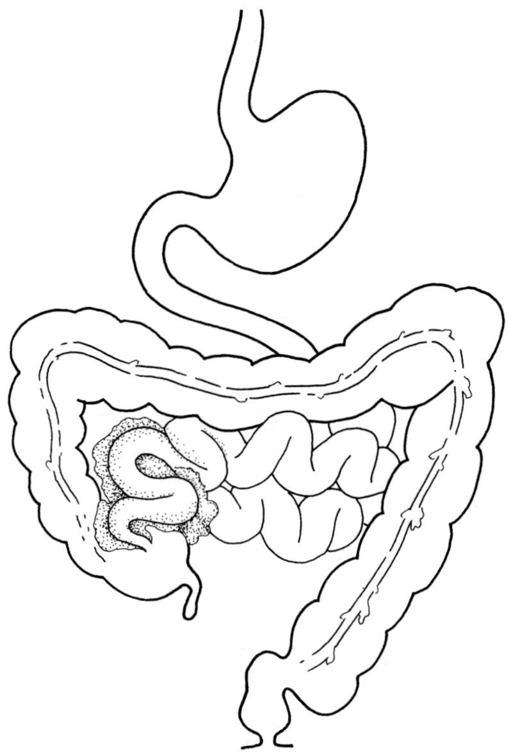

attempting to create a proximal diverting stoma when a strictureplasty has a high risk of leakage. I have successfully employed the principle of proximal diversion to protect multiple strictureplasties performed in the presence of gross distal sepsis and strictures. After 12 weeks' recovery the diverted loop of gut has been returned to "circulation" (Fig. 12.15). I once predicted that in the future strictureplasty would be superseded by balloon dilatation (Alexander-Williams 1982). I have since learned to be less fanciful in my predictions. I no longer think that balloon dilatation has more than a limited place. I think that the pharmacological manipulation of fibrosis is a long way off and that tissue glues are unlikely to make suture lines safer in Crohn's disease.

b

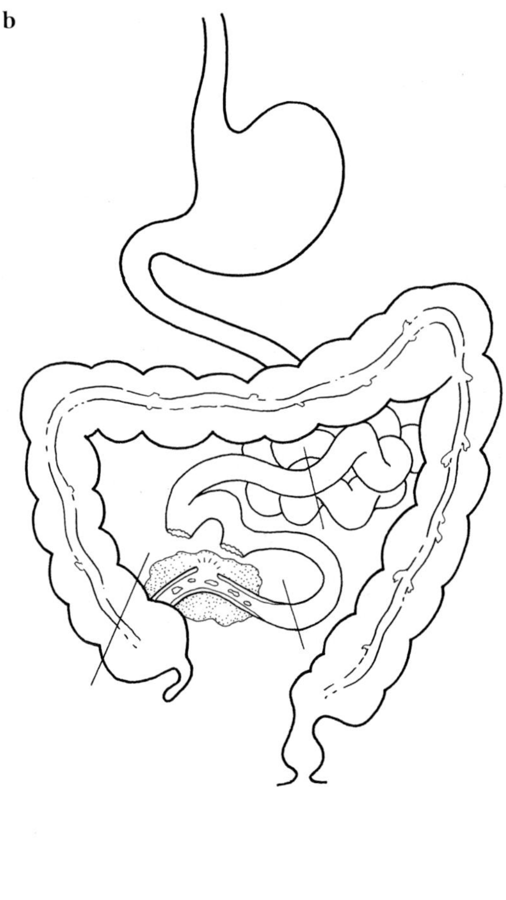

c

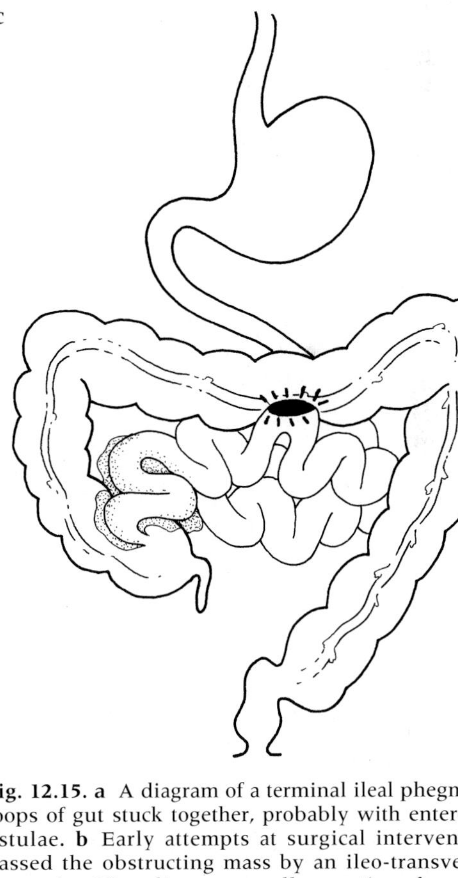

Fig. 12.15. a A diagram of a terminal ileal phegmon with loops of gut stuck together, probably with entero-enteric fistulae. **b** Early attempts at surgical intervention bypassed the obstructing mass by an ileo-transverse anastomosis. The disease usually continued and often progressed to an external fistula even though the obstruction was overcome. A technique used now only for severely compromised patients or by inexperienced surgeons. **c** Present-day approach is to dissect out the mass and separate from it adherent proximal loops, even those that have a fistula connecting with the main abscess/mass. The main acute ulcerated area is resected.

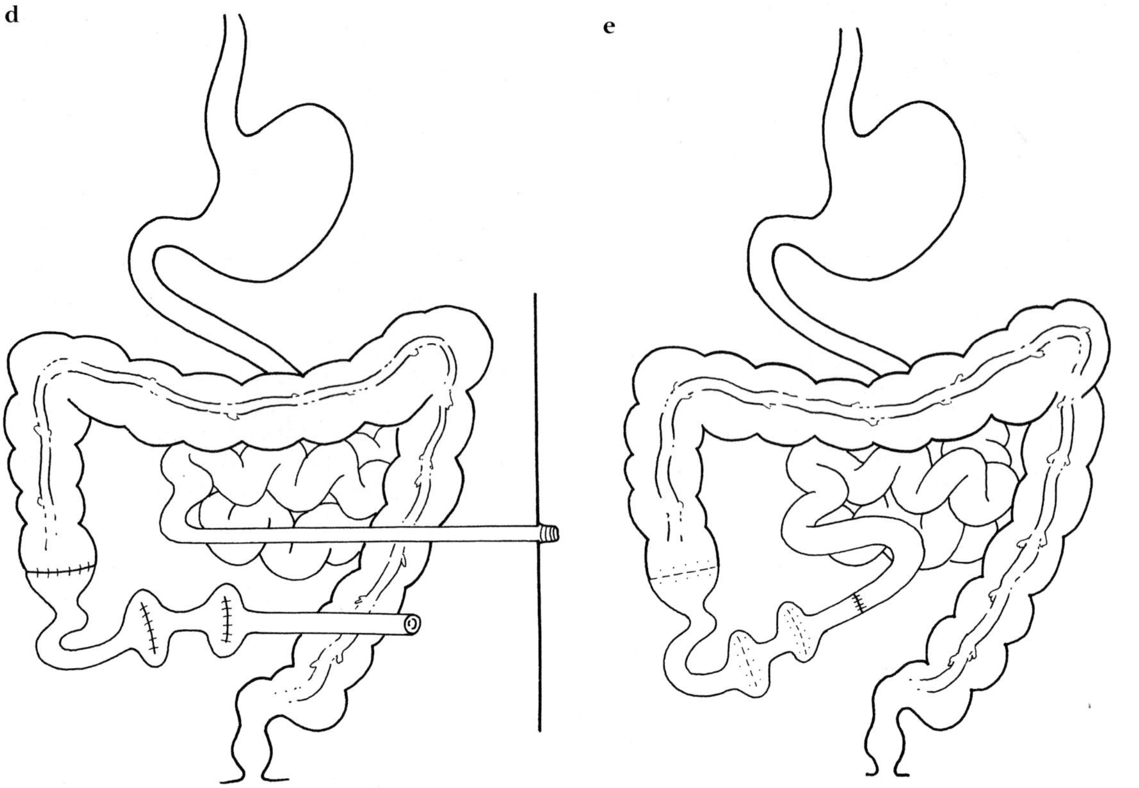

Fig. 12.15d The proximal skip area and sites of fistula were closed as a strictureplasty. Because there was a large local abscess, bowel continuity was not restored. A proximal defunctioning end ileostomy was created and the distal end brought out at the lower end of the laparotomy wound as a mucus fistula. **e** Twelve weeks later with the patient recovered and well nourished, continuity is restored by a simple operation.

References

Alexander-Williams J (1982) New directions for future research: surgical/clinical. In: Rachmilewitz D (ed) Inflammatory bowel diseases. Martinus Nijhoff, The Hague

Alexander-Williams J (1986) How I do it – the technique of intestinal strictureplasty. Int J Colorect Dis 1:54–57

Alexander-Williams J, Fornaro M (1982) Strictureplasty beim morbus Crohn Chirurg 53:799–801

Alexander-Williams J, Haynes IG (1985) Conservative operations for Crohn's disease of the small bowel. World J Surg 9:945–951

Alexander-Williams J, Allan A, Morel P, Hawker PC, O'Connor H (1986) The therapeutic dilatation of enteric strictures due to Crohn's disease. J R Coll Surg Eng 68:1–3

Andrews HA, Keighley MRB, Alexander-Williams J, Allan RN (1991) Strategy for management of distal ileal Crohn's disease. Br J Surg 78:679–682

Cabrol J. Griffiths C, Alexander-Williams J (1991) Carbon dioxide insufflation in gastrointestinal surgery. Br. J. Surg 78:499–500

Dehn TCB, Kettlewell MGW, Mortensen NJMcC, Lee ECG, Jewell DP (1989) Ten-year experience of strictureplasty for obstructive Crohn's disease. Br J Surg 76:339–341

Dunn WT, Cooke WT, Allan RN (1977) Enzymatic and morphometric evidence for Crohn's disease as a diffuse lesion of the gastrointestinal tract. Gut 18:290–293

Fazio VW, Galandiuk S, Jagelman DG, Lavery IC (1989) Strictureplasty for Crohn's disease. Ann Surg 210:621–625

Goodman MJ (1980) The case for conservative treatment. In Truelove SC, Kennedy HD (eds) Topics of gastroenterology, vol 8. Blackwell Scientific, Oxford

Greenstein AJ, Sachar DB, Pasternack BS et al. (1975) Reoperation and recurrence in Crohn's colitis and ileocolitis. N Engl J Med 293:685–690

Hamilton SR, Bussey NJG, Boitnott JV et al. (1981) Active inflammation and granulomas in uninvolved colonic mucosa of Crohn's disease resection specimen studies with an en-face histologic technique. Gastroenterology 80:1167

Hellers G (1979) Crohn's disease in Stockholm County 1955–1974. A study of epidemiology, results of surgical treatment and long-term prognosis. Acta Chir Scand (Suppl) 490:31–69

Heuman R, Boeryd B, Bolin T et al. (1983) The influence of disease at the margin of section on the outcome of Crohn's disease. Br J Surg 70:519–521

Katariya RN, Sood S, Rao PG, Rao PLN (1977) Strictureplasty for tubercular strictures of the gastrointestinal tract. Br J Surg 64:496–498

Kendall GP, Hawley PR, Nicholls RJ, Lennard-Jones JE (1986) Strictureplasty. A good operation for small

bowel Crohn's disease. Dis Colon Rectum 5:312–316
Kovelitz BI, Sommers SC (1977) Rectal biopsy in patients with Crohn's disease. Normal mucosa on sigmoidoscopy examination. JAMA 237:2742–2744
Lee, ECG, Papaioannou N (1980) Recurrences following surgery for Crohn's disease. Clin Gastroenterol 9:419–438
Lee ECG, Papaioannou N (1982) Minimal surgery for chronic obstruction in patients with extensive or universal Crohn's disease. Ann R Coll Surg Engl 64:229–232
Linares L, Allan A, Alexander-Williams J (1993) The influence of luminal content viscosity on the pressure and flow disturbance of gut obstruction. (In press)
Mekhjian HS, Switz DM, Watts HD, Deren JJ, Katon RM, Beman FM (1979) National cooperative Crohn's disease study: factors determining recurrence of Crohn's disease after surgery. Gastroenterology 77:907–913
Morel P, Alexander-Williams J, Rohner A (1990) Relations between flow-pressure diameter studies in experimental stenosis of rabbit and human small bowel. Gut 875–878
Murray JJ, Schoetz DH, Nugent FW et al. (1984) Surgical management of Crohn's disease involving the duodenum. Am J Surg 147:58–64
Ross TM. Fazio VW, Fromm RC (1983) Long-term results of surgical treatment of Crohn's disease of the duodenum. Ann Surg 197:399–406
Sayfan J, Wilson DAL, Allan A, Andrews H, Alexander-Williams J (1989) Recurrence after strictureplasty or resection for Crohn's disease. Br J Surg 76:335–338
Sharif H, Alexander-Williams J (1991) Strictureplasty for ileo-colic anastomotic strictures in Crohn's disease. Int J Colorect Dis 6:214–216
Silverman RE, McLeod RS, Cohen Z (1989) Strictureplasty in Crohn's disease. Can Assoc Clin Surg 32:19–22
Williams AJK, Palmer KR (1991) Endoscopic balloon dilatation as a therapeutic option in the management of intestinal strictures resulting from Crohn's disease. Br J Surg 78:453–454

13 The Management of Fistula

J. Alexander-Williams

Principles

An intestinal fistula is a granulation tissue-lined tract between the gut and an epithelial surface. An intestinal fistula should be expected to heal by the normal process of healing of granulation tissue. To understand the principles governing fistula healing and the management of a fistula it is useful first to understand the physiological mechanisms involved.

Defence mechanisms and repair

Primary defences

The body protects its sensitive and vital internal organs (mesoderm) from noxious external substances (chemicals and microbacteria) by two efficient defence mechanisms. The exterior of the body is covered by a thick layer of impervious scales (skin) that provide effective protection from invasion of chemicals or micro-organisms. An impervious internal layer of epithelium in the respiratory or alimentary tract would obviously be impractical because of the need for rapid exchange of gases, fluids and solutes. The internal cavities of the body are therefore lined by a different epithelium. In the gut this is mucous secreting; the production of large volumes of mucous and a rapid turnover of new cells provide a barrier against the invasion of micro-organisms. This is a higher energy system than the external squamous epithelium because the gut epithelium is active and rapidly replicating.

Secondary defences

Whenever these two epithelial defence mechanisms are breached as a result of loss of the epithelium by ulceration or trauma there is a potential for micro-organisms to gain access to internal organs. To combat this the body employs its secondary defence mechanism: the granulation tissue response. Granulation tissue is produced by the mesoderm in response to chemical or physical trauma. Granulation tissue is composed of outbudding of loops of young capillaries from adjacent vessels. These loops of capillaries are accompanied by immature fibrous cells, fibroblasts. The capillaries bring blood to the surface and with it the body's secondary defence mechanisms, the white blood cells. The granulation tissue exudes white cells and serum and as the immature capillaries are fragile they frequently also exude blood.

In complex intra-abdominal sepsis as the result of perforation of the gut, the contaminated mesoderm needed to create a granulation response can cover an area of up to 10% of the body surface and is physiologically as devasting as a third degree burn to a limb (Katz et al. 1986).

Granulation tissue is a high-energy system requiring a large calorie expenditure. The energy required to maintain an area of granulation tissue is so extravagant of the body's resources that the body must try to reduce the size of an area of granulation (Cato 1985). This mechanism involves the maturation of fibroblasts to fibrocytes. The efficacy of the contraction of granulation tissue as it matures can be seen dramatically when third degree burns of the skin heal and produce a tight scar. Similarly when a large cavity, such as the perineum after a rectal excision, is left to granulate, the initial large area is reduced to half or a quarter of its size within a week or two. Therefore it is clear that the contracting forces of healing are powerful. It is the process of contraction with the maturation of granulation that is the force primarily responsible for the healing of an intestinal fistula (Alexander-Williams and Irving 1982).

The natural history of an intestinal fistula

It is convenient to formulate four hypotheses or rules of fistula:

Rule 1. All fistulas heal

Rule 2. All fistulas heal, unless the pressure within the fistulous track exceeds the power of contraction of maturing granulation tissue

Rule 3. All fistulas heal unless epithelium joins to epithelium and there is no granulation tissue required to fill the gap. Therefore no further contraction occurs

Rule 4. Any fistula that has not healed by 12 weeks is unlikely to heal spontaneously

Rule 2 applies when there is a persistent biliary fistula due to distal obstruction by stone or tumour following the removal of a T-tube. Rule 3 applies when the epithelium of an ileostomy is sutured to the skin.

Classification of fistulas

We usually employ an anatomical classification, indicating the location of the epithelial surfaces that are connected by the granulation tissue-lined track. We refer to an entero-enteric, entero-cutaneous, entero-vesical or entero-vaginal fistula. Similar designations are applied to fistulas that arise from the colon, rectum and anus.

The anatomical classification gives no indication of the severity of the problem nor gives any guide to therapy. In an attempt to improve on this classification I used to teach that there were three sorts of intestinal fistula: 1, good news; 2, bad news; and 3, disaster. I now have a less evocative but perhaps more acceptable definition:

1. *Simple fistula.* A direct granulation tissue-lined track between one epithelial surface and the other without ramification. Examples of such a fistula are that existing between a common bile duct and the skin surface after removal of a T-tube from an unobstructed bile duct system or a fistula following the removal of a caecostomy tube. Such a fistula heals quickly and without complication.

2. *Complicated fistula.* This is when the tract does not run directly to the other epithelial surface but ramifies widely into surrounding tissues, usually within the abdominal cavity. Such a fistula occurs if there is a leakage from an intestinal anastomosis. The leak is first into a localised area in the abdominal cavity and then out through a drain site or a wound. The ramifications of the track within the abdomen make it complex. They also make it prone to develop satellite abscesses within some of the track complexities. Such satellite abscesses often require drainage before healing can occur.

3. *Obstructed fistula.* This occurs when there is some significant obstruction of normal distal flow along the intestine, forcing gut contents out through the fistula track rather than onward. Such an obstructed fistula is common in Crohn's disease, which is often proximal to an area of fibrous stenosis. Similarly fistulas complicating colonic carcinoma or diverticular disease are usually obstructed fistulas. There are some instances in which an obstructed fistula can be converted to a complex fistula such as when the obstruction is due to an ileus distal to the fistula due to sepsis which can be resolved simply by drainage.

Causes of fistula

The initiation of an enteric fistula is a breach of the mucosal defence of the gut. This may be either acute or chronic.

Acute

The common causes of an acute fistula are post-operative anastomotic failure or trauma.

Chronic

Chronic fistula may be due to chronic ulceration of the gut due to mucosal damage from drugs, malignancy or disease. The difference between an acute and a chronic fistula is that an acute breach of the bowel wall invariably leads to contamination of the entire peritoneal cavity with peritonitis, whereas a chronic, slowly progressive fistula first adheres and then penetrates. If an acute perforation into the peritoneal cavity drains externally by rupturing through the wound or a site of drainage it becomes a complex fistula. Chronic ulceration is usually preceded by adherence of the ulcerating gut to the parietal peritoneum or an adjacent organ. The chronic ulceration then penetrates locally either into the adjacent organ or through to the skin. A skin exit is most likely to occur where the gut is already adherent to the abdominal wall. In patients who have had abdominal operations, fistulas due to chronic ulceration often present through a wound.

Peculiarities of fistulas in Crohn's disease

Post-operative fistula (acute fistula)

This is invariably due to a post-operative anastomotic leakage. Anastomotic failure usually does not take place for 5–10 days after the operation and because of adhesions it is unusual for the dehiscence of an anastomosis to rupture free into the peritoneal cavity. It is more likely that, initially, there will be a localised abscess which almost invariably discharges itself through the operative wound. The physical signs of a post-operative leakage and abscess are often modified in Crohn's disease by the fact that the patients are receiving steroids. Although in our centre we often operate on patients who have never had a trial of therapy with steroids, in many centres patients with Crohn's disease have been treated with steroids for some weeks or months before the decision to operate is made.

Spontaneous fistula (chronic ulceration)

This occurs as a result of the slow penetration of a Crohn's disease ulcer through the wall of the gut to form a localised abscess. The inflamed wall of the gut has inevitably become adherent to other structures, either adjacent loops of the bowel, the bladder or the abdominal wall or vagina. For such ulceration to penetrate through the bowel wall and not be able to drain back into the lumen there has to be some distal obstruction. In all the intestinal fistula patients that we have seen with Crohn's disease the fistula has always initiated from an area of chronic fibrous stenosis.

Assessment

Clinical

It is usually possible to make an accurate assessment of a Crohn's disease fistula on simple clinical grounds. If shortly after an operation the patient has a septic illness and presents with an abscess in the wound which discharges, this is almost inevitably a post-operative fistula; as soon as gas appears in the discharge the diagnosis is certain. The differential diagnosis is a stitch abscess, which does not discharge air. However, a stitch abscess is likely to be infected with colonic organisms and therefore the discharge may have the appearance and smell of intestinal contents. If there is any doubt about the diagnosis and the patient is stable, it is possible to give a marker taken by mouth and to confirm that it is a fistula when the marker appears in the wound. This is not easy and many attempts with dyes have failed because the dye pigment may be altered by the enteric enzymes. In those rare instances when there is a reasonable doubt I have found that the best marker is a small quantity of poppy seeds by mouth. These are always recognisable as they appear in the wound. I tell my medical students that, if there is still doubt, they have to plant the seeds and wait for them to germinate!

Ultrasound

In my experience ultrasound has limited value in the initial assessment of fistulas in Crohn's disease. There is rarely any significant volume of pus in an associated abscess, even a complex fistula usually does not contain sufficient volume of pus to be recognised on ultrasonography. The principal value of ultrasound is in the later detection of satellite abscesses that are not draining adequately into the established track. Even these may be difficult to differentiate from adherent loops of thick wall bowel. The advantage of ultrasound is that it is non-invasive and can be repeated frequently. I regard ultrasound as an extension of the clinician's fingers. If an ill patient is being examined daily, changes in the ultrasound findings can be noted more easily than changes in the findings on palpation (Sonnenberg et al. 1982).

Contrast examination and computed tomographic scanning

Investigations involving radiation should always be limited to the minimum in patients with Crohn's disease. We should always bear in mind the future limits of the patient's radiation exposure with many decades of life ahead of them and the possibility of many future recrudescences that may require investigation. The advent of computed tomographic (CT) scanning has led to an increase in the amount of radiation exposure experienced by some patients with complicated Crohn's disease (Irving 1990).

When conventional contrast radiography is performed, it too should be limited and close collaboration with a specialist gastroenterological radiologist is vital. When employing contrast radiology it is important to consider precisely what is required from the investigation. I frequently reiterate the dictum that "all investigation should be limited to those tests, the results of which are likely to make a difference to management". This is particularly true of X-ray investigations, which are expensive, polluting and may have long-term dangers. The questions that may be answered by radiological contrast investigations in patients with intestinal fistulas are what is the cause, the location, complexity and prognosis of the fistula?

The cause of the fistula is rarely in doubt if the patient has had previous operations for histologically proven Crohn's disease. If it is a post-operative fistula then the site of the anastomosis is usually known and even if there have been multiple resections it is unlikely to make any difference to the management if we discover which of the anastomoses has leaked. Spontaneous fistulas, occurring from areas of recrudescence in Crohn's disease, are almost certainly going to require surgical management and at operation the site of fistula is easily determined. When I operate on a patient with recurrent Crohn's disease, in particular with a fistula, I always separate all adhesions to allow a complete assessment of the length of the remaining small bowel. Consequently, I rarely request orthograde contrast examination before operation as I achieve all the information that I need during the laparotomy dissection.

The complexity of the fistula track may need to be determined, although, in my opinion, it rarely makes any difference to the way in which it is managed. A patient with a complex fistula is usually ill and in need of further intervention only when part of the track is draining inadequately and so is behaving like a closed abscess. If this is so, it is usually not demonstrated by contrast radiology and is more likely to be detected clinically or by sonography, CT or magnetic resonance imaging (Irving 1990).

I believe that fistulography in Crohn's disease is an overused investigation. Although non-absorbable contrast gives a clear image its use cannot be justified in the assessment of a fistula track because residual non-absorbable contrast within a track seriously obscures further radiological or imaging investigations.

The demonstration of distal obstruction which may prevent healing, can have a place in the management. This is particularly important if a post-operative fistula, which might have been expected to heal spontaneously, has failed to do so by six or more weeks. Most intestinal fistulas that are going to heal spontaneously have done so by six to ten weeks. Once again we should avoid non-absorbable contrast because, if retrograde contrast studies of the large bowel are performed, residual barium may remain in the colon and limit or prevent future imaging. Furthermore, non-absorbable contrast leaking into complexities of a fistula track has the disadvantages already mentioned.

If surgical intervention is being considered, as it has to be in all spontaneous Crohn's disease fistulas, the surgeon should question whether the radiological findings are going to significantly affect his or her surgical approach. I know that many surgeons regard reintervention in a patient who has had a number of operations for Crohn's disease as a potentially difficult and hazardous operation. When this is compounded by a serious complication such as a fistula, they feel that they would like to be armed with all the obtainable information. I believe that this fear leads to what I would consider to be unnecessary investigations.

Nutrition

Post-operative fistula

Patients who have had an operation associated with an anastomotic breakdown with consequent sepsis and an eventual fistula, are usually ill and septic; particularly if the fistula is complex and the area of granulation large. They will have lost serum protein rapidly and will require a high calorie and protein intake to support the energy-expensive body defence mechanisms. For this reason I believe that one of the first requisites in the management of a post-operative fistula is the establishment of an adequate nutritional intake of over 200 $kJ/kg^{-1}/day^{-1}$ (50 $kcal/kg^{-1}/day^{-1}$) (Kovetz 1986; Heatley 1986; Pettit and Irving 1988). In these patients this is not achievable by oral intake and usually, because there is some associated ileus, not even by nasogastric drip feeding. Most patients will require total parenteral nutrition, which needs to be delayed until septicaemia has been corrected by adequate drainage of any associated sepsis (Matuchansky 1986). Patients with well-drained open wounds rarely have more than a low-grade pyrexia; a high fever is almost always an indication for surgical intervention to drain pocketing sepsis.

Once sepsis is controlled and parenteral nutrition initiated the bowel function soon returns. If the site of the fistula is in the distal alimentary tract, as it usually is in patients with Crohn's disease, it is possible to reinstitute early alimentary feeding without detriment to the patient. In my experience this normally occurs about one week after the initiation of treatment for the post-operative fistula and I have rarely found it necessary to continue total parenteral nutrition beyond 10 days. Failure to initiate oral feeding may be because there is still satellite sepsis producing ileus and so there is indication for another search to detect a focus of drainable sepsis.

Enteral nutrition should begin again gradually, as often the patient is disinclined to drink because of discomfort or nausea. We usually initiate oral feeding via a fine bore nasogastric feeding tube, which enables a slow infusion of liquid over 24 hours. Once it is clear that the infusion is not causing gastric distension or ileus, nutrients are introduced in increasing quantities and strengths (Rocchio et al. 1974). Once an oral intake of more than 50 $kcal/kg^{-1}/day^{-1}$ is achieved, total parenteral nutrition can be discontinued. As a complex fistula is a constant source of blood and protein loss transfusion may be required; we normally aim to keep the haemoglobin above 11 g/l.

Spontaneous fistula

Sometimes spontaneous fistulae occurs in chronically ill patients. As I have said before, I would regard this as neglected disease that should have had surgical intervention before the fistula had occurred. When presented with a sick, poorly nourished patient with a spontaneous fistula in Crohn's disease, there should be a "nutrition conference" when the patient's nutritional status and requirements are discussed (Mason and Rosenberg 1990). If the patient with spontaneous intestinal fistula is well nourished and in good condition there is often no reason to delay surgical intervention. As there is nothing that is a serious impediment to healing, the patient is likely to improve dramatically once the associated stenotic segment has been removed and normal oral intake can resume quickly. If factors such as a local abscess prevent immediate restoration of intestinal continuity, the patient will have to have a proximal stoma and even then normal oral feeding will begin early. Once the patient has fully recovered, usually after about 12 weeks, she or he is in a good nutritional state and intestinal continuity can be restored.

The questions we have to try to answer are:

1. Will the malnourished, hypoproteinaemic patient with a fistula due to Crohn's disease benefit from intestinal support, or will she or he be at any less risk if the nutritional status is improved?
2. Is it possible to significantly improve the patient's nutritional status before operation?

The obvious immediate response to both these question is "yes". However, in practice we have often found it difficult to make any significant change in the measurable parameters

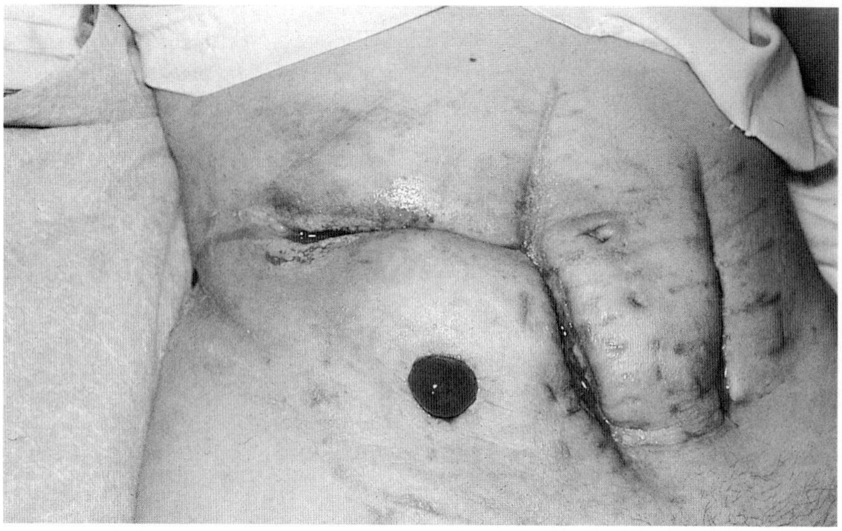

Fig. 13.1.a A complex obstructed duodenal fistula with an output of up to 6 litres per day followed the drainage of a subhepatic abscess after proctocolectomy for acute colitis. The fistula and sepsis were only controlled after laying open the abdomen and exposing the duodenal opening as a "laparostomy". The fistula has recently healed and the abdominal wall loosely reconstructed. The patient remains well with no incisional hernia 12 years later.

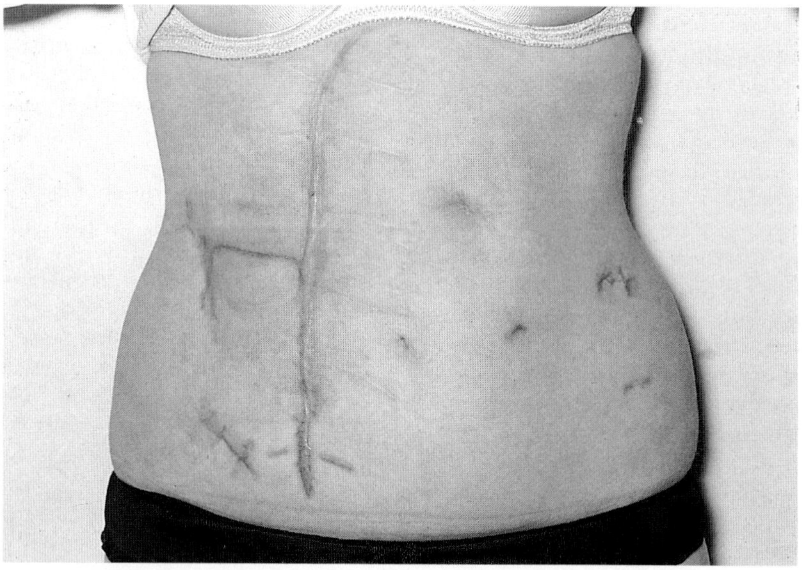

Fig. 13.1.b A reconstructed abdominal wall after extensive laying open for the intra-abdominal sepsis.

of nutrition, even by pre-operative total parenteral nutrition (Mason and Rosenberg 1990). Total parenteral nutrition is not without its dangers and sometimes persistence with parenteral nutrition is time-consuming and delays the patient's appropriate surgical treatment and return to good health. It has therefore been our practice in recent years to treat almost all patients with spontaneous fistula in Crohn's disease by early operation once their haemoglobin and serum electrolytes are at a satisfactory level (Higgens et al. 1984). When it is possible to give oral feeding while investigating and awaiting surgical intervention we usually employ fine bore, nasogastric drip feeding with high-calorie, high-protein preparations. The methods of delivery and the formulation of the feeding is a constantly changing field and the reader is referred to current specialised texts (Higgens et al. 1984; Heatley 1986; Kovetz 1986).

Surgical intervention

Post-operative fistula

The role of surgery is to eradicate septic foci that are not draining well. This usually involves the conversion of a complex fistula into a direct simple fistula by surgical exploration. It is safe, practical and usually advisable to open the abdomen widely. If necessary, this can be done with a T-shaped incision, knowing that the abdomen can be reconstructed later once the patient has recovered. It is usually possible to do this and achieve an acceptable cosmetic result (Fig. 13.1).

Sometimes it is necessary to reoperate to ensure that the fistula exit site from the gut is in such a position that it can be managed optimally by appliance fitting. A complex fistula that is draining in or near the groin defies good appliance fitting. I have often had to intervene at an early stage to establish access to the cavity at the point where the fistula leaves the gut so that an adhesive appliance can be applied to it directly.

Once closed sepsis has been eradicated, drainage established and distal obstruction has been excluded and the patient has been established on an adequate nutritional intake, it is best to wait for the natural healing processes of the granulation tissue reaction to occur. The fistula then usually heals spontaneously, often within six weeks. If the fistula has not healed by 12 weeks it is unlikely that it will do so. (See Rule 4 above.)

One of the causes of failure of complete healing that we have encountered is when the granulation tissue of a complex fistula track surrounds gut distal to the fistula. First the sepsis impairs the normal progression of peristalsis due to a local ileus and then as the granulation tissue matures and contracts, a distal fibrous obstruction prevents final healing. Under these circumstances I recommend leaving the patient at least 12 weeks before reoperation. Often they can be managed at home, providing there is good access to stoma care services. Even in those patients who require careful supervision I believe that it is important to consider their morale and we frequently allow patients in this state to go home on what we call "weekend leave". The length of the leave can be extended as they progress.

Spontaneous fistula

Early surgical intervention is usually indicated as described above. The aim of the operation is to eradicate the obstructing disease associated with the fistula. If it is a simple fistula with adherent thickened obstructed bowel stuck directly on to the parietal peritoneum, without a significant intra-abdominal abscess and if the patient is in a good nutritional state, primary resection and anastomosis is the quickest way to restore normal activity. Resection and anastomosis is usually achieved with a low risk of anastomotic complications. On two patients with short segments of relatively quiescent disease associated with a short simple fistula I have simply performed a strictureplasty; they enjoyed primary healing and long-term relief of symptoms. However, this combination of factors is likely to remain the exception rather than the rule.

I believe, as do others, that it is unwise to perform any intestinal suturing if there is significant intra-abdominal sepsis with extensive granulation within the abdomen, particularly with pocketing of pus (Pettit and Irving 1988). I then advise resection of the gut at origin of the fistula with an end ileostomy and either a mucous fistula or a closure of the end.

References

Alexander-Williams J, Irving MH (1982) Intestinal fistulas. Wright, Bristol

Cato ME (1985) Healing (repair) and hypertrophy. In: Anderson JR (ed) Muir's textbook of pathology, 12th ed. Edward Arnold, London, pp 51–59

Heatley RV (1986) Assessing nutritional state in inflammatory bowel disease. Gut 27:61–66

Higgens CS, Keighley MRB, Allan RN (1984) Impact of pre-operative weight loss and body composition changes on postoperative outcome in surgery for inflammatory bowel disease. Gut 25:732–736

Irving MH The management of surgical complications of Crohn's disease: abscess and fistula. In: Allan RN, Keighley MRB, Alexander-William J, Hawkins CF (eds) Inflammatory bowel disease, 2nd edn. Churchill Livingstone, Edinburgh

Katz S, Schulman N, Levin L (1986) Free perforation in Crohn's disease: a report of 33 cases and review of the literature. Am J Gastroenterol 81:38–43

Kovetz RL (1986) Nutritional support: how much for how much? Gut 27:85–95

Mason JB, Rosenberg IH (1990) Nutritional therapy of Inflammatory bowel disease. In: Allan RN, Keighley MRB, Alexander-Williams J, Hawkins CF (eds) Inflammatory bowel disease, 2nd edn. Churchill Livingstone, Edinburgh

Matuchansky C (1986) Parenteral nutrition in inflammatory bowel disease. Gut 27:81–84

Pettit S, Irving MH (1988) The operative management of fistulating Crohn's disease – experience with 100 consecutive cases. Surg Gynecol Obstet 167:223–228

Rocchio MA, Cha CM, Hass KF et al. (1974) Use of chemically defined diets in the management of patients with high output gastrointestinal fistulas. Am J Surg 127:148

Sonnenberg A, Erchenbrecht J, Pter P, Niederau C (1982) Detection of Crohn's disease by ultrasound. Gastroenterology 83:430–434

14 Colonic Crohn's Disease (Including Rectal Disease)

J. Alexander-Williams

Indications for surgery

Principles

Although small and large bowel disease often coincide in patients with Crohn's disease, the surgical management of colonic disease has many different indications and so is described separately. Colonic Crohn's disease is more likely to be associated with perianal lesions than is small bowel disease. Colonic disease less often obstructs and fistulates, although it may often have a fistula entering the sigmoid colon from associated ileal disease. Compared with small bowel Crohn's disease colonic disease is more likely to present with acute and chronic bleeding and, occasionally, it is subject to acute exacerbations, closely resembling acute attacks of ulcerative colitis.

Acute colitis

Acute colitis often occurs suddenly with no preceding history; a condition sometimes described as "fulminant colitis". Under these circumstances the differentiation from ulcerative colitis may be impossible before operation and can be difficult even after the colon has been removed and examined histologically. The management of acute colitis due to either of the two types of inflammatory bowel disease is essentially the same. The same initial medical treatment is used usually with bed rest, nil by mouth, intravenous therapy, steroids and antibiotics. For further details the reader is referred to the chapter on the same subject under "Ulcerative Colitis".

Surgical intervention is indicated if there is dilatation of the colon or significant deterioration after the first two or three days of medical treatment (Mortensen et al. 1984). It is customary for a decision to be made on or about the fifth day when patients who are still ill and have not responded are considered for colectomy. Often by five days there are some signs of improvement, in some the improvement continues but in others by 10 to 15 days there is a second decision crisis when the option of colectomy is reconsidered.

Chronic ill health

This is a common manifestation of colonic Crohn's disease. Minor degrees of ulceration in the large bowel are usually asymptomatic but if as much as a quarter of the large bowel is extensively ulcerated, there is a significant loss of water, sodium, potassium, proteins and blood through the ulcerated area. There is also the inevitability of invasion by microbacteria through the ulcerated mucosa, despite the granulation tissue defence.

It is worth considering surgical excision in any patient with chronic ill health who does not respond to medical therapy, usually with 5-ASA type of drugs and topical steroids either topically or parenterally. We use segmental excision for limited disease or total colectomy for extensive disease. Decisions about the timing of surgical intervention in colonic Crohn's disease is determined largely by the degree of involvement of the rectum. If the rectum is severely diseased then surgical excision is likely to mean loss of continence and to the creation of a permanent ileostomy. Therefore there is a natural tendency to persist with medical treatment rather longer than resort to surgical intervention. Whereas in a patient with a right-side colitis in whom a right hemicolectomy would be unlikely to result in a troublesome diarrhoea or loss of continence the threshold for surgical intervention would be lower.

Diarrhoea, urgency and incontinence

Diarrhoea, urgency and incontinence are frequent symptoms when there is extensive rectal involvement. Extensive rectal disease is also likely to be associated with a high incidence of perianal disease which may further impair faecal continence. Perianal disease will also mitigate against the success of sphincter-saving operations such a total colectomy and ileo-rectal anastomosis.

The relative importance of the three symptoms can be summarised by the axiom: "diarrhoea may be acceptable, urgency may be incapacitating but incontinence is devastating".

Patients can usually accept the symptom of diarrhoea, which is often defined as the passage of more than three stools a day, usually of watery consistency. It is sometimes surprising to surgeons that many patients prefer to have a stool frequency of 6–10 a day rather than resort to an ileostomy.

Urgency means that the sufferer is unable to voluntarily control the desire to defaecate for more than a minute, so that they have to interrupt whatever they are doing immediately and make for the nearest lavatory. Sufferers tend to check constantly on the availability of toilet facilities wherever they go, so that their social or business activities are often severely curtailed and the quality of their life is impaired.

Incontinence, if it is only a small volume, is often tolerated with remarkable fortitude. I am surprised how many patients with perianal Crohn's disease prefer to tolerate a small degree of incontinence with a little faecal discharge once or twice a day rather than have an ileostomy. However, significant incontinence with the lack of control and often lack of anal sensation is a devastating symptom and can ruin a patient's working and social life. Most sufferers will gladly exchange severe incontinence for a stoma or will be prepared to tolerate many or complex reoperations to try to restore continence.

Association of Crohn's colitis and diverticular disease

In some communities, particularly in developed countries, colonic diverticular disease is prevalent in the middle-aged and elderly. As Crohn's disease often occurs in the colon when it presents later in life, it is not surprising that the two diseases commonly coincide. It is not clear whether the presence of diverticular disease selects the sigmoid colon as an area of predilection in Crohn's disease but the association of the two diseases is common, particularly in the older patient. It seems likely that what some have described as "malignant diverticular disease" could well contain a number of patients with this association of diverticular disease and Crohn's disease (Small and Smith 1975). I am always particularly apprehensive when I recognise this coincidence of diseases in a patient. In my experience they can be difficult to manage and twice in our series we have had patients die as a result of progressive complications including perforation of gut wall (Allan et al. 1977). In both our fatal cases and in two others who have survived we have failed to realise the seriousness of the significance in patients who appeared to be treated correctly and conventionally for phlegmonous non-perforating diverticular disease. I felt that we had delayed surgical intervention too long until the patients had significant peritonitis from necrosis of the gut wall. I now have a lower threshold for surgical intervention than I had, although I realise that, almost inevitably, surgical intervention will necessitate at least a temporary stoma.

When the diagnosis is difficult and a patient has not been known already to have Crohn's disease, the diagnostic clue comes from the inflammation or ulceration of the mucosa at the sigmoid colon seen on endoscopy and sometimes on the presence of obvious perianal disease. I believe that, if the coincidence of Crohn's disease is recognised in anyone who needs to be operated on for presumed phlegmonous or perforated diverticular disease, the best emergency treatment is to excise the left colon and exteriorise the transverse colon as an end colostomy. If there is sufficient length of distal bowel available to bring it to the surface the safest management is a mucous fistula. I am never happy at having to close or bury a thickened or diseased rectal stump because of the high risk of pelvic sepsis. If pelvic sepsis does occur and the suture line of the rectal stump breaks down this can lead to serious and life-endangering septic complications. Sometimes these can only be overcome by performing a proctectomy. So worried am I at the potential risks of closing a rectal stump that, if it is particularly unhealthy or if there has already been some pelvic peritonitis, I am prepared to take a radical decision and to perform an emergency proctectomy at the time of the colectomy. If a proctectomy is necessary I use an intersphincteric technique and pack the perineal wound.

Dysplasia and carcinoma

As Greenstein and colleagues (1980) have pointed out it took many years for the malignant potential of Crohn's colitis to be appreciated and they felt that the number of reported cases was increasing, possibly because in earlier years the patients were being labelled as ulcerative colitis rather than Crohn's colitis. Large bowel cancer complicating Crohn's disease tends to occur 10 to 12 years younger than it does in the non-Crohn's disease general population and 60% of them are proximal to the splenic flexure (Zinkin and Brandwein 1980; Lightdale et al. 1975). We have observed a patient with multiple focal colonic cancer associated with Crohn's colitis (Keighley et al. 1975). We have also seen a cancer developing in a longstanding recto-vaginal fistula (Buchmann et al. 1980). The risk of cancer developing in patients with Crohn's colitis appears to be much greater than we once thought and is probably as great as that in ulcerative colitis. In our series of 413 patients with Crohn's disease there was a statistically significant excess of cancer in the large intestine (Gyde et al. 1980). This usually occurred at the site of macroscopic disease. In the New York series of 327 patients with Crohn's colitis Greenstein and colleagues (1980) found that the observed incidence of colonic cancer was seven times the expected incidence in their control population.

Although we are aware of the increased risk of cancer in patients with colonic Crohn's disease the effective surveillance of these patients presents even greater difficulties than it does in those with chronic ulcerative colitis. Macroscopically it is difficult to differentiate the appearance of severe ulcerated lesions in Crohn's disease from a flat plaque-like carcinoma. Early cancer symptoms such as bleeding and the passing of mucus per rectum are common in Crohn's disease and therefore the patient or the medical attendants are not alerted. Although we have long recognised that dysplasia may occur in both large and small bowel in patients with Crohn's disease (Fleming and Pollock 1975; Craft et al. 1981), this has proved to be an inefficient surveillance marker in our series (Gyde 1990).

Possibly because of the difficulties of early diagnosis, most of our patients have failed to survive five years, although three of the nine lived for eight or more years (Gyde et al. 1980). Two of our three patients with right-sided colonic cancer complicating Crohn's disease have had a permanent ileostomy and proctocolectomy. However, I have been able to treat one of them by total colectomy and ileorectal anastomosis (Cooke et al. 1980).

Surgical options

Excision

Segmental colectomy

Our definition of segmental colectomy is the excision of a length of diseased colon with re-anastomosis of colon to colon or colon to rectum. This is indicated when there is only a localised area of Crohn's colitis with the rest of the colon appearing normal. In our small experience segmental colectomy carries a high rate of recrudescence although not significantly greater than following total colectomy and ileo-rectal anastomosis (Allan et al. 1989). Although in the past we have protected such anastomoses between the large bowel by a proximal diverting ileostomy we now tend to perform an unprotected primary anastomosis if conditions are favourable. If they are not, the severely diseased segment of the colon is removed and an end ileostomy and mucus fistula performed awaiting later reconnection.

Total colectomy

Total colectomy is the commonest operation that we perform for Crohn's colitis. If conditions are favourable, the rectum is sufficiently compliant and there is no intra-abdominal sepsis, total colectomy will be followed by an ileo-rectal anastomosis. This operation will be described in detail in the next chapter.

The other option after total colectomy is to perform an end ileostomy and mucous fistula or, less satisfactorily, an end ileostomy and closure of the rectal stump.

Panproctocolectomy

We remove the rectum at the same time as the colon, when the rectum is severely diseased and fibrotic or when the anus is so severely diseased or damaged by surgical intervention that we think that the patient would have incapacitating urgency or incontinence following an ileo-rectal anastomosis. In my experience it is the association with severe perianal disease that is the principal indication for proctocolectomy as a primary definitive operation. In years past we used to perform a total colectomy and defunction the rectum in the hope that this would allow the gross sepsis in the pelvis to settle and make the subsequent proctectomy simpler. We were inevitably disappointed and so this option is now rarely applied; I now usually advise a proctocolectomy with a careful intersphincteric dissection of the rectum but with laying open of any ramifications of infected granulation tracks in the perineum.

Diversion

Ileostomy only

Ileostomy only can be performed either as a defunctioning loop ileostomy or as a "split ileostomy" with the two ends of the gut coming out through separate sites. Although split ileostomy has been popular in some centres we have now abandoned the technique (Truelove et al. 1965; Oberhelman et al. 1968; Lee 1975; Harper et al. 1982). Rarely it has a place in the temporary management of very severe rectal and perianal disease. We and others have used a temporary loop ileostomy in debilitated patients (Zelas and Jagelman 1980).

Colostomy only

Although in some centres good results have been reported following diverting colostomy for perianal Crohn's disease (Baker and Milton-Thompson 1974), our experience has not been favourable. We have had four patients referred to us with an already established colostomy in Crohn's disease; it has inevitably been associated with early recurrence in the colostomy. This, of course, could be a biased sample as these patients were often referred to us because they were in trouble. Nevertheless, colostomy is something we always try to avoid in Crohn's disease.

References

Allan R, Steinberg DM, Alexander-Williams J, Cooke WT (1977) Crohn's disease involving the colon: an audit of clinical management. Gastroenterology 73:723–732

Allan A, Andrews H, Hilton CJ, Keighley MRB, Allan RN, Alexander-Williams J (1989) Segmental colonic resection is an appropriate operation for short skip lesions due to Crohn's disease in the colon. World J Surg 13:611–616

Baker WN, Milton-Thompson GJ (1974) Management of anal fistulas in Crohn's disease. Proc R Soc Med 67:58

Buchmann P, Allan RN, Thompson H, Alexander-Williams J (1980) Carcinoma in a rectovaginal fistula in a patient with Crohn's disease. Am J Surg 140:462–463

Cooke WT, Mallas E, Prior P, Allan RN (1980) Crohn's disease: course, treatment and long term prognosis. Q J Med 195:363–384

Craft CF, Mendelson G, Cooper HS, Yardley JH (1981) Colonic precancer in Crohn's disease. Gastroenterology 80:578–584

Fleming KA, Pollock AC (1975) A case of Crohn's carcinoma. Gut 16:533–537

Greenstein AJ, Sachar DB, Smith H, Janowitz HD, Aufses AH Jr (1980) Patterns of neoplasia in Crohn's disease and ulcerative colitis. Cancer 46:403–407

Gyde SN, Prior P, Macartney JC, Thompson H, Waterhouse JAH, Allan RN (1980) Malignancy in Crohn's disease. Gut 21:1024–1029

Gyde SN (1990) Cancer risk in Crohn's disease. In: Allan RN, Keighley MRB, Alexander-Williams J, Hawkins C (eds) Inflammatory bowel disease. Churchill Livingstone, Edinburgh, p. 575

Harper PH, Kettlewell MG, Lee EC (1982) The effect of split ileostomy on perianal Crohn's disease. Br J Surg 68:608–610

Keighley MRB, Thompson H, Alexander-Williams J (1975) Multifocal colonic carcinoma and Crohn's disease. Surgery 78:534–537

Lee EC (1975) Split ileostomy in the treatment of Crohn's disease of the colon. Ann R Coll Surg 566:94–102

Lightdale CJ, Sternberg SS, Psner G, Sherlock P (1975) Carcinoma complicating Crohn's disease. Report of seven cases and review of the literature. Am J Med 59:262

Mortensen NJ McC, Ritchie JK, Hawley PR, Todd IP, Lennard-Jones JE (1984) Surgery for acute Crohn's colitis: results and long-term follow up. Br J Surg 71:783–784

Oberhelman HA, Kohatsu S, Taylor KB, Kivel RM (1968) Diverting ileostomy in the surgical management of Crohn's disease of the colon. Am J Surg 115:231–239
Small WP, Smith AN (1975) Fistula and conditions associated with diverticular disease of the colon. Clin Gastroenterol 4:171–199
Truelove SC, Ellis H, Webster CU (1965) Place of a double-barrelled ileostomy in ulcerative colitis and Crohn's disease of the colon. Br Med J i:150–153
Zelas P, Jagelman DG (1980) Loop ileostomy in the management of Crohn's colitis in the debilitated patient. Ann Surg 191:164–168
Zinkin LD, Brandwein C (1980) Adenocarcinoma in Crohn's colitis. Dis Colon Rectum 23:115–117

15 Technique of Total Colectomy and Ileo-rectal Anastomosis

J. Alexander-Williams

Pre-operative check

On admission the patient has blood taken for measurement of haemoglobin, haematocrit, serum urea and electrolytes and usually also of the serum proteins. The serum is also used for the cross-matching of two units of blood. A final psychological counselling session ensures that the patient knows precisely what is to be done and the reasons for doing so. The stomatherapist discusses with the patient the possibility of there being a temporary diverting stoma and marks the stoma site.

Depending on how recently there has been an assessment of the health of the rectal mucosa, I like to perform a final inspection of the rectum with a flexible sigmoidoscope just before operation.

Bowel preparation

The patient is given fluid only by mouth for 36 hours before the operation and has a saline cathartic bowel preparation, starting 24 hours before operation. Currently we use sodium picosulphate 10 mg with large volumes of clear fluid by mouth and repeated once after four hours. This preparation attracts large volumes of fluid into the gut and, despite drinking as much as they can, some patients become dehydrated. The urine output should be checked carefully before operation and the anaesthetist often gives an extra load of one litre of normal saline intravenously at the beginning of the operation. It is not our practice to use oral antimicrobial agents because we have found that, in themselves, they are not as efficient as parenteral antibiotics and, if parenteral antibiotics are used, there is no extra benefit from adding oral ones (Keighley et al. 1979). We use parenteral antibiotics effective against aerobic and anaerobic microbacteria. They are usually given intravenously on the induction of anaesthesia. However, I recognise that there are theoretical advantages in giving the initial dose two hours pre-operatively so that there are optimum tissue levels at the time of operative contamination. Our current preference is for metronidazole 500 mg and cefuroxime 1.5 g intravenously on induction. We prefer to continue the metronidazole intravenously, eight-hourly, until oral intake is resumed or for a total of five days. Oral cefuroxime is 750 mg eight-hourly until oral intake is resumed (Higgens et al. 1980; Hares et al. 1982).

Patient position and skin preparation

I usually perform this operation with the patient lying prone and occasionally I operate with the patient in the low Lloyd Davis position with the legs supported on stirrups.

In patients who are suitable for an anastomosis at a level between 15 and 20 cm from the anal verge, a handsewn anastomosis can be performed comfortably from within the abdomen. Although there is a slight advantage in the Lloyd Davis position in being able to position a second assistant between the patient's legs, our usual practice in patient's having this operation for Crohn's disease is for them to be in the standard prone position.

If the upper or mid part of the rectum has to be resected there are advantages in the Lloyd Davis position so that a stapled anastomosis can be performed. However, I rarely use this technique in Crohn's disease because I think that, if less than 12 cm of the rectum remains, it does not have sufficient storage or water absorption capacity to enable the patient to manage with an acceptable frequency of defaecation. Furthermore, if there is any thickening of the rectal wall, a stapled anastomosis is not always satisfactory.

My preference is for minimal shaving. In ladies there is usually no shaving or possibly one or two centimetres off the top of the pubic hair. Hairy men have only the area of the incision and stoma site shaved after the induction of anaesthesia.

The bladder is catheterised with a balloon catheter (14 f gauge) and the rectum is also catheterised with a balloon catheter (24–30 f gauge). The rectal catheter is connected to a sigmoidoscopy bellows which is positioned on the operating table at the side of the patient's left loin so that the surgeon can squeeze it through the drapes to inflate air into the rectum to test the anastomosis. Although I generally use CO_2 for gut inflation when I am dissecting the small bowel, I see no reason not to use the simpler, cheaper expedient of inflating the rectum with air to test the integrity of the ileo-rectal anastomosis. The skin is prepared with a spirit-based antiseptic (iodine or chlorhexidine).

Position of the surgical team

As a right-handed surgeon, I stand on the patient's left side for dissection of the sigmoid and upper rectum and move to the patient's right side for the dissection of the splenic flexure. The nurse and first assistant stand on the patient's right side. The first assistant exchanges position with the surgeon whenever he/she moves. In a teaching programme I often have a second assistant who stands beside the surgeon or between the leg if the Lloyd Davis position is employed. The scrub nurse stands towards the head of the patient and has instruments on a trolley positioned above the patient's chest and head.

Incision

Although I have a preference for transverse incisions, many patients have already had some abdominal operation so that it is usual to reuse the original incision. In young girls, who are particularly keen to have a good cosmetic result I perform initially a long curved suprapubic incision with the understanding that should I find mobilisation of the splenic flexure difficult I will make a central vertical extension. On many occasions it has been possible to perform a total colectomy through a suprapubic transverse incision with a good cosmetic result (see Fig. 10.1).

As in Crohn's colitis the colon is often shortened, there is relatively little difficulty in mobilising the splenic flexure, which is usually difficult in operations for cancer or diverticular disease. Therefore in Crohn's disease it is often not necessary to extend even a midline incision high above the umbilicus. If I have to extend, I do not incise through the umbilicus but prefer to curve around it to the left, as close to the umbilicus as possible.

The laparotomy

When the abdominal cavity is opened, all peritoneal adhesions to the parietal peritoneum are gently broken down. Usually this can be achieved by sweeping round with the hand the free parts of the peritoneal cavity and by encircling any adherent omentum and gut with the finger and gently teasing it away from the parietal peritoneum. I take care to avoid damage to the omental blood vessels. Where gut is firmly adherent to the parietal peritoneum I employ the "postage-stamp" technique described in Chapter 10 (Fig. 15.1).

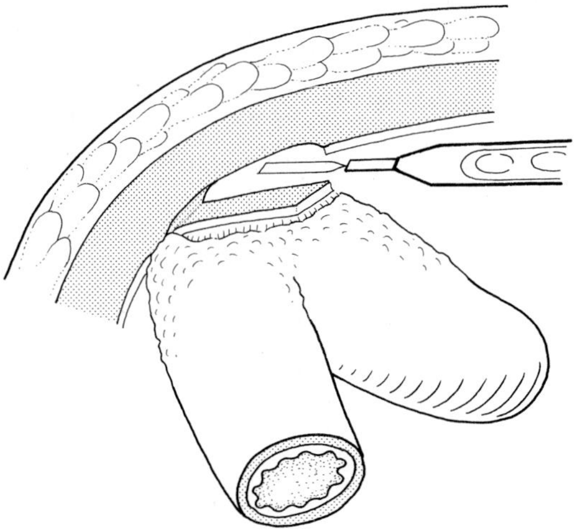

Fig. 15.1. A portion of the attached parieties is cut off with diathermy: the "postage-stamp" manoeuvre. (See also Fig. 10.6b.)

When I have divided all the adhesions to the parietal peritoneum of the anterior abdominal wall, a plastic wound drape and ring is inserted. The entire small bowel is "run" carefully between the forefinger and thumb to make sure that there are no skip lesions of Crohn's disease. If the small bowel is unaffected and entirely free, I frequently enclose the whole of the small bowel in a plastic bag with a draw-string, which is lightly tightened over a gauze swab. This plastic bag allows the small gut to be moved from side-to-side during the dissection, it prevents it being traumatised by being handled too much and keeps it warm and moist.

The other intra-abdominal organs are then palpated, particularly the liver and gall bladder. If stones are detected or their presence confirmed then I will always perform a cholecystectomy. If there is no history of jaundice and the liver function tests are normal I do not perform a routine operative cholangiogram.

If the gall bladder is distended, it is gently compressed to empty the bile so that any gallstones can be palpated more readily. As already mentioned the pre-operative work-up should have included ultrasound examination of the gall bladder. In my opinion this is a better way of detecting gall stones than is palpation at laparotomy. In the female the internal genitalia are inspected and palpated.

When the pathology of colonic Crohn's disease is maximal in the region of the splenic flexure and this is the area where dissection is most difficult, considerations of access are more important than those of a good cosmetic result. Under these circumstances I use a midline incision with a lateral left transverse extension beneath the costal margin. This gives excellent access to adherent large bowel in the left upper quadrant. Furthermore, if the transverse limb of the incision is placed in a skin crease it gives an acceptable cosmetic result.

Dissection of the upper rectum

For there to be an effective ileo-rectal anastomosis, it is necessary for most of the rectum to be retained to permit adequate fluid reabsorption. Consequently, I aim to make the anastomosis at the sacral promontory or above. The best way of determining the site for anastomosis is at a pre-operative flexible sigmoidoscopic assessment.

When considering an ileo-rectal anastomosis I never dissect the lateral ligaments of the rectum or divide the peritoneum in the pouch of Douglas as I do for low anterior resection of the rectum. The first incision is on the peritoneum on each side of the rectum close to the base of the mesorectum. The peritoneum is divided on each side, the rectum is pulled towards the anterior abdominal wall and the posterior soft tissue space immediately opens up. The space is usually easily amenable to blunt dissection with diathermy haemostasis to any small veins that may be put under tension or inadvertently torn. The ureters should be identified in this space at the base of the mesorectum at the pelvic brim. This rarely presents any difficulty but it is always worth waiting a moment or two to observe ureteric peristalsis to make certain that the correct structure has been identified. Always spare another moment to consider that there might be a double ureter.

My preferred point of resection of the rectum for an ileo-rectal anastomosis is about the level of the sacral promentary. At this point the mesorectum can be separated from the muscle wall of the gut without difficulty. When standing on the patient's left side I use my left hand to pinch the back of the muscular coat of rectum. Approximation of the index finger and the thumb with a pinching movement enables muscle wall to be identified reliably. I then dissect the soft tissue plane at this point to enable me to transfer the pinching movement to the mesorectum behind the rectum. The mesorectum at this level is a substantial piece of tissue containing branches of the superior haemorrhoidal artery supplying the upper part of the rectum. This is isolated and clamped with a cholecystectomy clamp. If it is a thick bunch of oedematous tissue then it has a suture ligation (see Fig. 10.8). However, often there is little inflammation at this level and it is simple to perform a standard haemostatic ligation of the pedicle.

Having divided the blood supply it is then possible to place a clamp across the upper rectum. I usually use two semicircular clamps (Potts) as used in vascular surgery but there is no reason why a crushing clamp should not be used on the proximal part of the bowel that is going to be resected. I then divide the bowel with scissors between the two clamps. It is advisable to wash out the lumen of the rectum from below with a weak aqueous antiseptic solution such as aqueous chlorhexidine or povidone-iodine. I then drain it thoroughly, leaving the balloon catheter in situ in the rectum.

As the anastomosis is high in the pelvis and relatively easy to perform by hand I do not feel that the extra speed of the circular stapling device is worth the money. Also, I feel happier suturing rather than stapling the slightly thickened bowel wall that one often finds in patient's with Crohn's disease.

The bowel, having been divided between the clamps, has three long tissue forceps (Allis) applied to the cut edge of the rectum to hold it open as the lower clamp is removed. Any remaining antiseptic solution in the rectal stump is sucked out. I usually insert a povidone-iodine soaked tampon into the rectum to be removed after the posterior row of sutures has been inserted.

Colectomy

The removal of the colon is often more difficult in Crohn's disease than it is in ulcerative colitis. As Crohn's disease is a transmural disease, the omentum may be firmly adherent to the inflamed bowel which also may be stuck to adjacent structures. Although I try to preserve the omentum wherever practical, it is often not possible in Crohn's disease if the anterior and posterior leaves of the omentum are stuck firmly together. Nevertheless I always make an attempt to preserve as much as possible and will try to prepare at least a tongue of viable omentum with a good blood supply that can be brought down later to cover the anastomosis.

Because there are so many small aberrant vessels in the peritoneum lateral to the ascending and descending colon, I perform much of the peritoneal dissection with diathermy; picking up the larger of the peritoneal vessels with tissue forceps and coagulating them before cutting. I try to divide the major colic vessels under direct vision but often this is not possible because of inflammatory thickening and fatty infiltration of the mesocolon. When this occurs I use the finger dissection technique described above. This relies on the fact that gentle finger pressure will separate fat and nodes but is not sufficient to tear major blood vessels. By this method it is possible to isolate each of the major vascular pedicles and clamp them with heavy duty curved artery forceps (cholecystectomy). When the vascular pedicle is short and fat or oedematous the technique of interlocking sutures described in Chapter 10 for small bowel resection is used.

In years past I have had to reoperate on patients who have had primary operations for inflammatory disease elsewhere when the major vascular pedicles were ligated with non-absorbable sutures such as linen thread. In many of these reoperations I found chronic abscesses within the abdominal cavity containing 2 or 3 ml of pus and unabsorbed suture. Therefore it is important to stress that only absorbable suture material should be used for these pedicle ligations. I normally use a braided 2/0 Polyglactin unless it is a very large or thick pedicle when I use 0 Polyglactin.

The ileo-colic artery is divided more peripherally than would be done if the operation was for malignant disease; the terminal ileum will receive a good blood supply through the arcade vessels. If the terminal ileum is thickened or affected with Crohn's disease this is resected as far back as necessary to leave macroscopically normal bowel. The drawstring of the plastic bag containing the small gut may have to be undone at this stage to release some gut. The ileum at the site chosen for resection is divided obliquely as described in Chapter 10 to give a luminal diameter as near as possible the same size as the divided rectum. A crushing intestinal clamp is applied to the end to be removed and Allis tissue forceps applied to the proximal end to be anastomosed. Any ileal content is sucked out and a povidone-iodine tampon inserted. The colon is then removed.

If there is any suspicion that there might be skip lesions in the terminal ileum I investigate this by carbon dioxide insufflation or balloon catheter and sometime by both. The quickest and simplest method is carbon dioxide insufflation (Cabrol et al. 1991). This involves placing the end of a plastic sucker tubing into the open end of the ileum and securing it gently by finger pressure so that it is gas tight. The other end of the tubing then leads from the sterile operating field to where it is connected to the laparoscopy carbon dioxide insufflator. Carbon dioxide is then inflated to distend the small bowel; this is done slowly until there is adequate gentle distension of small bowel. When the gut is inflated it is easy to inspect and palpate any possible thickened areas along the mesenteric border. If areas of skip lesions are detected the carbon dioxide is allowed to run out through the tube and a latex balloon catheter is inserted retrogradely up the bowel from the cut end to examine the skip area for narrowing (see also Chapter 12 on strictureplasty). I usually do not treat narrow areas unless they are 20 mm diameter or less but any area less than 20 mm is worthy of treating by strictureplasty.

The anastomosis

The obliquely cut end of the ileum and the cut end of the rectum are then placed close to each other to assess any size discrepancy. If the end of the ileum is still much smaller, a further relieving incision is made along the antimesenteric border. The rotation of the mesentery of the small gut is then checked to make sure that the rotation is no more than 90°. The mesenteric end of the oblique cut is then fixed to the right lateral edge of the rectum with a seromuscular suture, tied and held with a clamp. The antimesenteric border is then sutured to the left lateral aspect; I usually do this with a full length atraumatic 3/0 or 4/0 Polyglactin suture which has been lubricated to make sure it runs smoothly. I know that there are surgeons who prefer to use monofilament absorbable sutures because they run particularly smoothly when using a continuous suture. However, at present, these sutures are considerably more expensive than the braided ones and I am quite happy with the way that the oiled, braided Polyglactin "runs" and takes up any slack (see also p. 81).

With the two stay sutures at either end held apart, one further seromuscular stay suture is applied in the centre of the back row and usually one more a quarter of the way along the back row (Fig. 15.2). Using these stay sutures for gentle traction the assistant holds up the edges to be sutured at about 45° to the surgeon. The anastomosis is then performed with a running seromuscular stitch, knotting with each quarter stitch as it is reached. Once the back row is completed the iodine tampons are removed from the lumen at each end. Three more stay sutures are then placed along

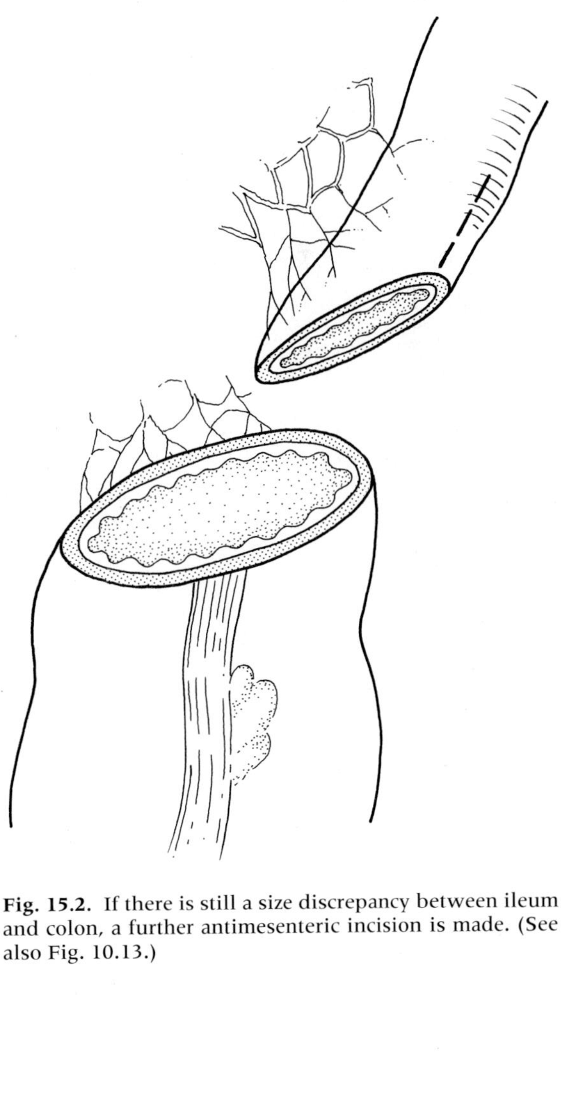

Fig. 15.2. If there is still a size discrepancy between ileum and colon, a further antimesenteric incision is made. (See also Fig. 10.13.)

each quarter of the anterior row and the seromuscular suture completed in the front row in the same manner.

If carbon dioxide has already been used for inflation, the small gut is reinflated with about 500 ml of carbon dioxide just before the last of the anterior row of sutures is placed. If gas insufflation has not been necessary before, the rectum is inflated with air via the balloon catheter to test the completed anastomosis. Air or gas distension stretches the suture line and takes up any slack in the continuous suture. Any persistent air leaks are detected and closed carefully, usually with a single horizontal mattress Polyglactin suture. The gas testing is repeated until the anastomosis is gas tight on gentle distension.

The peritoneal cavity is washed out with two litres of saline at 37 °C. The gap between the mesentery of the bowel and the mesorectum is sutured with continuous 3/0 Polyglactin to prevent gut herniating through it. The "tongue" of preserved omentum is then brought down and wrapped around the anastomosis. Usually it is secured with Polyglactin sutures.

Closure of the abdomen

The technique is the same as that for small gut resection described above. If an L-shaped incision has been used, I usually use two loops of PDS, one for each limb. As there has been no extra peritoneal space exposed or contaminated, I never drain the peritoneal cavity (Alexander-Williams 1988).

References

Alexander-Williams J (1988) Cholecystectomy: ironmasters and eggheads. Proc R Soc Med 81:560–561

Cabrol J, Griffiths C, Alexander-Williams J (1991) Carbon dioxide insufflation in gastrointestinal surgery. Br J Surg 78:499–500

Hares MM, Bentley S, Allan RN, Burdon DW, Keighley MRB (1982) Clinical trials of the efficacy and duration of antibacterial cover for elective resection in inflammatory bowel disease. Br J Surg 69:215–217

Higgens C, Allan RN, Keighley MRB, Arabi YM, Alexander-Williams J (1980) Sepsis following operation for inflammatory bowel disease. Dis Colon Rectum 23:102–105

Keighley MRB, Eastwood D, Ambrose NS, Allan RN, Burdon DW (1979) Incidence and microbiology of abdominal and pelvic abscess in Crohn's disease. Gastroenterology 83:1271–1275

16 Technique of Panproctocolectomy

J. Alexander-Williams

The colonic resection is identical to that in total colectomy described in Chapter 15.

Preparation and position of the patient

The pre-operative checklist is similar to that described in detail in Chapter 15. Psychological counselling and the stomatherapist visit are essential. The rectal mucosa does not have to be inspected and the large bowel does not have to be emptied with any purgation. The five-day antibiotic cover is the same as in Chapter 15.

The patient is positioned on adjustable Lloyd Davis stirrups that are set to give the correct compromise in not impeding the abdominal surgeon and also allowing adequate access to the perineum (Fig. 16.1).

The bladder is catherised. No purse string is used around the anus. The rectum is washed out with a bladder syringe containing aqueous povidone-iodine, a procedure that is repeated once the rectum has been clamped by the abdominal surgeon (see below).

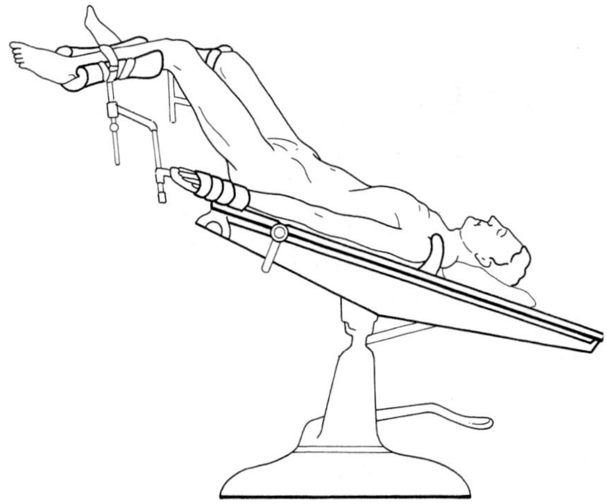

Fig. 16.1. Lloyd Davis "stirrups" supporting legs on a tilting table.

Rectal dissection from above

Unlike protectomy for malignant bowel disease the dissection is kept as close to the rectum as possible thus minimising the possibility of damage to the nerve supply to the pelvic floor and genitalia and also minimising the size of the resultant cavity. As we usually only remove the rectum when there is severe proctitis or severe perianal disease, the dissection close to the rectum has to be performed through thickened inflamed tissue. I dissect the mesorectum by pinching the fatty tissue with the forefinger and thumb and so isolating the blood vessels, as described in Chapter 15. If access to the pelvis is difficult, I often only apply one haemostatic clamp on the mesorectum leaving the blood vessels on the rectal side to be controlled by coagulation diathermy. Because of perirectal thickening it is often difficult to isolate the lateral pedicles of the rectum and these are often controlled first by electrocoagulation and then divided with scissors through the coagulated area.

Perineal dissection

The essential feature of this operation is that it is an intersphincteric dissection keeping as close to the bowel wall as possible. Furthermore, the rectum is often being removed because of severe associated perianal disease and sometimes with perirectal disease. For this reason the technique is fundamentally different from that of abdomino-perineal resection at the rectum for carcinoma.

As no anal purse string suture is used, contamination is minimised by the abdominal surgeon placing a clamp across the upper rectum as early as possible in the operation so preventing intestinal contents from descending into the rectum. The first task of the surgeon at the rectal end is then to repeat the wash-out to make the rectum as clean as possible and instil in it some povidone-iodine solution. The rectum is then excised "open" with inevitable microbacterial contamination.

When performing the perineal dissection I find it useful to insert the index finger of the left hand into the rectum to enable a close rectal excision to be performed. This is particularly useful when there is a perirectal granulation tissue from abscesses.

The essential feature of my technique of intersphincteric dissection involves the infiltration of spaces around the rectum with saline containing 1:100 000 adrenaline. I am not certain how much the adrenaline reduces the capillary oozing and I have no objective evidence of its value. However, I find invaluable the separation of the tissue planes by the injected saline. Using diathermy dissection I find that there is a good bloodless field that enables the muscles of the pelvic floor to be identified more easily than I used to find with scalpel or scissor dissection.

I begin with a circum-anal incision in the intersphincteric groove, incorporating where possible the exit of any fistula tracks if these are present. If there are so many fistula tracks that to excise them would mean too wide an excision of the perineum, I do not necessarily remove all the tracks but merely ensure that the granulation tissue area is draining satisfactorily.

Once the gap between the sphincters has been defined, the intersphincteric space can be developed leaving the external sphincters intact. I use tissue forceps on the rectal wall and on the external sphincter and pull them apart to provide distraction; so enabling the plane between them to be divided with diathermy. Using this technique it is easy to see the colour differentiation between the "white meat" of the rectal smooth muscle and the "dark meat" of the striated muscles of the pelvic floor.

Usually the posterior space is developed first and, once past the level of the coccyx, it is usually possible to make palpable contact with the tips of the fingers of the abdominal surgeon. The intervening tissues are then divided with diathermy as the rectum is held forward until contact is made between the two surgeons' hands behind the rectum. Once this space is opened up the perineal operator's fingers can enter the pelvic space and pull the pelvic floor downwards, enabling the muscular fibres of puborectalis to be divided from the rectum under direct vision. The middle rectal vessels are usually encountered and I almost always control these by diathermy coagulation.

The anterior space between the rectum and the vagina or the rectum and urethra and prostate is the most difficult and dangerous one to separate in patients with Crohn's proctitis. In this space I find saline separation of the tissue planes invaluable. In the female I place my left index finger in and press on the posterior wall of the vagina, this enables me to follow the track of the needle through which I am injecting saline so that it keeps close to but does not enter the vagina. When there is induration or acute inflammation in this space it often requires considerable pressure of saline injection to infiltrate the space; it is valuable to have a syringe into which the needle can be locked. When the space is well infiltrated with saline I cut through it with the diathermy; once again using my left index finger pressing against the posterior wall of the vagina for guidance (Fig. 16.2). Because the dissection is being performed with the rectum open and containing an antiseptic, it is not such a serious error to enter the rectal lumen as it would be in an operation for carcinoma. In the female, care is needed to avoid making a hole in the posterior wall of the

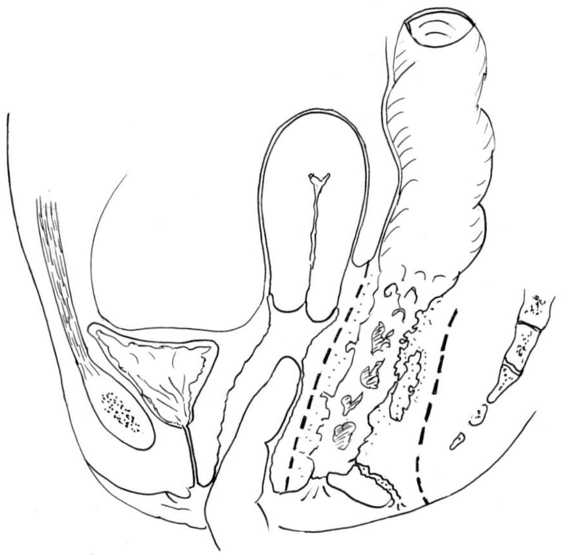

Fig. 16.2. Diagram of pelvic cross-section during an intersphincteric diathermy dissection for severe Crohn's disease of the rectum with fistula and post-rectal abscess. The lines of diathermy dissection shown as the rectum is "cored out". The perirectal tissues and the rectovaginal septum are infiltrated with saline and a finger in the vagina ensures that the dissection does not enter the vagina.

vagina and in the male, to avoid damaging the urethra. When the tissues are firmly adherent I err towards making the plane of dissection within the muscular wall of the rectum.

As the dissection progresses caudally, the plane of separation becomes easier. By the time the perineal surgeon has entered the loose connective tissue between the cervix and rectum or between the seminal vesicles and rectum, the abdominal surgeon will have divided the peritoneum in the pouch of Douglas; finger tip contact is then made between the perineal and abdominal surgeons. The completion of the separation of the rectum depends on close collaboration between the abdominal and perineal teams. I find it best to perform most of the dissection from the perineal end because the perineal surgeon has the option of inserting a finger into the rectum, and therefore is able to make blind sharp dissection close to the rectum.

It is important that if there are two surgeons working simultaneously, they do not compete with each other, one trying to pull the rectum up and the other pulling it down. When I am performing both ends of the excision myself, there is a stage in the operation in which I find it helpful to perform blunt dissection in the pelvis simultaneously from above and below. I stand near the patient's left hip with my right hand in the pelvis and left hand through the perineal space. This enables the appropriate tissue plane to be found by blunt dissection within the mass of inflammatory and fibrous tissue that is often encountered.

Once all the tissues close to the rectum have been freed the specimen is removed upwards or downwards. As there is usually a greater degree of contamination at the perineal end I usually pull the rectum through the perineum as far as possible. I then enclose it in a sterile glove, which is ligated at the cuff; then the colon and rectum are pulled back up into the abdominal wound.

The small space that is left behind after an intersphincteric incision is then packed with a moist gauze swab and left for a few minutes. When the pack is removed, the space is inspected from below under a strong light and a long narrow retractor to see whether any obvious bleeding points can be identified and, if found, coagulated with diathermy. Once the rectum has been removed it is remarkable how little bleeding there is into the small residual space. If the dissection has been close to the rectum one does not experience the troublesome bleeding that is sometimes found during perineal excision for cancer, when veins close to the sacrum may be torn or divided.

Management of the pelvic space

The space is small after intersphincteric dissection and the pelvic floor muscles are intact. In Crohn's disease with perirectal inflammation there is often a deficiency of pelvic peritoneum so a complete reperitonealisation of the pelvic space from above is not possible.

At the perineal end of the operation, the intact puborectalis is approximated by a single mattress, absorbable suture, which effectively closes the exit from the pelvis and prevents gut and omentum from prolapsing. Under these circumstances, which are the usual ones encountered after excision for Crohn's proctitis, I have separated the pelvic space into two compartments. The space above the pelvic floor is allowed to drain into the main peritoneal cavity; wherever possible a tongue of omentum is brought down to fill the pelvic space. Once the pelvic floor is closed, there is only a relatively small subcutaneous space in the perineum. I usually manage this by a small antiseptic pack which is removed after two days. However, when the space is small and dry, I simply apply a small plastic coated dressing for 24 hours and then manage the raw wounds by simple irrigation, usually in a shower or bidet.

I perform a primary suture of the perineal skin only in the rare event of there being little pararectal or perianal induration and no infection so that the pelvic space has little or no contamination. I then perform primary suture of the pelvic peritoneum with vacuum drainage evacuation of the extra peritoneal space. This is the same technique that I usually employ after rectal incision for carcinoma.

Creation of stoma

The division of the ileum is as described under ileo-rectal anastomosis in Chapter 15 except that the end of the ileum is closed with a special handle-less clamp. When the mesentery and vessels have been divided the muscle and mucosa of the ileum are clamped with a Zachary Cope, triple blade, crushing clamp (Fig. 16.3). After the blades of the clamp are locked, the central clamp is removed and the bowel divided where it is crushed between the outer two. The cut ends of the bowel in the detachable blades of the clamp are then covered with a finger cut from a latex glove and stretched over the ends. This latex cover minimises contamination and makes it easier for the end of the ileostomy to be brought through the hole to be created in the abdominal wall.

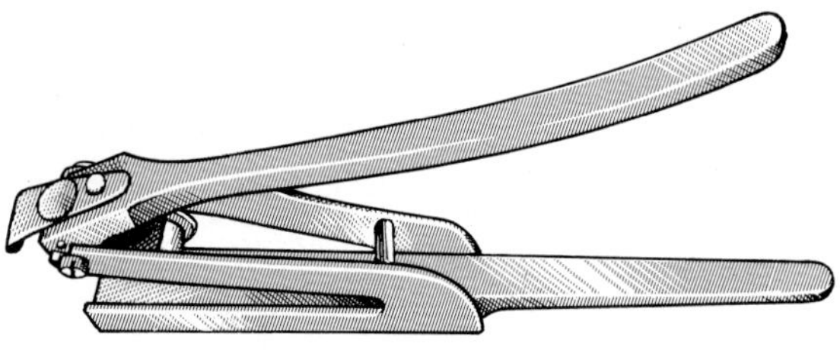

Fig. 16.3. A Zachary Cope triple blade crushing clamp.

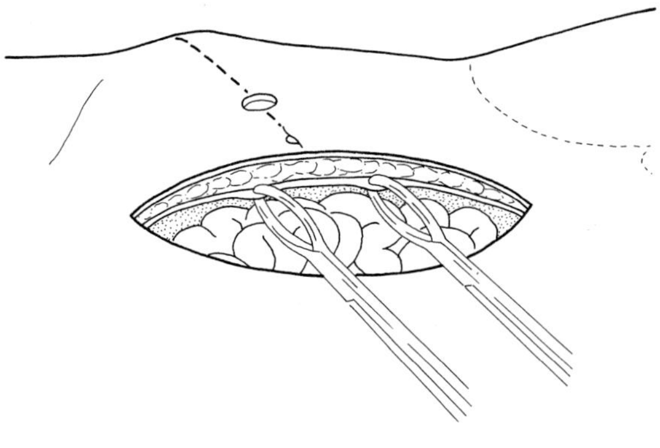

Fig. 16.4. The right side of the lower abdomen is put under tension by traction with tissue forceps and a diathermy trephine is made in the skin over the pre-marked stoma site.

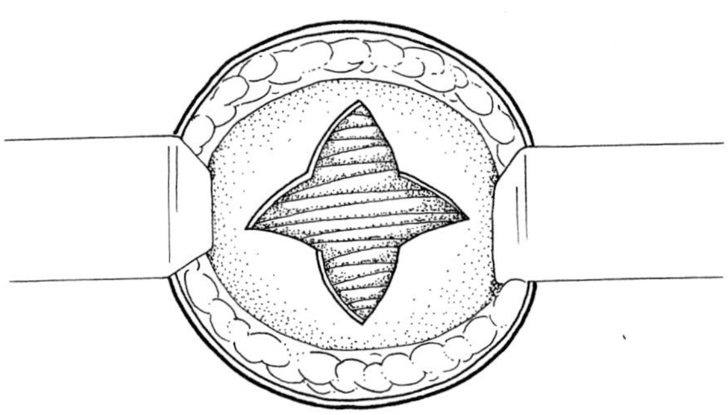

Fig. 16.5. A cruciate diathermy incision made in anterior rectus sheath while the fat is held apart by small retractors.

The stoma site has been marked before operation by the stomatherapist. However, as even indelible markers can become erased during the course of the operation, I usually mark the stoma site by touching the centre of it with a cutting diathermy so that it can be recognised easily at the end of the operation.

To make the skin excision at the stoma site two tissue forceps are applied to the full thickness of the abdominal wall so that it can be pulled towards the left and so place the skin of the abdominal wall flap under tension (Fig. 16.4). I aim to excise a disc of skin a little less than 2 cm in diameter using free-hand cutting diathermy. Haemostasis is achieved by diathermy and the fat of the abdominal wall is pushed aside by inserting the forefinger firmly down towards the fascia of the anterior rectus sheath. Occasionally some sharp dissection is required but usually it is quite easy to make a

a

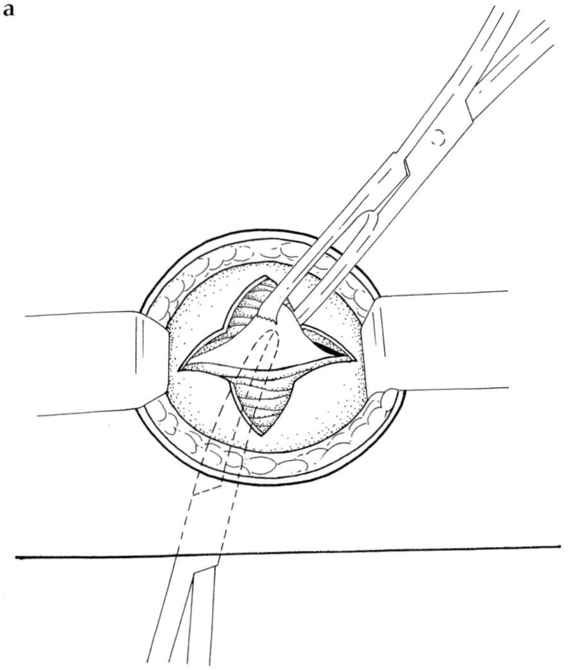

b

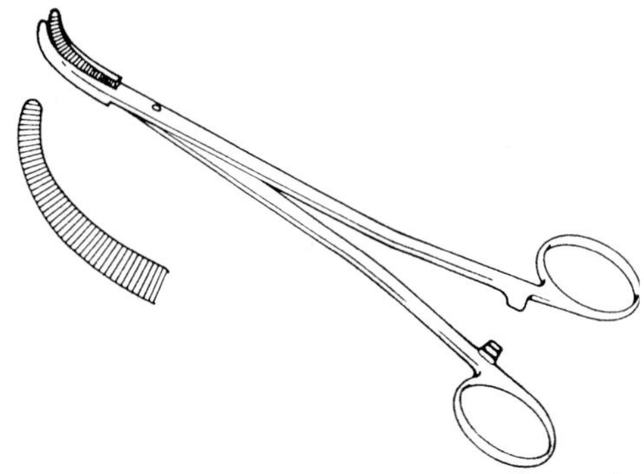

Fig. 16.6. a Cholecystectomy forceps (Moynihan; see **b**) push the posterior rectus sheath out through the muscle fibres where the apex of the tent is picked up with tissue forceps.

sufficient sized hole in the fat for two small retractors (Langenbeck or Czerny) to separate the fat and superficial fascia and so expose the fascia of the anterior rectal sheath. A finger from inside the abdomen pushes the rectus muscle and its sheath forward while the assistant retracts the fat. Using cutting diathermy I make a cruciate incision through the anterior rectus sheath; the limbs of the cross are just over a centimetre long (Fig. 16.5). A large curved artery forceps (cholecystectomy) is then inserted into the abdomen and pushes the posterior rectus sheath out to the surface separating the muscle fibres of the rectus abdominus as it does so. This tent of the posterior sheath pushed forward by the artery forceps, is then grasped with two tissue forceps and the posterior sheath incised with diathermy longitudinally. The cut edges picked up with two more tissue forceps and the posterior sheath is then incised transversely and two more tissue forceps pick up the edges of the posterior sheath so that it is pulled up into the wound (Fig. 16.6). Initially this hole is too small for the ileum to be brought out through it without tension, therefore, relieving incisions have to be made between each of the tissue forceps giving a stellate hole (Fig. 16.7). To ensure that this hole is now large enough for the ileum to be brought through comfortably I find that it is optimum to stretch it so it will just admit the tips of two fingers placed within the abdomen. These are pushed out through the hole that has been created in the rectus sheath (Fig. 16.8). This stretch can usually be achieved without detaching the tissue forceps from the posterior rectus sheath. When the hole is large enough the blade of the Zachary Cope clamp, covered with a latex glove finger is inserted from within the abdomen out through the ileostomy hole. The mesentery is then orientated so that it is directed cranially and sufficient of the ileum is brought out through the hole to form the eversion ileostomy. I find that the length outside the abdominal skin is approximately equal to the length of my index finger (Fig. 16.9). The posterior rectus sheath is still held by the tissue forceps and is then sutured to the serosa of the ileum or the mesentery of the ileum in each of the four quadrants. I use 3/0 absorbable Polyglactin sutures to fix the length of ileum that lies outside the abdomen. The eversion of the ileostomy is then left until the abdominal wall skin is closed. I make no attempt to close the

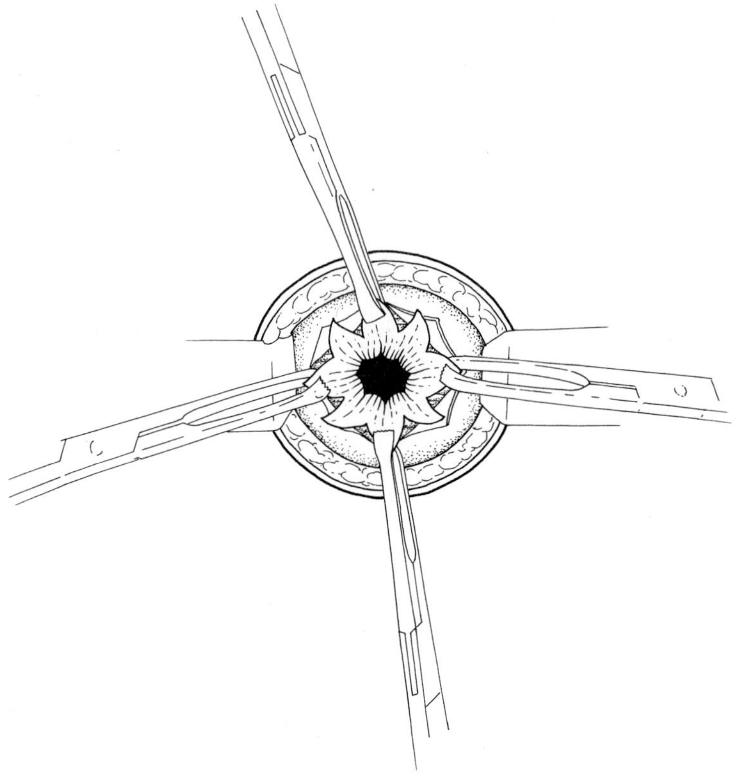

Fig. 16.7. To enlarge the hole in the posterior rectus sheath stellate cuts are made.

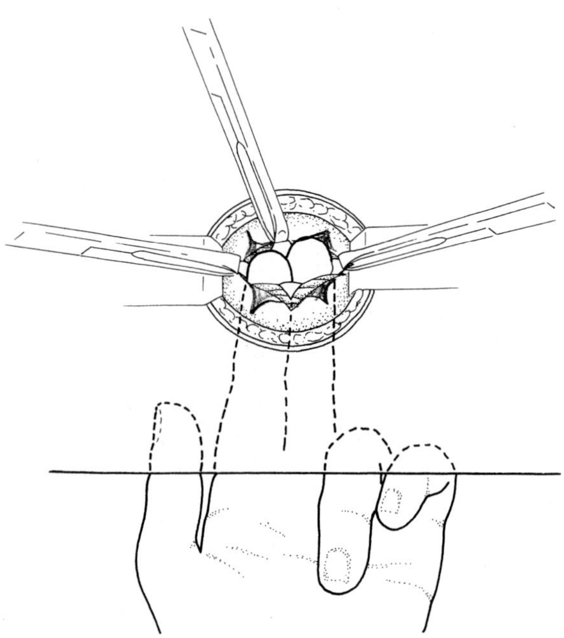

Fig. 16.8. The tips of two fingers should just be able to be pushed through the gap in the rectus muscle fibres.

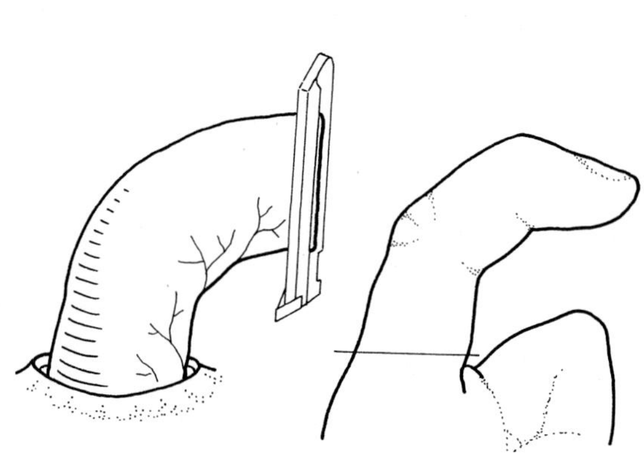

Fig. 16.9. Approximately 6 cm of ileum is required to project beyond the skin to ensure an optimum length stoma of 2 cm after eversion. This is approximately the length of the surgeon's index finger.

lateral gutter between the ileum and the right lateral abdominal wall but I anchor the root of the mesentery cranially for 4 or 5 cm with a running 3/0 Polyglactin suture. The abdomen is then ready for closure.

Abdominal closure

This is performed in the same way as previously described in Chapter 15. Once the skin layer is closed with a subcuticular stitch, the wound is sprayed with an impervious plastic spray. Once this is dry it is covered with a towel.

Eversion of the ileostomy

This is performed in the same manner as described in the section on ileostomy under ulcerative colitis (Fig. 16.10).

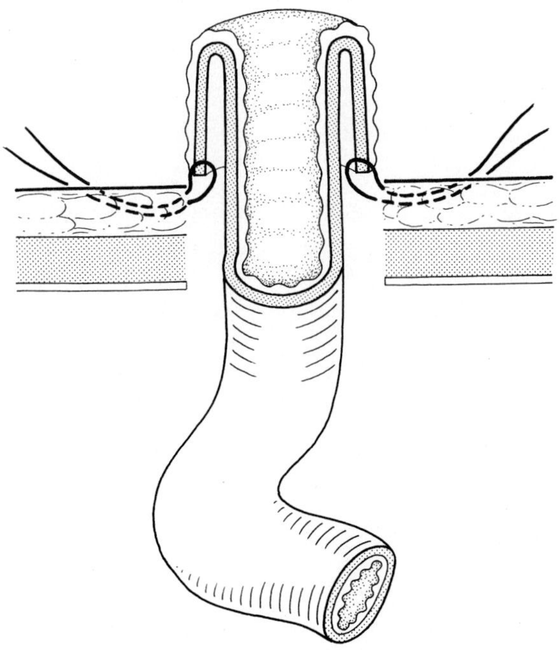

Fig. 16.10. A 2–2.5 cm eversion stoma is fixed with seromuscular sutures.

17 Post-operative Complication

J. Alexander-Williams

Early complications

The majority of patients who have had operations for the complications of Crohn's disease have a satisfactory and rapid recovery. They have resumption of normal oral feeding during the first post-operative week and are discharged home during the second week. However, in the early days after operation 10%–20% of patients experience some complication (Irving 1990). These complications can be categorised as fever, ileus, or peritonitis.

Fever

An elevated body temperature is a manifestation of the body's response to inflammation and is, in part, dependent on normal immune competence. Patients who are having immunosuppressive drugs including steroids may not be able to mount a normal response and so patients can be ill after operations for Crohn's disease without showing any of the normal signs such as fever, leucocytosis or abdominal signs of guarding or rigidity. In a patient who is able to mount a normal defence response, a post-operative fever can occur at any time between the first and tenth post-operative day. Different causes tend to manifest at different times after operation.

Chest infections

Chest infections are common after any operation in the abdomen. They are commoner in smokers, in patients with chronic bronchitis and possibly in those who are ill before operation. Fever from atelectasis, or failure to completely expand the alveoli after operation, is quite common in the first and second days after operation. It is not usually associated with serious systemic illness and usually clears spontaneously with the recovery of the patient's ability to take a deep breath; recovery is sometimes speeded by physiotherapy. In Crohn's disease the commonest age groups for operation are between 10 and 29. In them significant chest infection is not common and rarely causes concern. However, if there are serious respiratory problems in an obviously ill patient for four or more days after an operation this usually has a more serious significance. It is not safe to attribute a fever and systemic illness simply to chest infection. Any ill patient with serious respiratory problems more than four days after operation should always be suspected as having some serious intra-abdominal catastrophe such as an anastomotic dehiscence. These will be considered in detail below.

Fever due to local infection

Fever due to local infections does not usually manifest itself until the sixth to tenth post-operative day. Wounds of the abdomen or perineum that are left open to drain freely may discharge purulent material and serum but do not usually cause fever. It is usually pus under tension in either the wound or the perineum that gives rise to a fever. This is presumably due to micro-organisms entering the circulation. Localised intra-abdominal sepsis occurs in 5%–10% of patients after such procedures as strictureplasty and usually settles spontaneously (Alexander-Williams and Haynes 1987). It is presumed that this is due to a local infection adjacent to the suture line that resolves or possibly drains back into the gut. Persistent pyrexia towards the end of the first week after operation should suggest the complication of focal sepsis and is usually an indication for continuation of antibiotic therapy. In only a minority of cases does the clinical examination of the patient give localising information. Sophisticated imaging such as serial ultrasound or MRI scanning may be justifiable if the outcome of the investigation is likely to alter the clinical management.

Venous access sepsis

Venous access sepsis may be responsible for fever. The so-called three-day fever of peripheral line sepsis is well known and is usually clinically obvious. It is an indication for a change of peripheral venous access site. It is also a reflection on the standard of care of the peripheral line. In patients having total parenteral nutrition persistent fever may indicate line tip sepsis. Culture of blood withdrawn through the line rarely helps in the diagnosis but sometimes the presence of a continued unexplained sepsis is an indication to withdraw the central line and culture its tips.

Ileus

The normal "quiet abdomen"

The normal "quiet abdomen" response to the trauma of an intra-abdominal operation is anticipated particularly if there is an indication for surgical intervention of complex complications for Crohn's disease. Although electronic or pressure monitoring of the small bowel after operation shows that effective intestinal activity returns within a few hours, the clinical manifestations of return of bowel function (bowel sounds) usually do not appear until the second or third post-operative day. In the first 48 hours it is normal for the abdomen to be silent, often the patient is aware of the return of some intestinal movement earlier than is the attending physician. After an uncomplicated operation for complications of Crohn's disease it is usual for the patient to pass gas by the third or fourth day. The passage of a stool or effluent from a stoma occurs soon after. Any delay in the clinical manifestations of the return of bowel function beyond what is usual is considered to be pathological and is termed "ileus". Ileus may have a variety of causes from a minor inflammatory response of gut traumatised at operation, through such physiological disturbances as shifts of water, sodium and potassium, to peritonitis due to an anastomotic dehiscence. (Goligher 1984).

If bowel function has not returned by the expected time it is correct to question why this should be so. Furthermore, a gut that is not working physiologically should not be loaded and given work to do. The presence of ileus is generally taken as an indication for cessation of normal alimentary intake and the restoration of fluid and electrolyte balance via the intravenous route. In Crohn's disease I feel that there is never any indication for trying to stimulate alimentary activity by parasympathomimetic drugs. I think that electrolyte imbalances should be detected and where possible corrected. The alimentary tract should be put at rest and, if there are signs of inadequate gastric emptying, the upper gastrointestinal tract should be aspirated to prevent gastric distension. The policy then is of "wait and see". Once simple electrolyte disturbances have been excluded or corrected, persistent ileus is likely to indicate some focal complication. This may be simply a para-anastomotic inflammatory reaction or localised abscess. These complications are best left to resolve rather than attempting immediate surgical correction.

Diarrhoea

Diarrhoea often occurs with the resolution of either physiological or pathologically delayed ileus. There is frequently a copious watery loss either as diarrhoea or ileostomy flux. The patient may lose two or more litres per day through the alimentary tract. This loss may be critical if there is not adequate oral intake. It is a common observation that patients having an ileostomy for Crohn's disease have a higher volume of post-operative ileostomy output than do similar patients having ileostomy for ulcerative colitis (Steinberg et al. 1975). When patients have a larger than usual volume of alimentary fluid loss following operation for complications of Crohn's disease, there is often a dilemma as to whether or not to try to control this output by drugs such as opiates or loperamide. Our policy is to restore fluid and electrolyte losses and await natural resolution rather than trying immediately to reduce output by drugs.

Peritonitis (general or local)

Following operations for inflammatory bowel disease, even those in which there has been gross contamination of the peritoneal cavity, it is almost unknown for there to be a primary peritonitis. When generalised or localised peritonitis occurs it is almost always due to an anastomotic dehiscence or to an extra peritoneal collection of blood that has become secondarily infected and then bursts into the perineal cavity. In patients with Crohn's disease there may or may not be a general peritoneal cavity. In some patients there is such extensive and dense peritoneal adhesion that post-operative generalised peritonitis cannot occur. If peritonitis occurs it is, of necessity, localised by the adhesions and this may modify significantly the physical signs. It is a useful, general rule to say that any patient developing local or general peritonitis four or more days following an operation for complication of Crohn's disease should be assumed to have an anastomotic dehiscence and treated accordingly. The physical signs will often give a good impression of the severity of the complication of peritonitis and confirmatory localising investigations are only indicated if these are going to significantly alter the management.

Different clinical scenarios demand different reactions. If a patient who has hitherto had no significant intra-abdominal adhesions has had a total colectomy and ileo-rectal anastomosis for colonic Crohn's disease and on the sixth post-operative day suddenly develops signs of septicaemia and peritonitis it is likely that there has been an anastomotic dehiscence. If this is confirmed the appropriate immediate action would be laparotomy with an end ileostomy and closure or drainage of the rectal stump. Prompt re-intervention could make a difference between rapid recovery and prolonged illness. Therefore, immediate investigation by a low-pressure water-soluble contrast enema is indicated.

On the other hand a patient who has had many previous operations and has just undergone a series of complicated strictureplasties after the dissection of an almost totally obliterated peritoneal cavity, who then develops pain and fever with localised tenderness, probably has a localised anastomotic leak. However, reintervention is not essential and such patients are better managed expectantly with antibiotics and nil by mouth. Under these circumstances contrast X-ray examination to confirm the presence of a leak is not indicated. Another important consideration is the accepted value of imaging techniques under these circumstances. Ultrasound, CT or MRI are unlikely to give clear-cut indications of exactly what has occurred. Serial scanning is likely to be the most valuable and, at present, expense dictates this should be by abdominal ultrasound examination.

Intermediate

Subacute ileus

By the end of the first week after operation alimentary function should have returned sufficiently for the patients to be able to be given a light diet and for the stomach to empty normally. Sometimes patients fail to reach this milestone but more commonly they appear to reach it and then make little or no progress. Increasing the intake of solid or even liquids is accompanied by nausea, sometimes they vomit and sometimes there is a full-blown clinical picture of subacute intestinal obstruction. This state of subacute ileus occurs quite often but is always worrying. It appears to be due to a number of factors such as slow-to-resolve local sepsis, prolonged electrolyte imbalance particularly the disturbances of intra-cellular potassium and vitamin deficiencies in malnourished patients and low grade plastic peritonitis. This last entity of plastic peritonitis is well recognised by surgeons who for one reason or another have to reoperate in the early weeks after resection or strictureplasty for Crohn's disease. Loops of gut are more or less firmly stuck together by maturing fibrinous exudate. The bowel wall is often oedematous and is easily torn even with the most gentle of intra-abdominal dissection. Because subacute ileus is multi-factorial there is no easy or universal remedy. There are two schools of thought: those who advocate stimulating the gut and those who advocate resting. I belong to the latter group. I regard sympathomimetic drugs as potentially harmful and on the few occasions in which I have been associated with their use I have not been convinced of their efficacy (Catchpole 1969). I believe that resting the gut, providing adequate replacement of fluid, electrolytes and if necessary parenteral nutrition and trace elements and vitamins should also be given. In my experience most patients resolve on a conservative regime. In the past I have regretted early surgical intervention but I have not regretted delay.

Delayed sepsis

Intra-peritoneal or wound sepsis usually manifests in the second week. It usually presents clinically, it may discharge or is drained or resolves. In most patients in whom I have been persuaded to reintervene surgically I have often been impressed by how small is the volume of pus that is detected.

I have seen three patients who have presented with focal sepsis in the abdomen or the perineum between 12 months and seven years after major surgical intervention in Crohn's disease. In one of these patients the sepsis is due to recrudescence of the disease but in two it was clearly independent of any recrudescence of bowel disease. I refer particularly to delayed perineal sepsis where there is no connection between the deep-seated pelvic pus and any lesion of the bowel. I used to think that all such delayed focal sepsis was due to non-absorbable suture material but I have had two cases in which no such foreign body was ever detected but who still presented four to eight years after the operation.

References

Alexander-Williams J, Haynes IG (1987) Up-to-date management of small bowel Crohn's disease. Adv Surg 20:245–264

Catchpole BW (1969) Ileus: use of sympathetic blocking agents in its treatment. Surgery 66:811

Goligher JC (1984) Surgery of the anus, rectum and colon, 5th edn. Baillière Tindall, London

Irving M (1990) The management of surgical complications in Crohn's disease: abscess and fistula. In: Allan RN, Keighley MRB, Alexander-Williams J, Hawkins CF (eds) Inflammatory bowel disease. Churchill Livingstone, Edinburgh, pp 489–498

Steinberg DM, Allan RN, Brooke BN, Alexander-Williams J, Cooke WT (1975) Sequelae of colectomy and ileostomy: comparison between Crohn's colitis and ulcerative colitis. Gastroenterology 68:33–39

18 Perianal Crohn's Disease

J. Alexander-Williams

Introduction

In 1921 Gabriel described granulomas in non-tuberculous fistula tracks around the anus and in 1938 Penner and Crohn recognised perianal fistulae as a complication of regional ileitis: before Americans called the disease after Crohn or fistulae fistulas.

All authorities are agreed that perianal lesions or anal abnormalities are commonly seen in patients with Crohn's disease but there is debate and argument about their relative frequency with estimates ranging from 14% to 76% (Table 18.1). There is a consensus of opinion in favour of the belief that perianal lesions are more common when the other manifestations of Crohn's disease are in the large gut than when they are in the small gut without significant colonic involvement (Table 18.2). The different figures of incidence from different centres probably depends on a variety of factors. Surgical units with a bias towards coloproctology will be more likely to attract secondary referral of patients with perianal and colonic Crohn's disease and also will be likely to detect asymptomatic perianal Crohn's disease. Whereas gastroenterologists with a principal interest in nutrition may tend to have a secondary referral bias towards small bowel disease and, by training or inclination, may not be moved to a close or probing inspection of the asymptomatic anus (Fig. 18.1).

Table 18.1. Reported incidence of perianal complication in Crohn's disease

Authors	Date of publication	Percentage of perianal disease
Crohn and Yarnis	1958	14
Morson and Lockhart-Mummery	1959	50
Fielding	1972	76
Goligher	1984	45

Another reason for the apparent differences in the incidence of abnormality is related to the definition of normality. The normal anus and perianal region is something that is not defined precisely. In the human face we accept

Table 18.2. Incidence of perianal lesions related to the site of intestinal Crohn's disease (*n* = numbers of patients in series)

Series	Small bowel		Small and large bowel		Large bowel		Overall % incidence
	n	% incidence	*n*	% incidence	*n*	% incidence	
Loygue and Hugier (1971)	49	8	25	8	46	22	29
Fielding (1972)	118	76	35	94	14	92	80
Lockhart-Mummery (1975)	62	32	101	56	141	70	61

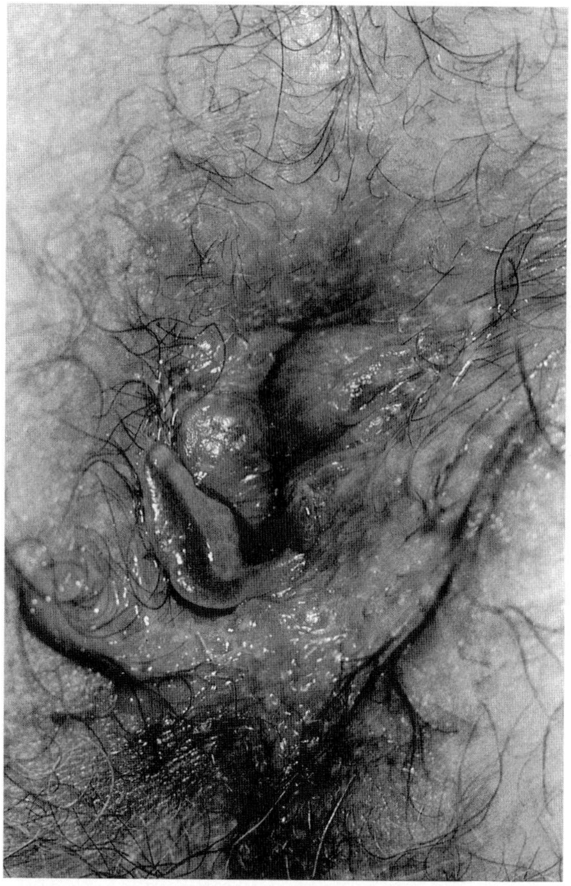

Fig. 18.1. A middle-aged general practitioner presented with intermittent vague colicky abdominal pain for three months. He was unaware of any anal symptoms. The photograph is of a typical perianal Crohn's disease eccentric acute painless ulcer. Ileal Crohn's disease was later confirmed.

changes in contour and expression as the normal accompaniment of the aging process; similarly we may need to qualify anal normality by sex and age, remembering that many women also have their perianal contour affected by pregnancies and episiotomies. Many observers would regard an anal skin tag as a normal finding whereas an oedematous skin tag would be regarded as abnormal.

Definition

The following definition and classification of perianal Crohn's disease (PACD) results from a working party report at the Rome '91 Conference (Alexander-Williams et al. 1992):

Definite perianal Crohn's disease can be diagnosed when there is a persistent, characteristic, pathological lesion adjacent to, or arising from, the anal canal in a patient known to have two of the following criteria for the diagnosis of intestinal Crohn's disease: clinical, radiological or histological.

Probable perianal Crohn's disease can be diagnosed in the absence of obvious clinical manifestations of intestinal Crohn's disease, providing there are typical perianal lesions showing histological evidence of granulomata in biopsies taken from skin tags, ulcers or abscess. The histological evidence must be reviewed by an experienced histopathologist who is able to exclude other granulomatous diseases such as foreign body granuloma, tuberculosis, etc.

When making a diagnosis of probable perianal Crohn's Disease it must be remembered that there are a number of diseases which are often mistaken for perianal Crohn's disease such as hidradenitis suppurativa (Fig. 18.2), chronic complicated anal crypto-glandular sepsis and tuberculosis.

Classification

Anatomical and pathological classification

Anorectal Crohn's disease is best understood in relation to anatomical and pathological factors (Hughes 1978).

Distal Crohn's disease can affect the colon, the rectum, the anal canal and the perianal skin. Perianal Crohn's disease is seen occasionally without demonstrable proximal bowel disease but usually occurs in association with ileal disease with a normal large bowel or in continuity with large bowel disease. Because the prognosis is said to be worse with concurrent, contiguous rectal disease, a classification of anal Crohn's disease should state whether there is associated disease of the small bowel, colon or rectum.

The pathological processes in perianal Crohn's disease are the same as seen in Crohn's disease of the ileum with superficial fissures or diffuse inflammation leading to a thickened bowel wall; or with ulcers penetrating through the bowel wall to induce a deep abscess and/or a fistula. These patho-

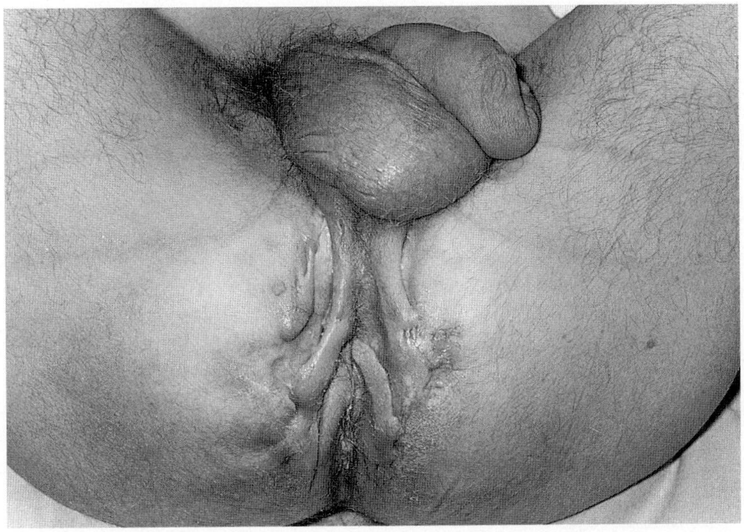

Fig. 18.2. The perineum affected by hidradenitis suppurativa. The patient had been referred with a diagnosis of Crohn's disease.

logical processes, occurring in the anal canal, give rise to three groups of characteristic clinical states associated with ulceration, fistula and strictures. Hughes (1978) has further subdivided the lesions into "active" and "inactive". When the Crohn's disease process is "active" the anal lesions have a swollen, translucent pink or bluish appearance usually with obvious ulceration (see Fig. 18.1). When the disease activity resolves the oedema is lost, the tissue becomes opaque and the ulcers heal with a fragile layer of epithelium. "Inactive" lesions may remain clinically significant because of the mechanical effects of the fistula or strictures. Active disease appears to be associated with poor wound healing, but wounds usually heal normally when the disease is inactive. Thus anal Crohn's disease can be classified on the basis of the 3 pathological groups of lesions, the state of disease activity and the presence of proximal disease. A classification based on these features was first published by Hughes (1978) as the "Cardiff Classification" and is now presented in a modified form (Table 18.3).

Simple clinical classification

The problems with the Cardiff Classification are its complexity, the need for examination under anaesthesia to assess fistulas accurately and the lack of objective data to show what is the observer error in assessing activity. These problems make it unsuitable for out-patient or office assessment. Therefore we have devised a clinical classification, not requiring assessment under anaesthesia; this is shown in Table 18.4.

Functional classification: index of activity

A subjective assessment of the effects of the disease on function can be provided by completing the questionnaire as shown in Table 18.5.

The measures included in the table may vary with time so that a time-scale needs to be added. A high score for one day only in the preceding month is less important than a perpetual dysfunction for the whole month. We have yet to decide whether these categories are sufficient and whether any are redundant. We could then decide the relative numerical value to be assigned to each. For example, severe incapacity in sitting would seem to warrant a higher score than a disinclination to make love. It is suggested that the first three categories of sitting, defaecating and walking might have twice the value of the second three categories (work, social and sexual).

The proposed index will need a prospective multi-centre evaluation to test its ability to differentiate success from failure in management. We need to enquire which of the functions is the most sensitive and whether some can improve on treatment while others do not.

Table 18.3. "Cardiff" classification of perianal Crohn's disease

1. Pathological group
- U. Ulceration
  1. Superficial fissures
     - a. posterior and/or anterior
     - b. lateral
  2. Penetrating ulcers
     - a. anal canal
     - b. lower rectum terminal 1 cm
  3. Oedematous skin tags
  4. Ulceration extending to perineal skin (aggressive ulceration)
- F. Fistula and/or abscess
  1. Low
     - a. Perianal
     - b. ano-vulval/ano-scrotal
  2. High
     - a. blind supralevator
     - b. high complex (horseshoe)
  3. Vaginal
     - a. ano-vaginal
     - b. recto-vaginal
  4. Severe anal pain – no sepsis identified
- S. Strictures
  1. Anal canal
     - a. spasm only (pseudo-stricture)
     - b. organic stricture
  2. Low rectal
     - a. shelf-like
     - b. extra-rectal

2. Disease activity
   1. Active
   2. Inactive
   3. Uncertain

3. Proximal intestinal disease
   - 0. No proximal bowel disease
   - 1. Small intestine
   - 2. Colon – rectal sparing
   - 3. Contiguous rectal disease

Table 18.4. Clinical classification of perianal Crohn's disease (suitable for office or clinic use without examination under anaesthesia)

O. Observed pathology (on inspection)
- U Ulceration: granulation tissue or slough
- F Fistula: visible independent skin opening
- T Tags: larger than variation of normal irregularity

I. Induration of perianal skin (assess by gentle palpation with lubricated finger)
- I 0. No induration detected
- I 1. Firm or oedematous areas
- I 2. Woody hard

(I 1 and I 2: Qualified by extent of circumference involved 25%, 50%, 75%, 100%)

S. Stenosis of anal canal (assessment by gentle rectal examination without anaesthesia)
- S 0. No detectable stenosis
- S 1. Examination hurts the patient
- S 2. Full digital examination impossible

Example of assessment: 0 F; I 1, 25%; S 1.
From Alexander-Williams et al. 1992

Pathology

The primary pathological lesion in perianal Crohn's disease is chronic ulceration, to which all the other protean manifestations seen in this disease are secondary. The severity of the disease tends to be related to the depth of the penetration of the ulceration, to the effects of secondary infection and the extent of secondary healing. The anatomical variations of the tracking of the secondary infection are related to the position of the ulceration in the ano-rectum.

As with Crohn's disease ulceration elsewhere in the gut, ulceration in the rectum and anal canal can be superficial or deep and transmural. The early lesions, which are commonly seen in the rectum, are in the form of apthous ulcers. These are seen as patchy oedema with small central areas of ulceration, which may extend through the mucosa and submucosa.

In addition to suffering from characteristic Crohn's disease ulceration, patients having chronic inflammatory bowel disease with associated diarrhoea, tend to be prey to non-specific ailments of the anal and perianal region. These may present as a common-or-garden infected anal crypt or anal gland which may progress to a perianal, intersphincteric or ischio-rectal abscess. Such a common-or-garden

Table 18.5. Functional classification of perianal Crohn's disease

	Score
Effects on life (score: 0 = no effect, 1 = some disability, 2 = severe disability)	
Effect on essential activities	
Sitting	
Defaecating	
Walking	
Effect on quality of life	
Ability to work	
Ability to enjoy life (social relationship)	
Sexual relationship	
Sickness index profile (SIP)	
Symptoms of incontinence (score: 0 = none, 1 = occasional use of pads, 2 = pads night and day)	
Soiling	
Drugs (score: 0 = never, 1 = occasionally, 2 = most days)	
Pain-relieving medications	
Antibiotics	

From Alexander-Williams et al. 1992.

abscess discharging to the surface will become a fistula-in-ano. These may be difficult to differentiate from perianal abscesses or fistulae originating from a transmural Crohn's disease ulcer. The principal difference being that the Crohn's disease ulcer can occur anywhere in the anorectum whereas a common-or-garden fistula apparently always begins from an abscess in an anal gland that opens into the anal canal at the level of the dentate line. Rarely a deep pelvic abscess from ileal or colonic Crohn's disease can point through the pelvic floor to the perianal skin. This is likely to elude detection until the originating disease necessitates a laparotomy or until scanning or fistulography identifies the high origin of the fistula.

Fistula, skin tags and ulcers

The most easily recognised chronic perianal lesion in Crohn's disease is a fistula, often with multiple skin openings, associated with much fibrosis and often with oedematous hypertrophied skin tags. Sometimes the hypertrophied tags make perianal hygiene difficult and so a fistula may be complicated by perianal dermatitis. Even such an apparently unequivocal diagnosis has a reported incidence varying from 6% to 34%.

Sometimes there are shallow anal canal ulcers undermining the skin edges, which may coalesce leaving skin bridges between.

Characteristically these lesions, although they look and feel grossly abnormal to the observer, are relatively little trouble to the patient (Buchmann and Alexander-Williams 1980). Because they cause such little trouble when they are draining freely, they easily escape detection, unless there is meticulous inspection with a good light. Inspection must be accompanied by adequate retraction, careful palpation and often by probing of tracks (Fig. 18.3). To be completely certain that a patient does not have perianal Crohn's disease it is often necessary to examine thoroughly under general anaesthesia (Fig. 18.4). Therefore it is not surprising that, in some series, the incidence of lesions is reported as being low because some lesions are missed. In some series lesions such as oedematous tags of skin and cracking of macerated skin associated with perianal dermatitis may not be reported as they are not considered to be a specific disease; particularly in someone who is suffering from diarrhoea. In some series, there has to be

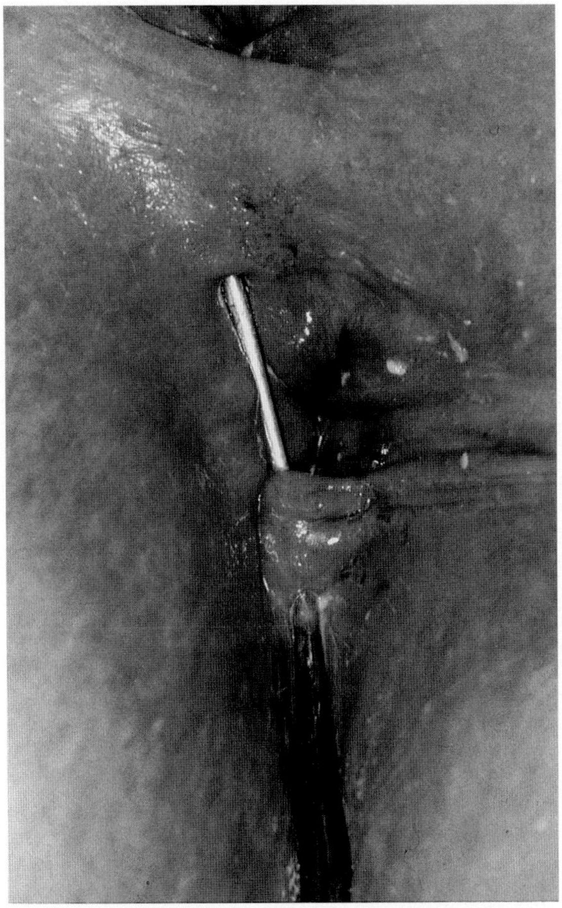

Fig. 18.3. Simple cryptoglandular superficial fistula-in-ano in Crohn's disease. Quiescent disease: only detected on probing.

a fistula track present or at least a large chronic ulcer before the diagnosis of perianal Crohn's disease would be accepted. In some reports, such as that of Fielding (1972) from our unit, every deviation from normality was recorded as perianal Crohn's disease; hence the high incidence.

In my opinion the only perianal findings that are unequivocally abnormal in patients with Crohn's disease are abscess, fistulae and ulceration, whereas skin tags, tissue oedema and split or excoriated skin are all such common lesions in the general population and particularly in those suffering from diarrhoea that they do not necessarily qualify for definition of perianal Crohn's disease.

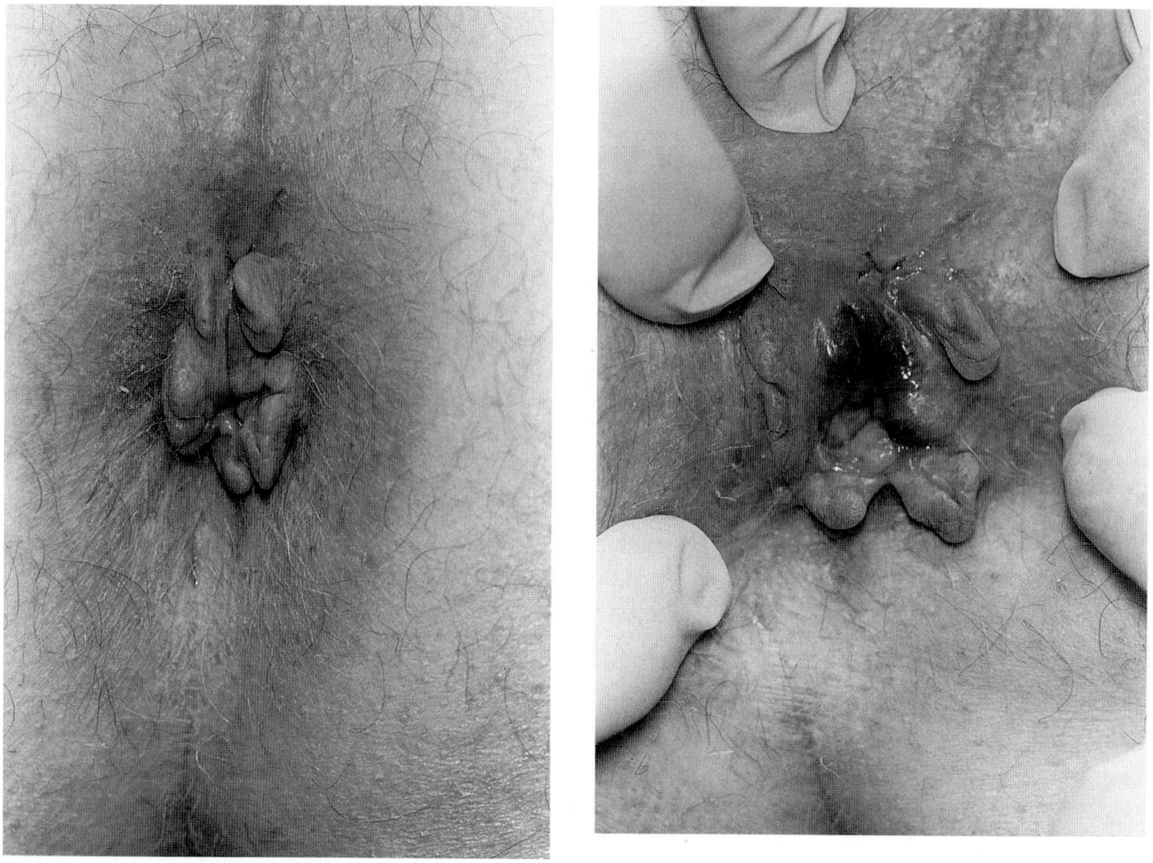

Fig. 18.4.a "Quiescent" asymptomatic skin tags in a patient with Crohn's disease. **b** Traction of the skin revealed active ulceration within the anal canal.

Symptoms and signs

Perianal Crohn's disease is often relatively painless. Painful Crohn's disease almost invariably indicates a complication such as pus under tension or severe fibrous stenosis. Pus under tension usually occurs in a patient who already has a fistula and in whom the external opening has healed sufficiently to prevent free drainage: an abscess then develops within the fistula track. The tissue tension in the abscess usually produces severe pain. If the abscess tracks widely in the fat under the skin, this extension often relieves the tension so that the pain is then not so acute. There now tends to be a more constant low-level pain with tenderness and induration. Such patients often experience an ill-defined malaise that is often not recognised until it is cured by appropriate treatment.

Fibrous stenoses are often not acutely painful but may give constant low-intensity pain, often with exacerbation after defaecation.

The discharge from an abscess or a fistula may soil the patient's underclothes, necessitating the wearing of an absorptive pad. Perianal itching or sore skin is usually due to perianal dermatitis caused by a variety of reasons already discussed above.

Bleeding is relatively rare in perianal Crohn's disease but may occur from trauma to the granulation tissue lining an ulcer. It often is only noticed on the tissue when the anus is cleaned after defaecation.

Patients will often complain of lumps protruding from the anus but these are rarely due to the protrusion of true intra-anal canal swellings. These lumps are usually skin tags, originating from the external part of the anal canal. Patients complaining of swelling or "piles" often have only skin tag oedema.

Table 18.6. Comparison between characteristic anal lesions in common-or-garden fissure-in-ano and anal fissure/ulcer in Crohn's disease

Common-or-garden fissure-in-ano	Anal fissure/ulcer in Crohn's disease
Fissure	Ulcer
Single	Multiple
Midline	Any quadrant
Painful	Not very painful
Narrow	Broad
Muscle fibre at base	Healthy granulation tissue base
Hard straight edges	Undermined irregular edges

Differentiation from common-or-garden anal disease

In the general population who do not have Crohn's disease, it is not uncommon to find lesions such as perianal abscess, fissure-in-ano, haemorrhoids, perianal dermatitis and skin tags; they are even more common in patients with chronic diarrhoea. Common-or-garden fissures are a midline split of the anoderm overlying the tight lower end of the internal sphincter, usually induced by constipation or diarrhoea (Table 18.6). Abscesses and fistulae are usually due to infection of anal glands which penetrate part or all of the lowermost fibres of the internal sphincter. Perianal dermatitis is a common complaint usually due to inadequacies in perianal hygiene, often associated with skin irregularities and soft tenacious faeces. Crohn's disease may predispose to these common-or-garden perianal conditions simply because it frequently causes diarrhoea.

Differentiation from specific anal ulceration

Primary chancre of the anus is commoner in, but not confined to, homosexual males. Chancres are not always easy to recognise but will be more likely to be suspected if an accurate history of sexual practices is obtained in all cases – an omission that is too common even in specialist proctological units. The chancre is usually single and more painful than ulcers in Crohn's disease.

Tuberculous ulcers are also more painful and more often associated with disorders of continence than are Crohn's ulcers. In my experience tuberculous ulcers of the anus are always initially misdiagnosed as Crohn's disease unless they occur in patients from parts of the world where tuberculosis is endemic.

Establishing the diagnosis

The diagnosis can sometimes be made on the typical appearances; particularly of the anal ulcers. The multiplicity of fistula openings is sometimes suggestive. In making a diagnosis the most important part is the history of Crohn's disease elsewhere in the alimentary tract which is present in 95% of cases. In only about 5% of our series was the anal disease the first clinical manifestation of Crohn's disease. (Alexander-Williams 1976). Rarely it is the only manifestation for years or even decades.

Multiple fistulas may be mistaken for hidradenitis suppurativa, though in my experience it is commoner for patient with hidradenitis to be diagnosed incorrectly as having Crohn's disease (see Fig. 18.2). In hidradenitis there is no track connecting the abscesses with the anal canal, though there is often a track connecting one abscess to another. Careful examination under anaesthesia may be required to differentiate and, even then, it may not be simple. Secondary or iatrogenic connection with the anal canal can occur in hidradenitis. Manifestations of hidradenitis in other apocrine-bearing skins (axillae and groins) may also aid in diagnosis of hidradenitis.

Crohn's disease anal fissures are rarely painful; in contrast to anal epithelioma, anal tuberculosis and primary chancre of the anus. When there is doubt about the diagnosis, biopsy, culture and, where appropriate, serological testing for syphilis are indicated.

Whenever it is necessary to operate on a patient with perianal lesions in Crohn's disease, such as draining an abscess or excision of redundant skin tags, tissue should be sent for histological examination. Disappointingly, the histological appearance of excised tissue is rarely absolutely characteristic. Typical granulomatous lesions are seen in only about 25% of the tissue removed from patients with Crohn's disease of the anus and, conversely, foreign body giant cell systems can be found in tissue from many patients with simple fistulas or fissures. Therefore, it appears that there is little justification for removing a piece of tissue simply to establish a histological diagnosis of Crohn's disease. It is probably more important to perform a mucosal biopsy from any abnormal areas seen coincidentally on rectoscopy (Dyer et al. 1970). However, it has not yet been determined which tissue biopsy gives the greater chance of an accurate histological diagnosis of Crohn's disease.

Bacteriological differentiation of the pus in abscesses or from fistulae is rarely of value and I do not recommend its routine use. It has been established that skin organisms predominate in primary follicular sepsis, such as hidradenitis, while bowel organisms predominate in abscesses originating from the interior of the anal canal (Grace et al. 1978). Nevertheless, this bacteriological differentiation is rarely of value in the diagnosis of patients with chronic lesion.

Natural history of the disease

Untreated disease

The disease often runs a benign course with occasional acute exacerbations but with little serious deterioration over decades. In 1968 Fielding performed a consecutive survey on 156 patients attending our Crohn's disease follow-up clinic (Fielding 1972). He classified 109 of these as having either fissures or fistulae. We monitored the natural history of these patients during the subsequent ten years, reassessing them in 1973 and 1978. During the decade of review 14 patients had died, some of them as a result of serious Crohn's disease elsewhere in the gut and a few from unrelated conditions. None died as a direct result of their perianal disease. Ten of the 109 required a protectomy but in all of them the principal indication for operation was the serious associated rectal disease and not the perianal disease itself.

We invited the remaining 85 patients to have further ano-rectal investigation in 1978 but 24 declined, stating that they were wholly symptom-free. The 61 patients who were fully investigated after 10 years were mostly found to have improved. Of the 54 patients who originally had fissures, only 10 still had active fissures 10 years later. However, of those who had fissures originally, 27 had progressed to develop chronic induration or stenosis of the anal canal; sometimes making it difficult to exclude with certainty the presence of a small fissure. Of 21 patients who had fistula-in-ano in 1968, eight appeared to have healed completely 10 years later. However, five new fistulas had arisen in patients judged not to have a fistula in 1968. During the course of the ten years, occasional surgical intervention had been needed because of acute abscesses, most of whom were treated by simple unroofing (Buchmann and Alexander-Williams 1980).

From these experiences we conclude that:

1. In most patients with perianal Crohn's disease it runs a benign course
2. Troublesome symptoms occur only as a result of complications
3. Most complications can be managed medically or with minor surgical intervention

Other clinics where large numbers of Crohn's disease patients are followed have recorded a similar view about the relatively benign natural history of perianal disease (Goligher 1984).

Prognostic factors

Perianal lesions are generally accepted as more common in patients with colonic Crohn's disease than in patients with Crohn's disease involving only the small intestine. Similarly perianal Crohn's disease with colonic disease is often more severe and usually responds less favourably to the conventional surgical treatment.

Favourable prognostic factors include:

1. Absence of symptoms (careful studies of the natural history of perianal Crohn's disease reveal that it is often surprisingly indolent)
2. Absence of overt ano-rectal Crohn's disease
3. Favourable and rapid response to medical treatment (including metronidazole and elemental diet)
4. Favourable and rapid symptomatic response to surgical drainage

Poor prognostic factors include:

1. Presence of persistent ano-rectal Crohn's disease especially in continuity with the perianal lesions
2. Failure to respond rapidly to medical treatment, surgical drainage or proximal diversion (with persisting presence of painful symptoms)
3. Pelvi-rectal abscess and/or high suprasphincteric fistula

4. Recto-vaginal fistula
5. High complex fistula with perineal involvement
6. Incapacitating incontinence
7. Development of carcinoma within the tract of a chronic fistula

Assessing the extent and anatomical location

Clinical assessment

Attempts at objective measurement by palpation of induration, oedema, fibrosis and muscle loss are notoriously inaccurate and subject to observer error. Such measurements are influenced greatly by the patient's anxiety and tolerance of discomfort.

Endo-rectal sonography

Endo-rectal sonography (ERS), in which a rotating or linear echo probe is positioned in the rectum, provides a picture of the rectal wall, the anal sphincters and adjacent structures. This investigation is usually performed to study the anal canal and lower rectum. For the less accessible parts of the large bowel the ultrasound endoscope has greater potential, although experience in its use is still limited. It is an operator-dependent investigation, the photographic images are difficult to interpret (Fig. 18.5).

Using ERS sepsis is imaged as an anechoic or hypoechoic cavity while a fistulous tract appears as a duct-like structure in the perianorectal tissues. By recognising the layers of the rectal wall, the internal and external sphincter and the levatores ani muscles, ERS can define the location and extent of sepsis in relation to the pelvic floor muscles. A fistulous tract between the rectum and vagina can be more clearly shown trans-vaginally than trans-rectally. Severe PACD can be defined as ERS evidence of sepsis involving two or more anorectal quadrants. Unfortunately ERS cannot be performed in patients with tight anal strictures; nevertheless, this simple, relatively inexpensive examination allows objective measurement of pathological anatomy. The lack of radiation and side effects make ERS ideal for follow-up. It is invaluable in the study of the natural history of the disease and to evaluate response to treatment.

Contrast radiology

Traditionally we employ subjective assessment of perianal Crohn's disease by inspecting the perineum, performing a rectal digital examination and, where possible, a proctoscopy. During acute exacerbations of perianal Crohn's disease the perineum is often

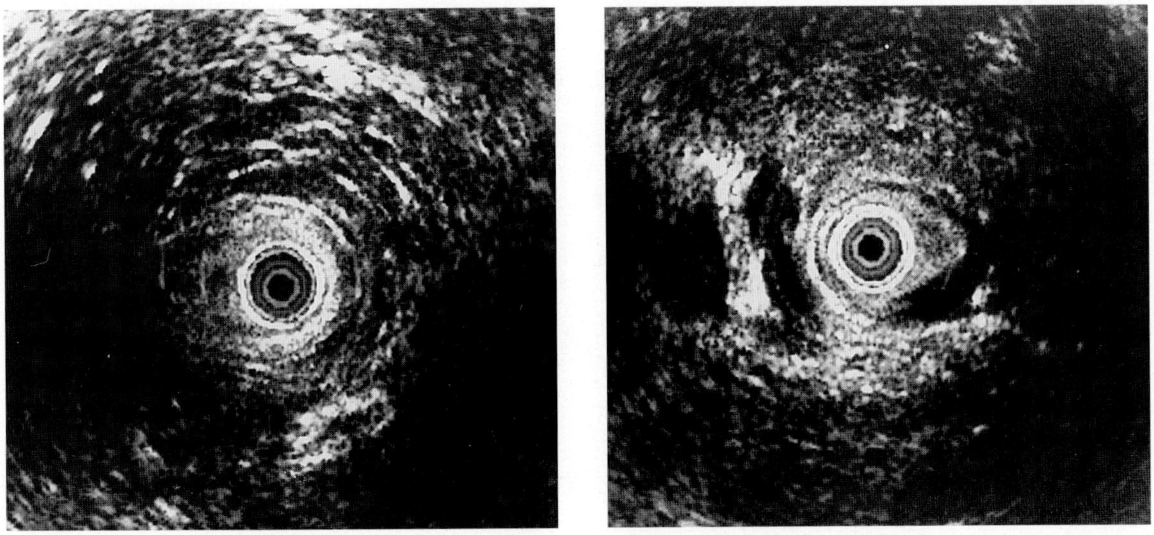

a b

Fig. 18.5.a Endo-rectal ultrasound of intact lower anal canal. **b** ERS image higher in anal canal showing horseshoe correction of ischio-rectal abscess.

painful which limits assessment. Much more information can be obtained from palpating the anus under general anaesthesia with complete relaxation. However, even this examination is largely subjective and logistically cumbersome because anaesthesia is required. Nevertheless under anaesthesia induration can be appreciated early and pressure can be exerted until pus is observed to be exuding through fistula tracks.

Barium enema examination is expensive and extravagant of radiation. It will only detect gross strictures and large fistulas both of which are usually readily appreciated by other examination. Fistulography without anaesthesia is uncomfortable and provides less information than can be obtained with examination under anaesthesia and probing. We believe that barium enema and fistulography are rarely, if ever, required.

Defaecography is a dynamic radiological investigation performed during voluntary evacuation of the rectum. In perianal Crohn's disease it provides a good measurement of function showing both impaired emptying and incontinence. It is, however, expensive and extravagant of radiation. It is not suitable for repeated follow-up investigation (Fig. 18.6).

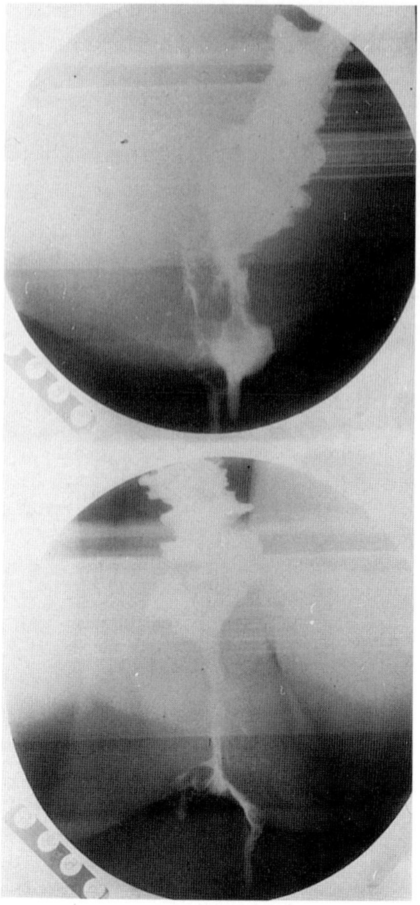

Fig. 18.6. Radiograph of defaecography.

Computed tomography

Computed tomography (CT) is a sensitive means of examining the perirectal and perianal regions in patients with Crohn's disease. The major abnormalities seen on CT include

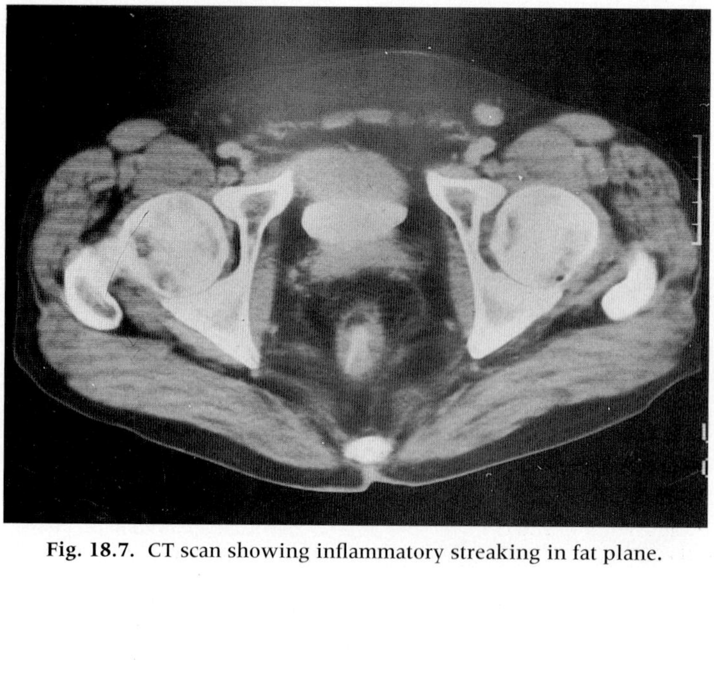

Fig. 18.7. CT scan showing inflammatory streaking in fat plane.

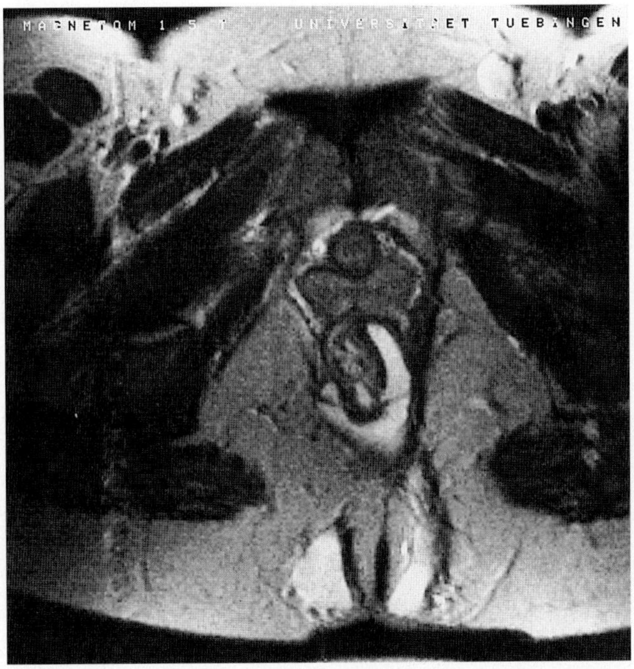

a

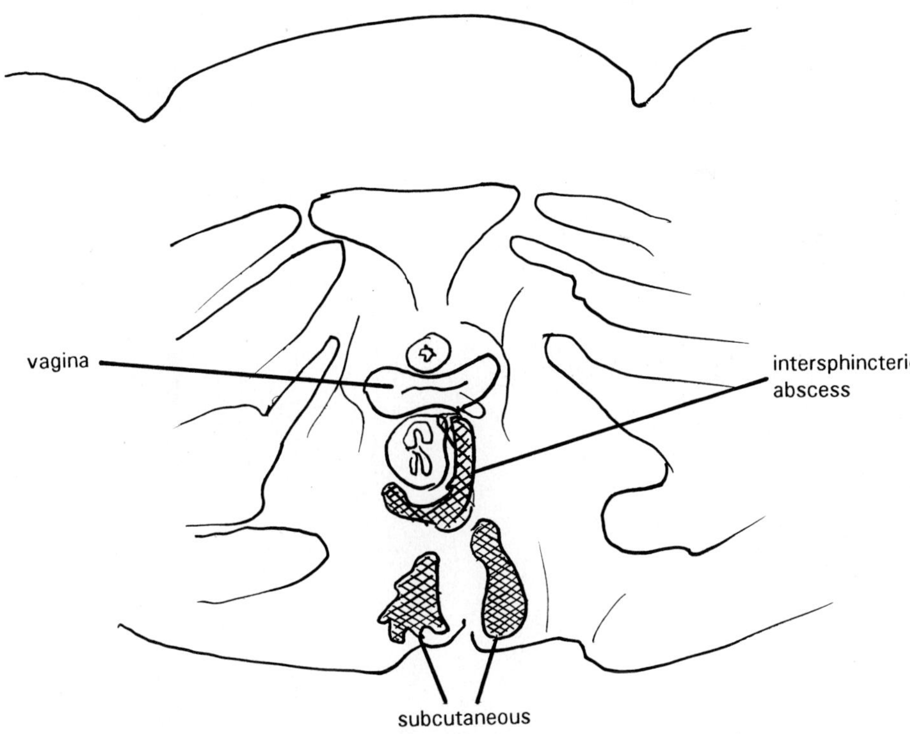

b

Fig. 18.8a,b. MRI. Transverse section of female pelvis. Shaded areas show subcutaneous abscess posteriorly and horseshoe intersphincteric abscess. (T2 weighted SE 2500/90.) (**a** reproduced with permission of the Department of Surgery, University of Tuebingen.)

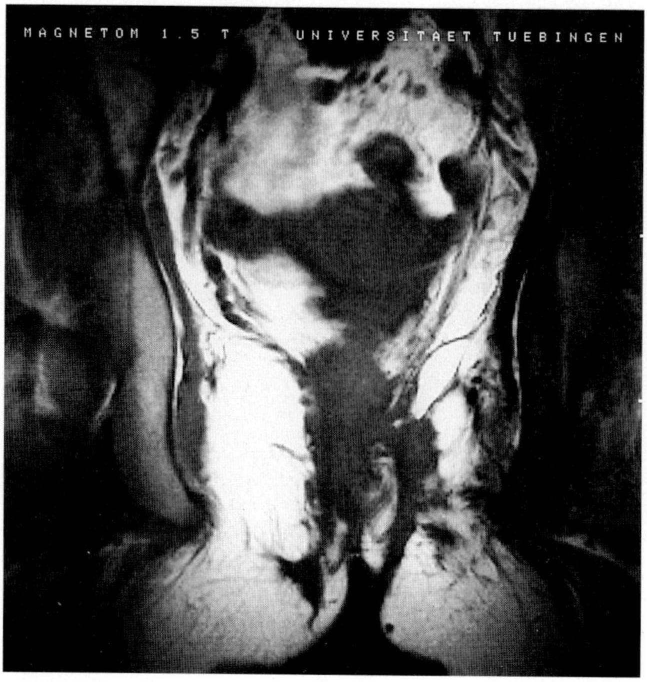

a

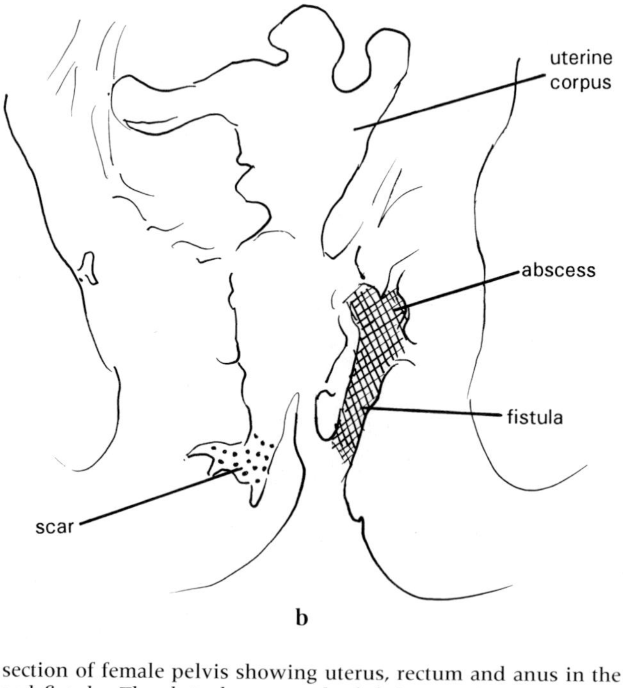

b

Fig. 18.9a,b. MRI. Vertical section of female pelvis showing uterus, rectum and anus in the midline. The shaded area on the right is an abscess and fistula. The dotted area on the left is scar tissue. (T1 weighted coronal SE 600/15) (**a** reproduced with permission of the Department of Surgery, University of Tuebingen.)

inflammatory thickening of the rectal wall, abscess, fistula and sinus tract. A typical CT manifestation of PACD is inflammatory streaking of the fat plane (Fig. 18.7); a finding that is better shown by CT than ERS. CT can localise sepsis below or above the levatores and can show clearly when sepsis originates from the peritoneal cavity above. CT imaging is limited to the axial plane in the pelvis. It is costly and involves significant radiation exposure.

Magnetic resonance imaging

Magnetic resonance imaging (MRI) has been studied in a small number of patients with Crohn's disease. The advantages of this cross-sectional imaging technique in the pelvis are its superb contrast resolution and its flexible multi-planar capability which provides accurate anatomical localisation of abnormalities. The supra- and infra-levator compartments are well seen in coronal MR images (Figs. 18.8 and 18.9). At present MRI is slow, expensive and susceptible to artifacts but it has the great advantage that patients are not exposed to radiation. As major advances develop in MRI technology, its use is likely soon to supersede that of CT (Lunnis et al. 1992).

Examination under anaesthesia

It is often difficult to assess clinically the complexity of subcutaneous sepsis and to discover loculations of pus. The presence of pain and tenderness usually indicates that there is loculated pus, but this pus may be difficult to localise, even when examining under anaesthesia.

I have made great use of examination under anaesthesia with opening up of ramifying tracks after probing with a firm curved probe. Under anaesthesia and antibiotic cover, I squeeze the indurated areas and "unroof" any cavity that can be shown to exude pus. I find that even severely symptomatic patients can be rendered asymptomatic by this process of "gardening" under general anaesthesia. The different investigation techniques with the relative merits and costs are summarised in Table 18.7.

The management of perianal Crohn's disease

Medical management

The three pillars of medical management of perianal Crohn's disease are:

1. Measures directed at improving the patient's general resistance to the disease
2. The use of antibiotics to overcome secondary infection
3. Anti-inflammatory and immunosuppressive drugs to treat the inflammatory aspects of the disease and control the immune response.

Improving resistance

Anything that improves the patient's state of nutrition and general well-being is likely to have a beneficial effect on healing. Many patients with severe symptomatic complications of perianal disease tend to undergo natural resolution if they are admitted to hospital and put on bed rest with improved nutrition, if necessary with iron and vitamin supplements. In some cases the resolution is dramatic. The possible beneficial effect on perianal disease of treating complicated Crohn's disease elsewhere in the gut by operation will be discussed below under the section on surgical therapy.

Table 18.7. Relative merits and costs of the different investigation techniques

	Inspection & palpation	ERS	Contrast radiology	Defaecography	CT	MRI	Exam. under anaesthesia
Sensitivity							
Endoluminal	++	++	+	++	+	+	++
Extraluminal	+	++	++	+/−	+++	+++	+++
Patient compliance	++	++	+	+	+++	+++	+
Radiation exposure	−	−	+	+++	++	−	−
Cost	−	+	+	++	+++	+++	++

ERS, endo-rectal sonography; CT, computed tomography; MRI, magnetic resonance imaging.

Antibiotics

Antibiotics, particularly the broad spectrum type and those that control the growth of anaerobic microbacteria, are effective in treating the localised secondary infection that often complicates perianal Crohn's disease.

There are many anecdotal reports of short-term beneficial effects of a variety of broad spectrum antibiotics. Particular attention has been paid to the use of metronidazole. One of the first of many reports on the value of metronidazole in the management of Crohn's disease was by Ursing and Kamme in 1975. Since then there have been some reports of a favourable response in Crohn's disease of the large bowel; many of these reports have commented favourably on the effect of metronidazole on perianal disease (Ursing and Kamme 1975; Allan and Cooke, 1977). Perhaps the most enthusiastic report was that of an uncontrolled study by Bernstein et al. (1980): they reported 21 patients with severe symptomatic perianal disease, ten of whom had failed to heal despite receiving previous medical treatment, including prednisolone. Seventeen patients had undergone previous surgical treatment; with one or more previous perineal operations in ten. The 17 patients were given a large dose of metronidazole (20 mg/kg per day) orally. The authors stated that the initial response to metronidazole was objectively and subjectively striking. Nineteen of the 21 patients reported decrease in pain and tenderness within one to two weeks. At the time of the report, 17 of the patients had been maintained on continuous metronidazole for from five to 21 months. On this regime fistulas healed, ulcers epithelialised and abscesses resolved. Metronidazole had to be discontinued in only three of the 21 patients, one who developed a neuropathy and two who failed to comply. The authors were convinced and enthusiastic about the beneficial effect of metronidazole. They postulated three possible mechanisms of action, an antimicrobial effect, an immunosuppressive effect and a direct effect on tissue healing. They thought that the effect on the microbacterial flora was not enough to account for all the benefits experienced, particularly as they had only succeeded in reducing the contamination with anaerobic microbacteria and then not universally. Some patients had persistent anaerobic micro-organisms isolated, despite long-term therapy. These authors thought that metronidazole might suppress cell-mediated immunity, especially granuloma formation. However, the drug showed no other significant changes in cell-mediated immunity, as shown by anergy screening or in vivo lymphocytes stimulation tests. Nevertheless, they found that the circulating immune complexes were decreased after metronidazole therapy. The third mechanism they postulated was an, as yet, unproven effect on wound healing. So enthusiastic were these authors about the beneficial effects of metronidazole that they questioned whether a controlled trial would be morally justified. However, in an editorial in the same issue of *Gastroenterology* Sachar (1980) points out the fallacies in drawing conclusions from such an uncontrolled trial. He emphasised that the criteria of the evaluation were mostly subjective and the very act of inclusion into a study with a "new drug" would be likely to cause a "placebo" improvement. Sachar concluded that it was morally unjustifiable not to conduct a controlled trial, yet so far no such controlled study has been reported.

In a small prospective study from our institution, Allan and Cooke (1977) failed to support the enthusiasm for long-term use of metronidazole; a view supported by Goligher (1984) who also quotes L.E. Hughes as holding similar views.

Immunosuppressives

Azathioprine has been advocated in the treatment of perianal Crohn's disease particularly for persistent anal fistulae (Brooke et al. 1976). We have a limited anecdotal experience of uncontrolled studies of apparent benefit after azathioprine. However, it is important to remember that we are studying a disease with a natural tendency to remission. The immunosuppressive effect of steroids is used commonly in the management of Crohn's disease but there is no documented controlled prospective evidence that steroids beneficially effect perianal Crohn's disease. My own impression is that they have no effect.

Surgical treatment: evolution of our present policy

Traditional approach

In early decades after 1932 the approach in our unit in Birmingham to perianal complications, such as fistulas and chronic fissures was traditionally oriented. The indications for intervention were similar to those advocated by McKay and McMaron (1972) and Lockhart-Mummery (1975). In 1976 I reported an audit of our management of patients with perianal Crohn's disease in a total series of 408 patients with Crohn's disease under review in our follow-up clinic (Alexander-Williams 1976). For perianal complications we performed 96 operations in 68 patients; including 25 drainage of abscesses and 52 laying open of fistulas. There were three who had wide excision of fissure, five a manual dilatation, seven excisions of deep fistulae and four haemorrhoidectomies. As a result of this policy there were a number of serious complications, including stenosis in 11 and incontinence in 16.

Changes in the light of our early experience

These experiences, combined with our study of the natural history of perianal Crohn's disease, brought about a change in our surgical policy from radical to conservative. For the past 15 years the incidence of operation for perianal disease in our unit has fallen dramatically. There have been only 16 operations for laying open of superficial fistulae, no deep fistulae have been treated surgically and six abscesses have been treated by simple drainage.

Present policy

It is now our policy to limit surgical intervention in perianal Crohn's disease to the following five complications:

1. Pain as a result of pus under tension. This is treated by simple unroofing (Fig. 18.10.).
2. Symptomatic anal stenosis which is treated by gentle dilatation. Initially we used to do this with one finger but now it is performed with a 20 mm coaxial balloon.
3. Rarely incontinence or recto-vaginal or recto-urethral fistulas can be treated by a definitive surgical repair, providing the local Crohn's disease is quiescent. The repair is usually protected by a temporary faecal diversion (Fazio 1987).
4. Large fleshy skin tags may be excised if they are causing great difficulty in perianal hygiene. There should be minimal excision of the base of these skin tags and, if possible, the incision should not encroach on anoderm, to minimise the risk of stenosis (Fig. 18.11).
5. Persistent complex fistulas that repeatedly heal at skin level and cause recurrent tension and pain are managed by a simple drainage Seton as advocated by Kuijpers (1984). I use polypropaline while others use Silastic (Williams et al. 1991b).

It is possible that superficial fistulas that undermine the superficial fibres of the internal sphincter heal more rapidly if they are treated by dividing the superficial fibres than they will if left alone. However, there is no prospective trial evidence to support this view.

Patients with Crohn's disease rarely suffer from true haemorrhoids and we now believe that haemorrhoidectomy is never indicated. Alarming results of haemorrhoidectomy in patients with Crohn's disease have been reported (Jeffrey et al. 1977). They suggested that 30% of their patients eventually underwent proctectomy largely because of the complications of haemorrhoidectomy, where-

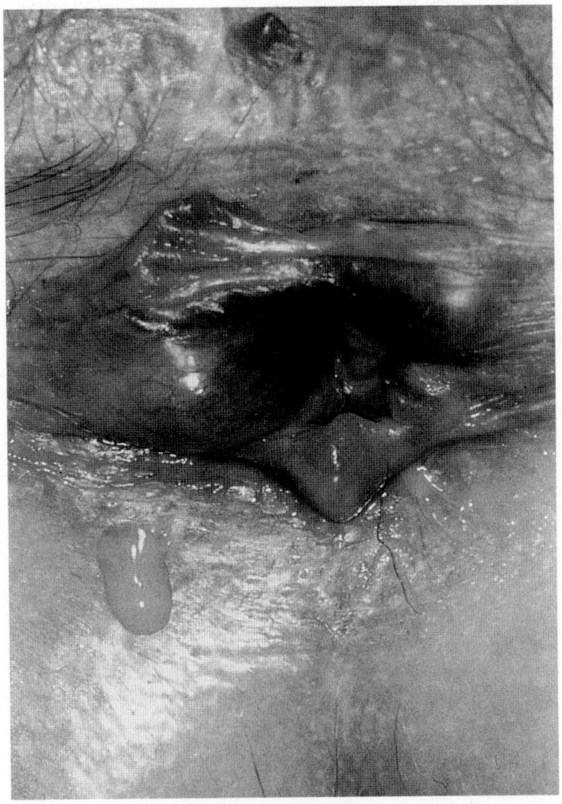

Fig. 18.10.a Previously painless complex perianal Crohn's disease with anterior (superior) fistula opening and posterior (inferior) chronic ulcer. The disease has recently become painful because pus has become under tension due to inadequately draining fistulous opening through which pus is beginning to exude. Simple unroofing of the abscess rendered the patient symptom-free once again.

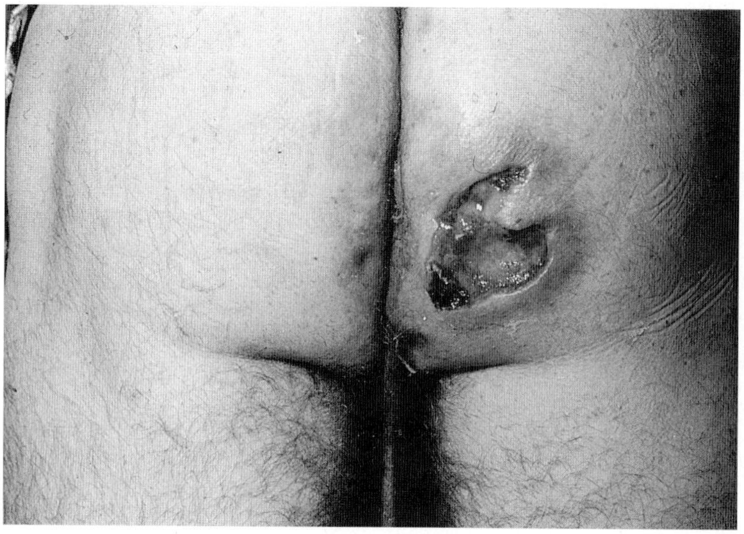

Fig. 18.10.b One week after simple unroofing of huge subcutaneous buttock abscess complicating complex fistulating Crohn's disease. The main fistula tracks have not been opened up but the patient is now symptom-free.

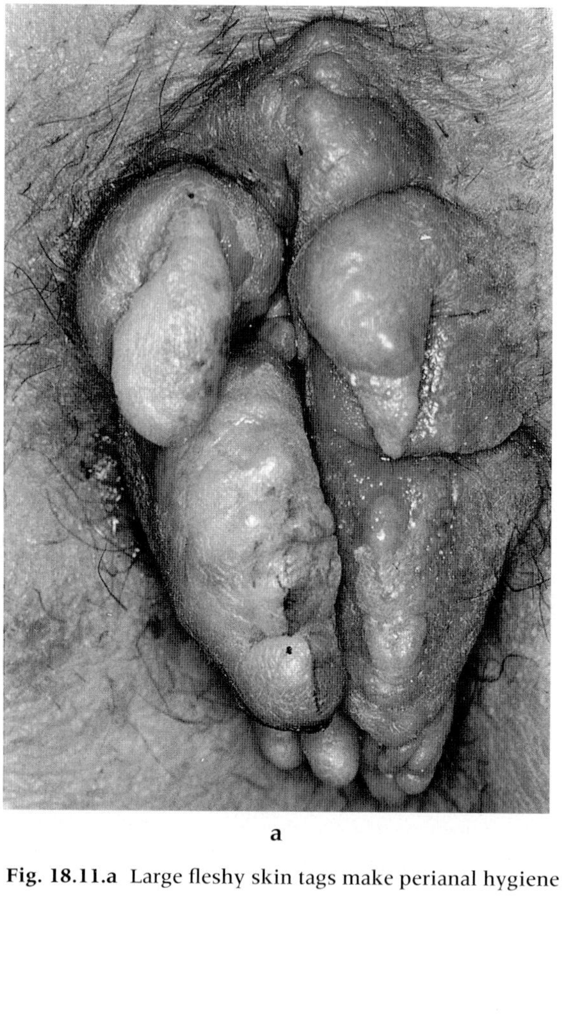

a

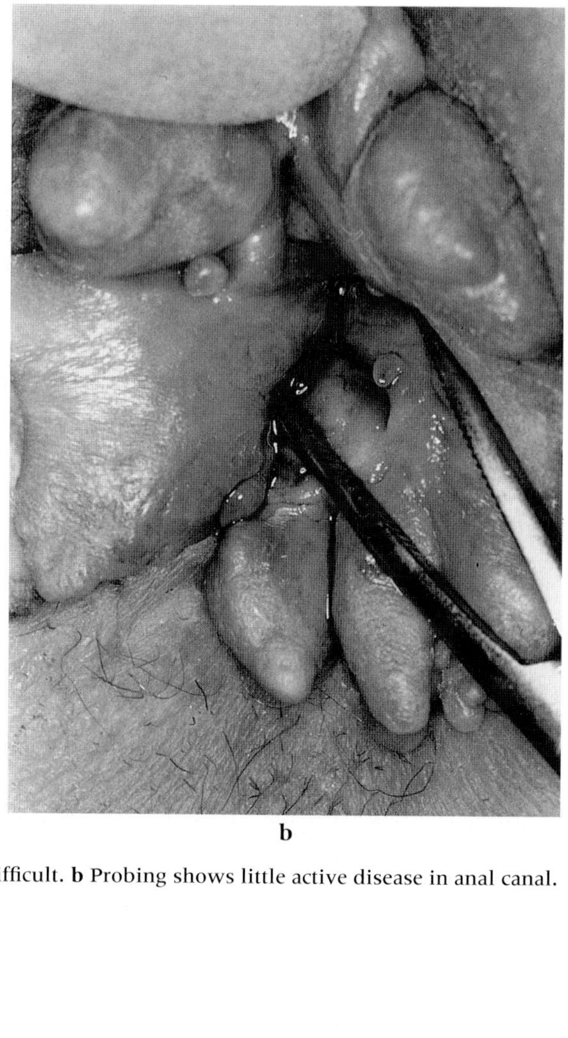

b

Fig. 18.11.a Large fleshy skin tags make perianal hygiene difficult. **b** Probing shows little active disease in anal canal.

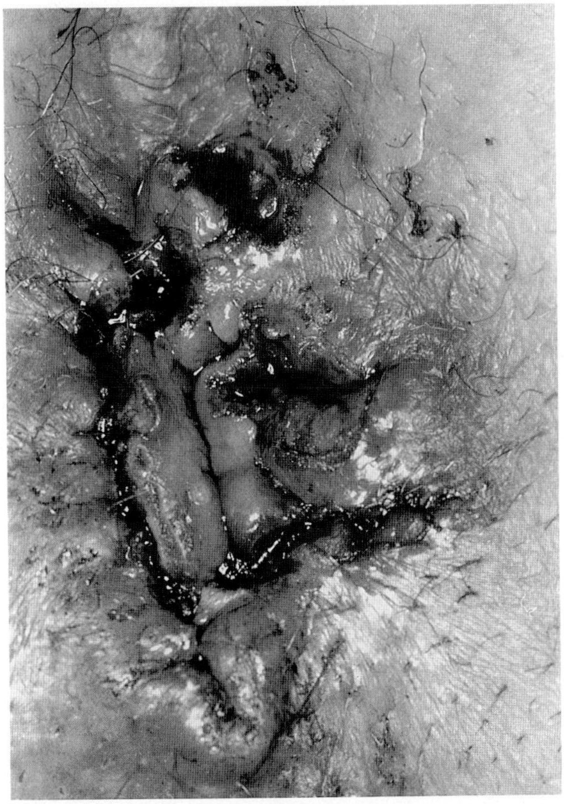

c

Fig. 18.11.c After tags excised with diathermy. Note that the anal verge is not removed. There was good rapid healing.

as it was more because of the extent of the associated rectal Crohn's disease.

Hughes and colleagues (1988) describe the condition of acute local painful lesions in Crohn's disease that are not associated with pus under tension. They advocate local injection of methylprednisolone into the painful area. I have tried this on three occasions with good pain relief in one and temporary relief in another. I do not understand the pathology.

Some unanswered questions

Should we first treat all associated intestinal lesions surgically?

Tradition or surgical folklore decrees that, when perianal Crohn's disease is associated with an active proximal intestinal lesion, the proximal lesion should be treated first. It is thought that then a certain proportion of the perianal lesions will clear spontaneously (Goligher 1984). Hellers and colleagues (1980) surveyed 184 patients with anal fistula and found that only 43 of them had been treated initially by primary intestinal resection of the underlying disease. In 20 of these 43 (47%) so treated, the anal fistula healed. However, in seven of the 20 of the fistulas, once healed, recurred within two and a half years. In the absence of a controlled study we do not know what proportion of the original fistulas would have healed spontaneously as part of the natural tendency of the disease to undergo remission. The reports by Hellers et al. (1980) give a clear indication that, in terms of rectal and anal preservation fistula-in-ano associated with rectal Crohn's disease carries poor prognosis. However, they also show that a fistula associated with underlying small bowel disease, but without rectal disease, carries a good prognosis. What these and all other retrospective surveys do not tell us is whether or not proximal ileal or ileo-colic disease should be

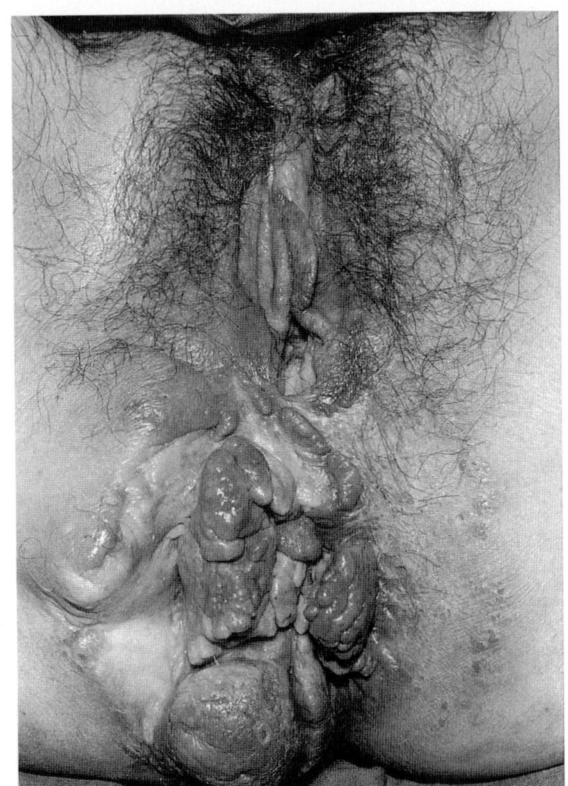

Fig. 18.12.a Complex symptomatic perianal Crohn's disease after many surgical interventions. It is now painful and discharging

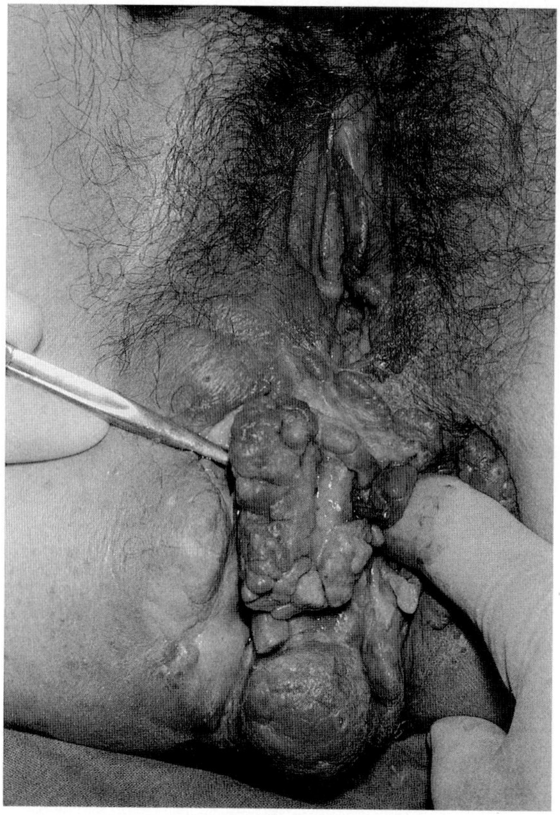

b

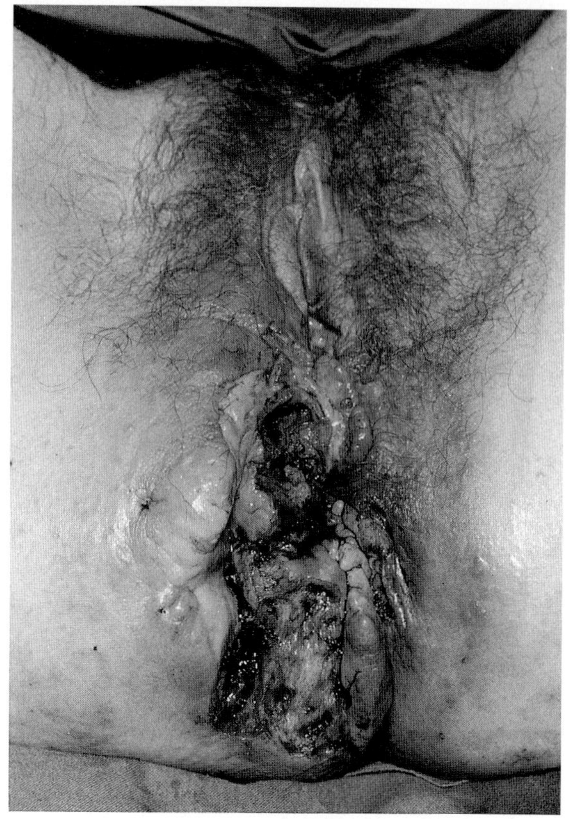

c

Fig. 18.12. b Probing shows a subcutaneous abscess and a fistula entering the anal canal above the dentate line. **c** The abscess cavities were unroofed and the deep fistulous track encircled with a polypropaline Seton to ensure continued drainage. Two year follow-up shows continued symptomatic improvement with no need for proctectomy.

treated before we undertake surgical treatment perianal disease. I believe that resection of proximal disease should not be performed, solely in the hope of curing perianal disease. (Simi et al. 1990).

Is the classical unroofing of a fistula-in-ano ever justifiable in Crohn's disease?

There are a number of reports of success in the management of superficial fistulas (Hughes and Jones 1983; van Dongen 1984; Hughes and Taylor 1990; Williams et al. 1991a). However, there are no reports of controlled comparative studies and many believe that if fistulas are left alone they often heal or at least become asymptomatic (Buchmann and Alexander-Williams 1980). I believe a controlled clinical trial should be planned to try to answer both these important questions. It would need both a multi-centre study to provide sufficient numbers to give reliable answers and a reproducible method of classification of disease and assessment of severity (Fig. 18.12).

Is it ever justifiable to perform faecal diversion by ileostomy or colostomy, solely to treat severe perianal disease?

In the Oxford series of Truelove and colleagues (1965) they included some patients with severe perianal disease in whom the disease of the anus resolved symptomatically after diversion (Lee 1976). However, many of these patients had areas of severe proximal disease excised at the same time. Lockhart-Mummery (1975), referring to severe destructive perianal lesions, states that "experience has shown that diversion of the faecal stream alone, that is by establishment of the colostomy or ileostomy without excising the diseased bowel, does not usually result in improvement or healing of the perianal destructive lesions". This view of the poor results of diversion was substantiated by our own findings (Burman et al. 1971). These conflicting opinions show how important it is to try to introduce some objective criteria of assessment of perianal disease in patients having faecal diversion for Crohn's disease. Nevertheless, I think that it would be difficult to answer this particular question by a prospective controlled trial.

How should we treat complex symptomatic abscesses?

In the local treatment of abscesses and fistula tracks once the abscess is decompressed, Lockhart-Mummery (1975) advocated carefully curetting of all the granulation tissue of tracks. It is not clear what is the rationale for removing granulation tissue nor is there any objective evidence of its efficacy. I believe that, once tension is relieved, granulation tissue is better left intact rather than removed by curetting; I believe that granulation tissue is part of Nature's defence mechanism. Perhaps there is room for yet another clinical trial!

The way ahead

More objective data are needed

As Sachar said in his editorial in 1980, "much of the recorded evidence about natural history and response to treatment in Crohn's disease is supremely subjective". We need objective measures of severity and patient disability; these are sadly lacking in most reports in the literature. Some generally agreed criteria for defining anal symptomatology should be devised. Anal canal diameter could be measured, possibly under an anaesthetic, to reduce any error due to muscular spasm. It might be possible to devise some measure of anal induration and possibly also to measure tissue tension. Refinement and easy availability of MRI should allow us to make precise reproducible records of anatomical extent. If some objectivity could be introduced into the subject, there would be opportunity to confirm or refute previous studies relating to the natural history of untreated disease. We could also assess the effect on the natural history of perianal lesions of medical or surgical treatment of underlying proximal disease. Also it might be possible to measure precisely what is the cause of symptoms and to verify or refute the dogmatic statements that I have made earlier in this chapter, such as the view that pain is always due to increased tissue tension.

With more objective measures to control our studies we should re-evaluate, in prospective control trials, the effects of anti-aerobic and anti-anaerobic antibiotics and also the role of anti-inflammatory or immunosuppressive drugs.

I believe, that until we have reliable prospective evidence of the superiority of one form of treatment over the other, the onus of proof is on those who advocate the more aggressive forms of therapy, particularly surgical therapy.

References

Alexander-Williams J (1976) Fistula-in-ano. Management of Crohn's fistula. Dis Colon Rectum 1976; 19:518–519.

Alexander-Williams, Hellers G, Hughes LE, Minnervini S, Speranza V (1992) A classification of PACD. Gastroenterol Int 5: 216–220

Allan RN, Cooke TW (1977) Evaluation of metronidazole in the management of Crohn's disease. Gut 18: A422

Bernstein LH, Frank MS, Brandt LJ, Boley SJ. Healing of perineal Crohn's disease with metronidazole. Gastroenterology 1980 79:357–365

Buchmann P, Alexander-Williams J (1980) Classification of perianal Crohn's disease. Clin Gastroenterol 9:323–330

Burman JH, Cooke WT, Alexander-Williams J (1971) The fate of ileo-rectal anastomosis in Crohn's disease. Gut 12:432

Crohn BB, Yarnis H (1958) Regional ileitis, 2nd edn. Grune and Stratton, New York

Dyer NH, Stansfield AG, Dawson AM (1970) The value of rectal biopsy in the diagnosis of Crohn's disease. Scand J Gastroenterol 5:491–494

Fielding JF (1972) Perianal lesions in Crohn's disease. J R Coll Surg Edinb 171:32–37

Gabriel WB (1921) Results of an experimental and histological investigation into seventy-five cases of rectal fistulae. Proc Soc Med 14:156–161

Goligher JC (1984) Crohn's disease. In: Surgery of the anus, rectum and colon, 5th edn. Baillière Tindall, London

Grace RH, Harper IA, Thompson RG (1978) Anorectal infection the relationship between the infecting organism, the finding of fistulas and the recurrence rate. Gut 19:A485

Hellers G, Bergstrand O, Eswerth S, Holmstrom B (1980) Occurrence and outcome after primary treatment of anal fistulae in Crohn's disease. Gut 21:525–527

Hughes LE (1978) Surgical pathology and management of anorectal Crohn's disease. J R Soc Med 71:644–651

Hughes LE, Jones IRG (1983) Perianal lesions in Crohn's disease. In: Allan RN, Keighley MRB, Alexander-Williams J, Hawkins CF (eds) Inflammatory bowel disease. Churchill Livingstone, Edinburgh, pp 321–333

Hughes LE, Taylor BA (1990) Perianal lesions in Crohn's disease. In: Allan RN, Keighley MRB, J Alexander-Williams, C Hawkins (eds) Inflammatory bowel diseases. Churchill Livingstone, Edinburgh

Hughes LE, Donaldson DR. William JG, Taylor BA, Young HL (1988) Local depo methyl-prednisolone injection for painful anal Crohn's disease. Gastroenterology 94: 709–711

Jeffery PJ, Ritchie JK, Parks AG (1977) Treatment of haemorrhoids in patients with inflammatory bowel disease. Lancet i:1084–1085

Kuijpers JHC (1984) Use of Seton in the treatment of extrasphincteric anal fistula. Dis Colon Rectum 27: 109–110

Lee E (1976) Results of split ileostomy in Crohn's colitis. In: Weterman IT, Pena AS, Booth CE (eds) The management of Crohn's disease. 1976; Excerpta Medica, Amsterdam, pp 220–223

Lockhart-Mummery HE (1975) Crohn's disease: anal lesions. Dis Colon Rectum 18:200–202

Loygue J, Huguier M (1971) Le traitement chirugical des localisation ano-rectales de la maladie de Crohn. Arch Fr Mal Appar Dig 60 (Suppl):29–33

Lunnis PJ, Armstrong PA, Phillips RKS (1992) Imaging anal fistula with MRI. Gut 33 (Suppl):564

McKay JL, McMahon W (1972) Crohn's disease of the anal region. Northwest Med 71:11–112

Morson BK, Lockhart-Mummery HE (1959) Anal lesions in Crohn's disease. Lancet ii:867–873

Penner A, Crohn BB (1938) Perianal fistulae as a complication of regional ileitis. Ann Surg 108:867–873

Sachar D (1980) Editorial comment on paper by Bernstein et al. (1980). Gastroenterology 79: 393–395

Simi M, Leardi S, Minnervini S, Pietroletti R, Schietroma M, Speranza V (1990) Early complications after surgery for Crohn's disease. Neth J Surg 42:105–109

Truelove SC, Ellis H, Webster CD (1965) The place of a double-labelled ileostomy in ulcerative colitis and Crohn's disease of the colon: a preliminary report. Br Med. J. i:150–152

Ursing B, Kamme C (1975) Metronidazole for Crohn's disease. Lancet i:775–777

van Dongen LM (1984) Controversies in Crohn's disease. MD thesis, University of Nijmegen, Netherlands

Williams JG, Rothenberger DA, Neurer FD, Goldberg SM (1991a) Results of aggressive surgical treatment. Dis Colon Rectum 34:378–384

Williams JG, Macleod CA, Rothenberger DA, Goldberg SM (1991b) Seton treatment of high anal fistulas. Br J Surg 78:1159–1161

19 Associated Diseases

J. Alexander-Williams

Because Crohn's disease and ulcerative colitis begin usually in young patients and in most of them the disease continues into their 60s or 70s it is not surprising that other diseases affect the patients during their lifetime. Some of these diseases will be closely related and some entirely coincidental. These associated diseases can be categorised as:

1. Those that may be aetiologically related to inflammatory bowel disease such as arthritis or dermatitis
2. Those that may have some aetiological relationship and whose surgical treatment is likely to have a direct bearing on the management of the inflammatory bowel disease or vice versa
3. Those which, by affecting the patient's lifestyle, mobility or dexterity, seriously affect their ability to manage the chronic disease, such as heart disease or neuropathy.

The first two categories tend to be more of a problem when the patient has Crohn's disease than when the diagnosis is ulcerative colitis.

Extra-intestinal manifestations

Extra-intestinal manifestations have relatively little bearing on the surgical management of inflammatory bowel disease and so will be discussed only superficially. They are dealt with in greater detail elsewhere (Kern 1980; Mayer and Janowitz 1990).

Extra-intestinal manifestations have long been recognised. Crohn (1925) wrote about the association of ocular lesions and ulcerative colitis even before he and his colleagues described the disease that bears his name.

Musculo-skeletal manifestations

These are reported in between 2% and 23% of patients with inflammatory bowel disease. They can be characterised as "colitic arthritis", which is a migratory, asymmetrical, arthritis, mostly affecting the large joints and the lower extremities and ankylosing spondylitis or sacro-iliitis, which is indistinguishable from idiopathic sacro-iliitis (Mayer and Janowitz 1990).

In many patients these manifestations are purely incidental and have no bearing on management. However, in those patients who have to have an ileostomy they may seriously impede stoma appliance management, because of the patient's difficulty in seeing the stoma and because of the folds of the abdominal wall that make it difficult to find an appropriate stoma site. I have had to resite the stomas of two patients with ankylosing spondylitis to make them more easily accessible for the patient.

Hypertrophic osteoarthropathy and finger clubbing. These occur in both ulcerative colitis and Crohn's disease but are more common with Crohn's disease where the incidence from our unit has been reported as 32%–58% (Fielding and Cooke 1971).

Skin diseases

The incidence of skin and buccal mucosa disease is reported as between 5% and 10% in patients with inflammatory bowel disease (Basler 1980). The common conditions are erythema nodosum, pyoderma gangrenosum and aphthous ulcers of the mouth.

Erythema nodosum is common and may be in part drug-related. It often responds to appropriate treatment of the inflammatory bowel disease and may disappear after appropriate surgical therapy.

Pyoderma gangrenosum is particularly troublesome in patients with ulcerative colitis, with an incidence of between 1% and 5% (Basler 1980). Severe pyoderma gangrenosum can be associated with acute colitis and in our series, has been a principal indication for total colectomy in two patients. Removal of the colon often, but not invariably, results in rapid healing of the pyoderma gangrenosum.

Aphthous ulcers may be regarded simply as early manifestations of Crohn's disease in the uppermost part of the alimentary tract. Their presence tends to parallel disease activity of Crohn's disease elsewhere.

Ocular manifestations

Uveitis and episcleritis are reported in between 3% and 4% of inflammatory bowel disease patients; being particularly common with Crohn's disease of the colon (Greenstein et al. 1976).

Iritis and uveitis are less common but more serious. Uveitis is not generally regarded as an indication for colectomy although Bilson et al. (1967) reported 17 patients in association with ulcerative colitis of whom eight responded well immediately after colectomy.

Renal diseases

Renal stones are reported as being commoner in patients with Crohn's disease (6%–10%) than in those with ulcerative colitis (2%–3%) (Mayer and Janowitz 1990). The incidence is particularly high in those parts of the world where nephrolithiasis is ordinarily more common, such as Eastern Europe. Nephrolithiasis tends to be particularly common in patients who have had surgical treatment complicated by sepsis-prolonged recumbency; often with a low urine output. Other factors include the effect on calcium metabolism, of bed rest and corticosteroid therapy and the excess losses of magnesium and citric acid and the low urinary sodium that occurs in all ileostomy patients. The increased risk of nephrolithiasis is important to consider when patients who have inflammatory bowel disease present with otherwise unexplained attacks of acute abdominal pain. Renal pain may be mistakenly diagnosed as an intestinal complication.

Renal amyloid used to be a common manifestation in patients who were chronically ill from inflammatory bowel disease. In the early decades of our experience it was a reported cause of death (Steinberg et al. 1978). It now appears to be less common.

Haematological and vascular manifestations

Chronic blood loss is common in both ulcerative colitis and Crohn's disease.

Autoimmune haemolitic anaemia is less common and is usually related to drug therapy.

Disorders of coagulation. Deep vein thromboses have been reported in between 6% and 39% of autopsy studies in patients with inflammatory bowel disease, although clinical deep vein thromboses are less common (1% to 7%) (Dennis and Karlson, 1952).

Metabolic manifestations

Metabolic manifestations are particularly common in children and have serious consequences before the age of skeletal maturation. They are reviewed in detail elsewhere (Evans and Walker-Smith 1990).

Severe growth retardation in children should be an important consideration when making a decision about the appropriateness of surgical treatment. In my experience, young children often do not associate the inability to eat normally with abdominal discomfort after meals. I have been involved in the treatment of two children with multiple jejunal strictures in Crohn's disease, whose appetite and nutritional intake improved dramatically after strictureplasty with rapid increase in height and weight (Booth and Harris 1984).

Associated diseases

Hepato-biliary disease

On our unit we have documented the incidence of hepato-biliary disease in in-patients with both ulcerative colitis and Crohn's disease (Eade 1970; Eade et al. 1971). The early histological changes are peri-portal inflammation progressing to fibrosis. The commonest management problem is that posed by primary stenosing cholangitis, sometimes complicated by cholangiocarcinoma. The natural history of these liver diseases does not appear to be affected favourably by surgical therapy for the intestinal disease.

Gall stones

An increased incidence of gall stones appears to occur in patients with Crohn's disease of the small bowel; especially those who have had a terminal ileum resection. Heaton and Read (1969) reported a 25% incidence of gallstones with small bowel Crohn's disease whereas in those with ulcerative colitis and colonic Crohn's disease alone the incidence was only about 5%, which does not differ significantly from that in the general population.

There is such a high incidence of gall stones in patients with terminal ileal Crohn's disease that, in them, I always wish to have an examination by ultrasonography before all primary operations and reoperations. At laparotomy I always make a point of inspecting and palpating the gall bladder carefully, whenever this is feasible. I believe that even asymptomatic gall stones, in a patient with Crohn's disease, is an indication for cholecystectomy. At one time I would always perform an intra-operative cholangiogram at the time of cholecystectomy; both to investigate for stenosing cholangitis and to exclude common duct stones. However, I think that, as cholangiography increases radiation exposure, it is unjustifiable as a routine. I do not use it in patients who have normal liver function tests and normal diameter bile ducts on ultrasonography.

Peptic ulcer disease

Crohn's disease can occur in the stomach and duodenum and the diagnostic differentiation from peptic ulceration is often difficult. The difficulties occur both with barium meal examination and on endoscopy. The presence of concurrent disease both in the antrum and the duodenum tend to be suggestive of Crohn's disease. Although, in theory, multiple biopsies should be helpful in making a diagnosis of antral or duodenal Crohn's disease, in our limited experience we have rarely found typical histological findings on endoscopic biopsy.

There may be some association between extensive ileal resection and gastric hypersecretion (Fielding et al. 1970). It is possible that the presence of acid–peptic hypersecretions is an adverse factor in preventing the normal healing of Crohn's disease ulceration in the antrum or duodenum. Therefore it seems reasonable to treat patients with symptomatic ulceration of the stomach or duodenum by antacids or H_2 receptor blockers or proton pump inhibitors. In 1990 we had one patient who had a fatal duodenal haemorrhage from a giant Crohn's disease ulcer in the second part of the duodenum (Fig. 19.1). This was apparently totally unresponsive to therapy with omeprazole and the ulceration continued after vagotomy and antrectomy.

Murray et al. (1984) reported 47 operations for gastroduodenal Crohn's disease performed at the Lahey Clinic. Twenty-four had a gastroenterostomy (17 without vagotomy). Seven had an antrectomy with a gastrojejunostomy and three an antrectomy with gastrojejunostomy. They reported a marginal (stomal) ulcer rate of approximately 25% if vagotomy was not performed. Dobbins (1989) recommended vagotomy as an adjunct to gastrojejeunostomy drainage and, although observing that most patients who had had vagotomy were not troubled by diarrhoea, nevertheless recommended that the vagotomy should be "highly selective".

Because of our experience of two patients with stomal ulceration after gastrojejunostomy for stenosing duodenal Crohn's disease, I used to "protect" a gastrojejunostomy by a truncal vagotomy (Fielding et al. 1970; Ross et al. 1983) (Fig. 19.2). However, this appears to be unnecessarily physiologically aggressive in patients who have potential abnormalities of small intestine function. I now prefer to treat duodenal stenosis by strictureplasty wherever possible.

Gastrointestinal cancer

The colonic cancer risk in ulcerative colitis is well known and well described elsewhere (Gyde 1990a).

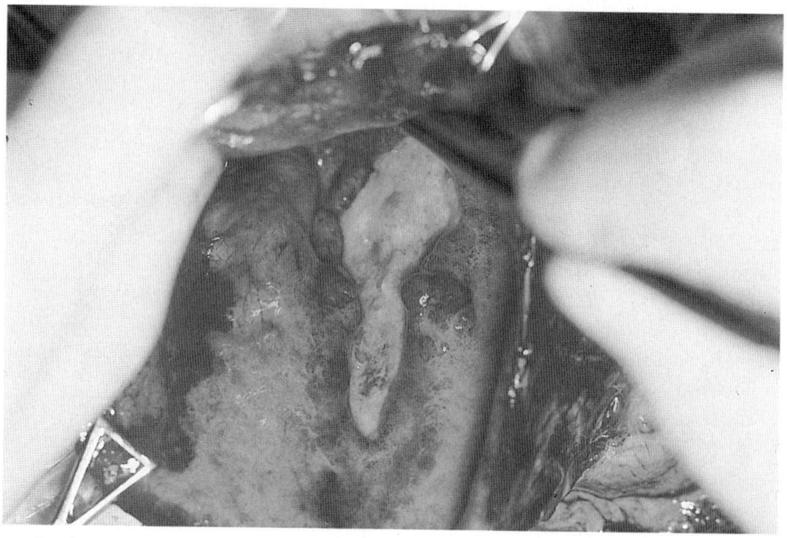

Fig. 19.1. Giant ulcer in the second part of the duodenum in a patient with Crohn's disease. There was a later fatal gastrointestinal bleed.

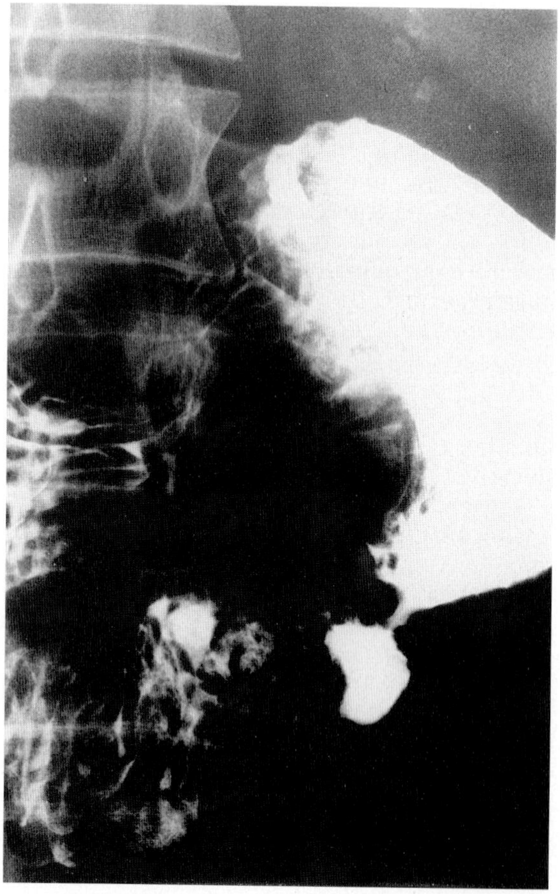

Fig. 19.2. Radiograph of barium meal showing large jejunal ulcer just distal to gastrojejunal stoma in a patient with Crohn's disease bypassed for duodenal stenosis.

In the Birmingham General Hospital series of 513 patients with Crohn's disease a total of 18 cancers were detected, nine colorectal and one was in the small bowel (Gyde 1990b). A ratio of observed to expected cancers (in the general population) was 4.0. We concluded that cancer is a rare complication of Crohn's disease and not often seen in clinical practice, despite a large relative risk of cancer when making comparisons with the risk as it occurs in the general population. The significance of the increased risk of colonic cancer in colonic Crohn's disease means that a similar surveillance programme should be organised for patients with colonic Crohn's disease as for those with ulcerative colitis. However, the problems of surveillance are greater as Crohn's colitis is a patchy disease and it is more difficult than it is in ulcerative colitis to recognise a plaque lesion or distorted gut wall. These difficulties make it almost impossible to direct target biopsies. We now question the practical value of colonoscopic surveillance in patients with Crohn's disease of the colon. Having had one patient develop a small bowel cancer after strictureplasty, we have been concerned that this procedure might lead to the same level of cancer risk as experienced after entero-enteric bypass in the Mount Sinai experience. As yet this risk does not appear to have any practical significance.

In my experience the occurrence of small or large bowel cancer in Crohn's disease has been

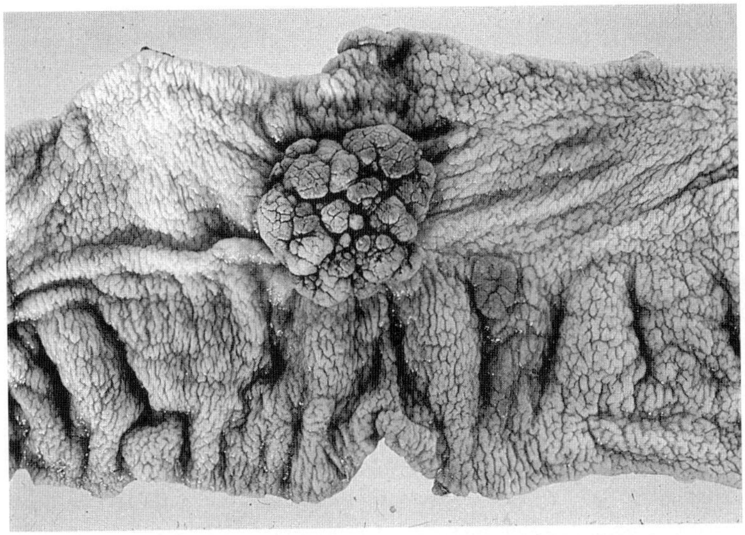

Fig. 19.3. Colonic cancer in a patient with quiescent Crohn's disease with only minimal colonic involvement. Probably a coincidental cancer; detected on X-ray contrast study. The only long-term survivor in our series.

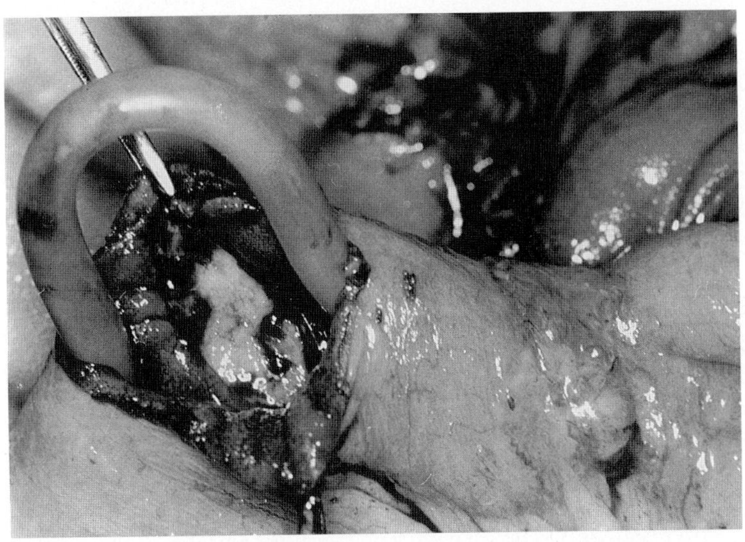

Fig. 19.4. Malignant jejunal stricture detected during operative balloon pull-through review for multiple strictures. It looks almost identical to benign small bowel ulceration. This was rapidly fatal.

almost uniformly disastrous. I have been involved in the management of four colonic and one jejunal cancer and only one has survived more than one year (Figs. 19.3 and 19.4).

References

Basler RSW (1980) Ulcerative colitis and the skin. Med Clin North Am 64:941–954

Bilson FA, de Dombal FT, Watkinson G. Goligher JC (1967) Ocular complications of ulcerative colitis. Gut 8:102–106

Booth IW, Harris JT (1984) Inflammatory bowel disease in childhood. Gut 25:118–202

Crohn BB (1925) Ocular lesions complicating ulcerative colitis. Am J Med Sci 169:260–267

Dennis C, Karlson KE (1952) Surgical measures as supplements to the management of idiopathic ulcerative colitis: cancer, cirrhosis and arthritis as frequent complications. Surgery 32:892–912

Dobbins WO (1989) Gastroduodenal Crohn's disease. In: Bayless TM (ed) Current management of inflammatory bowel disease. Philadelphia, B.C. Decker, pp 218–220

Eade MN (1970) Liver disease in ulcerative colitis. I. Analysis of operative liver biopsy in 138 consecutive patients having colectomy. Ann Intern Med 72:457–487

Eade MN, Cooke WT, Alexander-Williams J (1971) Liver disease in Crohn's disease. A study of 100 consecutive patients. Scand J Gastroenterol 6:199–204

Evans CM, Walker-Smith JA (1990) Inflammatory bowel disease in childhood. In: Allan RN, Keighley MRB, Alexander-Williams J, Hawkins C (eds) Inflammatory bowel disease, 2nd ed. Churchill Livingstone, Edinburgh, pp 523–546

Fielding JF, Toye DKM, Beton DC, Cooke WT (1970) Crohn's disease of the stomach and duodenum. Gut 11:1101–1006

Fielding JF, Cooke WT (1971) Finger clubbing in regional enteritis. Gut 12:442–444

Greenstein AJ, Janowitz HD, Sachar DB (1976) The extra-intestinal complications of Crohn's disease in ulcerative colitis. A study in 700 patients. Medicine 54:410–412

Greenstein AJ, Sachar D, Pucillo A et al. Cancer in Crohn's disease after diversionary surgery. A report of seven carcinomas occurring in excluded bowel. Am J Surg 135:86–90

Gyde SN (1990a) Cancer risk in ulcerative colitis. In: Allan RN, Keighley MRB, Alexander-Williams J, Hawkins C (eds) Inflammatory bowel diseases, 2nd ed. Churchill Livingstone, Edinburgh, pp 563–574

Gyde SN (1990b) Cancer risk in Crohn's disease. In: Allan RN, Keighley MRB, Alexander-Williams J, Hawkins C (eds) Inflammatory bowel diseases, 2nd Churchill Livingstone, Edinburgh, pp 575–580

Heaton KW, Read AE (1969) Gall stones in patients with disorders of the terminal ileum and disturbed bile salt metabolism. Br Med J iii:494–496

Kern F (1980) Extra-intestinal complications of chronic ulcerative colitis and Crohn's disease of the colon. In: Kirsner JB, Shorter RG (eds) Inflammatory bowel disease. Lea and Febiger, Philadelphia, pp 217–240

Mayer L, Janowitz HD (1990) Extra-intestinal manifestations. In: Allan RN, Keighley MRB, Alexander-Williams J, Hawkins C (eds) Inflammatory bowel diseases, 2nd ed Churchill Livingstone, Edinburgh, pp 501–511

Murray JJ, Schoetz DJ, Nugent FW et al. (1984) Surgical management of Crohn's disease involving the duodenum. Am J Surg 147:58–64

Ross TM, Fazio VW, From RG (1983) Long-term results of surgical treatment of Crohn's disease of the duodenum. Ann Surg 197:399–406

Steinberg DM, Allan RN, Brooke BN, Cooke WT, Alexander-Williams J (1978) Sequelae of colectomy and ileostomy: comparison between Crohn's colitis and ulcerative colitis. Gastroenterology 68:33–39

Section III

20 Ulcerative Colitis: Indications for Surgical Intervention

D. Kumar

The most significant morbidity and mortality of ulcerative colitis occurs in patients with severe attacks. It is the management of a severe attack and the ability to recognise when surgical intervention is required that determines the outcome and patient's survival. Most patients with ulcerative colitis do not need an operation; in the Oxford series only approximately 25% of patients required one (Truelove 1988). The crucial factor is to know when surgical intervention is needed and to have clear guidelines to allow optimal decision making. The decision to operate should be made jointly by a surgical and medical team.

The timing of an operation can be classified as elective, urgent and emergency. The decision about when to perform an emergency or urgent operation has been made easier since Truelove and Witts (1954) suggested an objective definition of severe disease. A commonly used definition in clinical practice describes a "severe attack" as the passage of six or more stools daily with blood, a temperature greater than 37.5 °C, tachycardia greater than 90/min, anaemia of 75% of the normal haemoglobin and an erythrocyte sedimentation rate (ESR) greater than 30 mm/h (Truelove and Witts 1954).

Some indications for surgical intervention for complications such as perforation, haemorrhage, presence of carcinoma, are relatively straightforward and do not require much discussion. However, it is often difficult to decide when to perform an elective operation. The most difficult decision is when a patient shows a favourable response to medical treatment initially and then stops improving further. The usual reaction under these circumstances is to continue medical treatment until there is further deterioration. In my opinion such patients should be considered for operative treatment as soon as it becomes evident that the response to medical therapy is inadequate. A "sit and wait" policy under these circumstances will often lead to a situation when urgent or emergency operative intervention is required.

Indications for urgent surgery

Severe attack

Most patients with severe attacks of ulcerative colitis will respond within the first few days of intravenous corticosteroid therapy with a reduction in diarrhoea, tachycardia and pyrexia and an increased feeling of general well-being (Jewell et al. 1991). After five to seven days the treatment is changed to oral steroids and the patients usually continue to show an improvement. A favourable response is judged on clinical assessment rather than by endoscopic or histological criteria. Patients who are said to have failed medical therapy either fail to improve within five to seven days or show signs of deterioration and develop a complication. The decision to operate on this group of patients is relatively easy. It is more difficult to

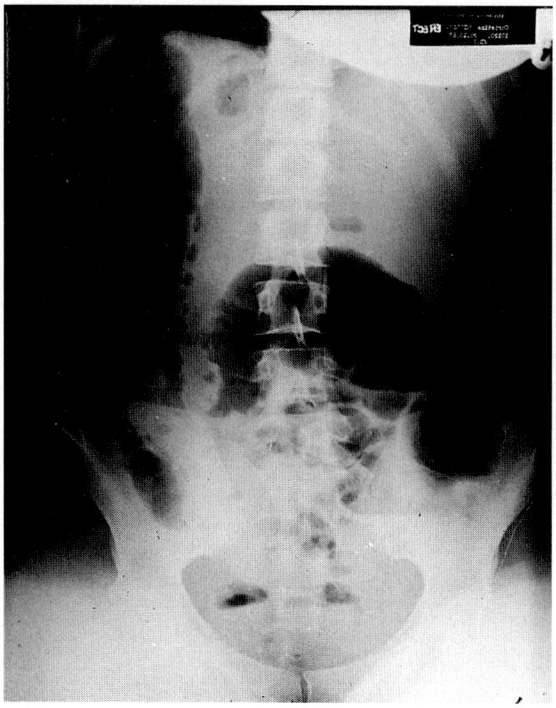

Fig. 20.1. Plain radiograph showing severe ulcerative colitis and extensive mucosal loss evident by the presence of mucosal islands.

make a decision to operate on those who show improvement but persist with many of the original symptoms and signs.

There are some useful radiological signs. If the lumen of the large bowel measures more than 5 cm in any area it suggests impending perforation (Bartram 1981). However, dilatation alone in the absence of other signs of a severe attack may not be an indication for surgical intervention. The presence of mucosal islands (Fig. 20.1), which indicates extensive mucosal loss due to ulceration and inflammation indicates severe disease and should be treated surgically.

Lennard-Jones and colleagues (1975) looked at the predictive value of a large number of clinical variables using a stepwise linear descriminant analysis. The most useful predictors for surgical intervention were diarrhoea more than nine times in 24 hours, a pulse rate greater than 100/min, temperature greater than 38 °C and serum albumin less than 30 g/l. In another study it was noted that a poor response to medical treatment could be predicted by the presence of extensive disease, a short history (Fig. 20.2), stool frequency of greater than 10/day, haemoglobin of less than 12.3 g% and an ESR greater than 30 mm in an hour (Meyers et al. 1987). Others have claimed that changes in C-reactive protein predict the outcome of medical treatment. Low values of C-reactive protein in the presence of a severe attack usually signify a distal colitis and are associated with a favourable response (Prantera et al. 1988). A rise in arterial pH is said to signify impending toxic dilatation (Vernia et al. 1979).

To decide when to operate we consider it essential that the patient is reviewed by a surgical and medical team twice daily. We monitor the following variables:

1. Four hourly measurements of pulse and temperature
2. Frequency and consistency of stools
3. Presence of blood with stools
4. Abdominal tenderness
5. Presence and the nature of bowel sounds

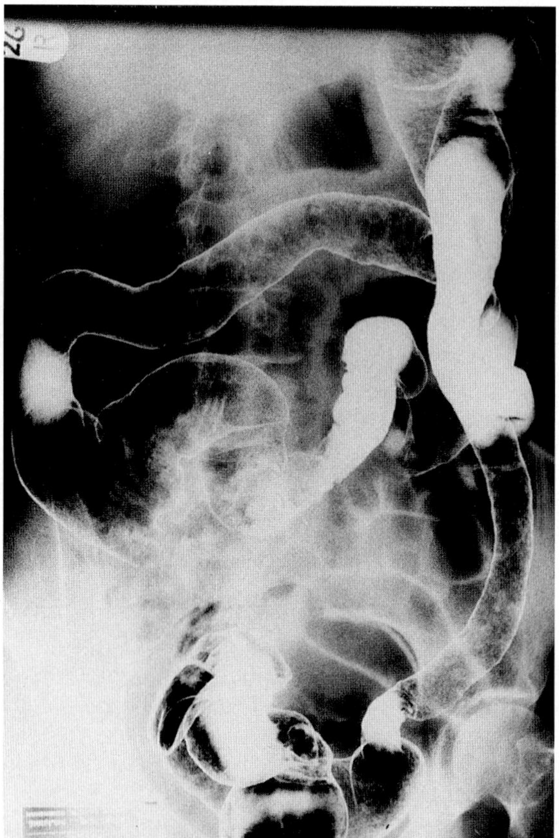

Fig. 20.2. An air contrast study showing extensive severe disease. The whole colon shows mucosal ulceration and loss of haustration. (Courtesy of Dr J.R. Lee.)

6. Daily electrolytes and haemoglobin estimation
7. ESR and/or C-reactive protein measurements on alternate days
8. Plain abdominal radiographs daily or until such time that clinical improvement is well established. This is a better indicator of dilatation of the colon than measurements of abdominal girth

Severe attack with complications

The decision to operate is easy in the presence of acute severe disease with complications. The complications that may occur are toxic megacolon, perforation and haemorrhage.

Toxic megacolon

Despite improved medical measures for the management of an acute severe attack toxic dilatation or toxic megacolon remains an important indication for surgical intervention. The term toxic megacolon is used when the diameter of the colon is greater than 5.5 cm on plain radiographs. The transverse colon appears to be maximally affected and this may be due to the fact that this part of the colon lies anterior to the rest of the colon in the supine position (Williams 1990). Patients with toxic megacolon often have extensive and severe disease and also show evidence of a fall in arterial pH and acidosis (Vernia 1979). However, transient episodes of toxic dilatation may be seen during the early part of medical treatment. If this remains less than 5.5 cm and the patient responds well clinically it may be sufficient to continue careful monitoring with plain abdominal radiographs without surgical intervention. It is important to remember that the operative mortality rates for toxic megacolon and other complications of an acute severe attack remain high. In a specialist centre in New York the in-hospital mortality rate for emergency operations for toxic megacolon was 16% (Greenstein et al. 1985).

Perforation

Perforation of the colon usually occurs whilst the patient is undergoing a trial of medical management for an severe acute attack. Due to high dose steroid therapy the classical signs of perforation are often masked. Because of the difficulties in diagnosing this condition the possibility of perforation must always be borne in mind during medical management. A rising pulse rate and absence of bowel sounds is often suggestive of perforation. An erect chest radiograph or decubitus abdominal film will usually show the presence of free gas in the peritoneal cavity (Fig. 20.3). Under these circumstances emergency surgical intervention is essential.

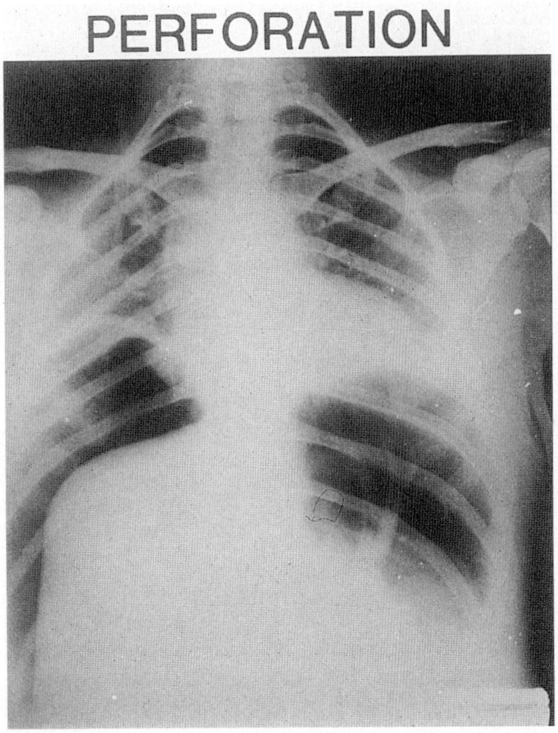

Fig. 20.3. Plain radiograph showing free gas in the peritoneal cavity due to perforation of the colon.

Haemorrhage

Minimal to moderate amounts of bleeding per rectum are common during an acute attack. Severe haemorrhage during an acute attack is rare but surgical intervention is mandatory when it occurs. Any patient who needs more than 6 to 8 units of blood within the first 24 to 48 hours and is still bleeding should have a colectomy.

In most patients a colectomy with an ileostomy and a mucus fistula will control the haemorrhage. Occasionally, in some cases the bleeding may come from the severe rectal ulceration. In such cases, removal of the rectum may also be required.

Elective surgery for ulcerative colitis

The indications for elective surgery for ulcerative colitis have changed since the introduction of restorative procedures. Since restorative proctocolectomy eliminates the need for a permanent ileostomy many centres have reduced their threshold of indication for elective operation.

Surgical intervention for uncomplicated disease

The most common indication for operation is the failure of medical treatment to control symptoms. However, there is no generally accepted meaning of the term "failure of medical treatment". For some, an improvement in symptoms dependent upon the continued need for steroid treatment may be regarded as success whereas others see it as a relative failure. I believe in the importance of the patient's opinion in making a decision for elective surgical intervention. It is the patients who can decide whether or not a certain level of frequency of defaecation and/or diarrhoea is acceptable to their life-style. Some clinical guidelines are helpful in deciding on an elective operation such as:

1. Frequent exacerbations of disease requiring intensive treatment, particularly repeated courses of steroids
2. When the disease is interfering with the patients career, social life or education
3. In children when repeated courses of steroids may result in growth retardation
4. Patients with associated disorders such as peptic ulcer where high-dose steroid therapy is likely to produce complications.

Surgical intervention for disease with complication

Carcinoma

Carcinoma is a common colonic complication of chronic ulcerative colitis. Once the patient has developed a carcinoma, surgical treatment is mandatory. In the past prophylactic colectomy was advised for many patients with longstanding ulcerative colitis as the risk of developing cancer increased with time. The reported incidence of cancer in ulcerative colitis varies from 1.7% to 4.4% of all patients with the disease (Butt et al. 1980, Whelan 1980; Butt and Morson 1981, Johnson et al. 1983). Lennard-Jones and colleagues (1980) have reported a 23-fold increase in the risk of developing cancer in patients who had the disease for 10–19 years and a 32-fold increase in those having the disease for 20–30 years. Patients with extensive disease or total colitis are at a greater risk of developing cancer.

In patients with colonic cancer in ulcerative colitis, a proctocolectomy with ileal pouch-anal anastomosis is the operation of choice. In older patients, a total colectomy and ileo-rectal anastomosis is an acceptable alternative; the bowel function is better than after a pouch and the rectum can be kept under simple sigmoidoscopic surveillance. Patients with advanced colorectal cancers usually have a panproctocolectomy and ileostomy.

Dysplasia

It is easy to decide when to operate in a patient with total colitis with symptoms refractory to medical treatment. It is more difficult when the disease is well controlled by medical means but the patient has had the disease for ten years or more. In such patients the presence of mucosal dysplasia may be a useful indicator for surgical intervention. The absence of dysplasia is not a reliable contraindication for operation because the distribution of dysplasic areas may be patchy and, therefore, may be missed on sampling. Nowadays, there is an increasing tendency to advise regular colonoscopy surveillance rather than offer prophylactic surgery. We tend to offer colectomy only to those patients with extensive disease in the presence of high-grade dysplasia, patients with low grade dysplasia in association with a raised lesion or if changes of high-grade dysplasia develop in a flat lesion with low-grade dysplasia elsewhere.

Several other markers of pre-malignant change in ulcerative colitis in addition to dysplasia are currently under investigation. These include abnormalities of goblet cell mucin (Boland et al. 1984), epithelial marker antigens (Allen et al. 1985) and DNA analysis by flow cytometry (Hammarberg et al. 1984).

Extra-intestinal manifestations

The commonest extra-intestinal manifestations in ulcerative colitis are skin disorders. These are present in approximately 20% of patients and include pyoderma gangrenosum, erythema nodosum and exfoliative dermatitis (Greenstein et al. 1976). Occasionally a colectomy is required before the skin manifestations settle down.

Another important extra-intestinal manifestation of ulcerative colitis is arthritis. It is seen in approximately 10% of patients. Commonly the arthritis is monoarticular and affects the knee joint. It often subsides when the disease remits but occasionally a colectomy is indicated if the arthropathy persists.

Eye problems occur in approximately 5% of patients with ulcerative colitis. Uveitis in particular, may be disturbing to the patient and usually responds to colectomy.

It must always be emphasised to the patient that although the extraintestinal manifestations may subside following a colectomy the remission is not always permanent.

References

Allen DC, Biggart JD, Pyper PC (1985) Large bowel mucosal dysplasia and carcinoma in ulcerative colitis. J Clin Pathol 38:30–43

Bartram C (1981) How useful is the plain abdominal x-ray? World Med 16:51–54

Boland CR, Lance P, Levin B, Riddell RH, Kim YS (1984) Abnormal goblet cell glycoconjugates in rectal biopsies associated with an increased risk of neoplasia in patients with ulcerative colitis: early results of a prospective study. Gut 25:1364–1371

Butt J, Morson B (1981) Dysplasia and cancer in inflammatory bowel disease. Gastroenterology 80:865–868

Butt J, Lennard-Jones JE, Ritchie J (1980) A practical approach to the cancer risk in inflammatory bowel disease. Med Clin North Am 64:1203–1220

Greenstein AJ, Janowitz HD, Sachar DB (1976) The extra-intestinal complications of Crohn's disease and ulcerative colitis. Medicine 55:401–412

Greenstein AJ, Sachar DB, Gibas A et al. (1985) Outcome of toxic dilatation in ulcerative colitis and Crohn's disease. J Clin Gastroenterol 7:137–144

Hammarberg C, Rubio C, Slezak P, Tribukait B, Ohman U (1984) Flow cytometric DNA analysis as a means for early detection of malignancy in patients with chronic ulcerative colitis. Gut 25:905–908

Jewell DP, Caprille R, Mortensen N, Nicholls RJ, Wright JP (1991) Indications and timing of surgery for severe ulcerative colitis. Gastroenterol Int 4:161–164

Johnson W, McDermott F, Hughes ESR, Pihl E, Milne B, Price A (1983) The risk of rectal carcinoma following colectomy in ulcerative colitis. Dis Colon Rectum 26:44–45

Lennard-Jones JE, Ritchie JK, Hilder W, Spicer CC (1975) Assessment of severity in colitis: a preliminary study. Gut 16:579–584

Lennard-Jones JE, Morson BC, Ritchie JK, Shove DC, Williams CB (1980) Cancer in colitis: assessment of the individual risk by clinical and histological criteria. Gastroenterology 73:1280–1289

Meyers S, Level PK, Feuer EJ, Johnson JW, Janowitz HD (1987) Predicting the outcome of corticoid therapy for acute ulcerative colitis. Results of a prospective randomised double-blind trial. J Clin Gastroenterol 9:50–54

Prantera C, Davoli M, Lolenzetti, Pallone F, Marcheggiano A, Iannoni C, Mariotti S (1988) Clinical and laboratory indicators of extent of ulcerative colitis. J Clin Gastroenterol 10:41–45

Truelove SC (1988) Medical management of ulcerative colitis and indications for colectomy. World J Surg 12:142–147

Truelove SC, Witts LJ (1954) Cortisone in ulcerative colitis. Preliminary report on a therapeutic trial. Br Med J ii:375–378

Vernia P, Colaneri O, Tomei E, Caprilli R (1979) Intestinal gas in ulcerative colitis. Dis Colon Rectum 22:346–349

Whelan G (1980) Cancer risk in ulcerative colitis. Why are results in the literature so varied? Clin Gastroenterol 9:469–476

Williams NS (1990) Ulcerative colitis: indications for emergency and elective surgery. In: Allan RN, Keighley MRB, Alexander-Williams J, Hawkins CF (eds) Inflammatory Bowel Diseases. Churchill Livingstone, Edinburgh, pp 423–428

21 Surgical Options

D. Kumar

Total colectomy and mucus fistula

Total colectomy and mucus fistula is the operation of choice when definitive restorative surgery is contraindicated as a primary procedure. If a severe acute attack does not respond to medical treatment, total colectomy and mucus fistula is the safest option for ensuring the patient's swift recovery. It is also the operation of choice in the presence of complications such as toxic dilatation, perforation and haemorrhage. Total colectomy and mucus fistula also has a place in elective surgery for ulcerative colitis, particularly when there is doubt about the diagnosis or when it is uncertain that the patient will accept restorative surgery; it allows time for full patient counselling and preparation for definitive surgery.

Patients who are on high doses of steroids may look deceptively well and may give the surgeon a false sense of security when deciding on a major definitive operation. Often these patients on high-dose steroids are at most risk of developing complications and therefore, in them the safest option is colectomy with a mucus fistula and ileostomy. Some decades ago a split ileostomy and blow hole colostomies were recommended in the management of acute fulminating disease (Turnbull et al. 1970). In my opinion such procedures have no place in the management of ulcerative colitis. With present-day anaesthesia and post-operative management facilities, it is always safe to perform a colectomy and mucus fistula.

The reported results of sub-total colectomy and mucus fistula confirm the safe nature of this procedure. At St Mark's Hospital, London, 101 patients underwent this operation between 1963 and 1986 and four died. In contrast seven of 62 (9%) patients who had a panproctocolectomy died (Hawley 1988). Flatmark et al. (1975) had no mortality in their group of 63 patients who underwent total colectomy. Greenstein et al. (1985) reported total colectomy for toxic dilatation in 75 patients of whom 12 died. The most significant factor affecting mortality in their group was the age of the patient. The mortality was 30% in those of 40 years and over and only 5% in those under 40; it was 44% in those with an associated perforation. Another important determinant of outcome was the timing of the surgery which reflected the severity of disease. Patients who required surgery in the first five days did worse than those who had an operation later (Greenstein et al. 1985).

Panproctocolectomy and permanent ileostomy

Surgeons once regarded panproctocolectomy and permanent ileostomy as the best operation for ulcerative colitis. Some still do; considering it to be the 'gold standard' against which all other operations for ulcerative colitis are judged.

Panproctocolectomy has the advantage that all diseased tissue is removed and so the risk of malignancy is eliminated. Furthermore, morbidity and mortality from this operation are low, and for patients who want to return to normal activity as quickly as possible, this is an attractive option (Spence and Wilson 1983). However, despite all the above advantages, it also has disadvantages, the most important of which is the presence of a permanent stoma which some patients cannot accept. Another disadvantage is the slow healing of the perineal wound which may result in a permanent discharging sinus (Baudot et al. 1980). There is a theoretical disadvantage of impairment of sexual function as a result of injury to the pelvic nerves (Nicholls and Lubowski 1987). However, since adopting close perimuscular dissection we have not encountered this complication.

The commonest indication for elective panproctocolectomy is in patients with chronic illness, which has responded poorly to medical therapy or frequent relapses interfering with work and/or social life. A less common indication is for carcinoma in ulcerative colitis or as prophylaxis against colorectal cancer in longstanding extensive colitis. The need for prophylactic colectomy for longstanding ulcerative colitis has been modified due to colonoscopic surveillance. These days colectomy is only recommended for patients with severe mucosal dysplasia (Morson 1985; Fossard and Dixon 1989).

Today panproctocolectomy is only recommended in patients who are unsuitable for restorative resection. These include patients with weak anal sphincters who may be incontinent and those who are unwilling to undergo the more complex surgery and risk a slightly higher morbidity. It is also the final operation in patients who develop complications from pouch surgery and require excision of the pouch (Vasilevesky et al. 1987). The mortality from this operation is less than 2% in most modern series (Berry et al. 1986; Jones et al. 1987). Post-operative morbidity following this operation is also low and may include stoma stenosis, prolapse or parastomal herniation, all of which may require stoma revision or re-siting. Transient episodes of ileostomy obstruction may also occur but resolve spontaneously with conservative treatment.

Ileo-rectal anastomosis

Ileo-rectal anastomosis was once a popular choice of operation for patients who had relatively mild disease in the rectum. The advantage is that the patient avoids a permanent stoma but the greatest risk is that of malignant change in the rectum. Despite regular sigmoidoscopic surveillance, early malignant change may be missed due to the difficulty in clearing liquid stool from the rectum. With the increasing popularity of restorative proctocolectomy, ileo-rectal anastomosis is not performed so often these days. I believe that it still has a place in older patients with relative rectal sparing and in some children when it is thought that a stoma may be too high a price to pay.

Early complications of colectomy and ileo-rectal anastomosis include diarrhoea and urgency. Rectal function usually improves with time but may take six months or more before an improvement is obvious; therefore, early reassurance is important. Those having an ileo-rectal anastomosis more than six months after an initial colectomy and mucus fistula usually have poor results, possibly due to irreversible contraction of the rectal stump which is non-compliant and cannot function as a reservoir (Parc et al. 1985).

After ileo-rectal anastomosis it is important to emphasise the need for regular endoscopic follow-up and mucosal biopsy and to avoid the operation on any patient who is thought unlikely to comply with this advice. Some patients attend for follow-up in the first few post-operative years only and several years later present elsewhere with a carcinoma. Surgeons used to recommend total colectomy and ileo-rectal anastomosis for the very young patient because it avoided the associated psychological morbidity of a permanent stoma and the possible risk of sexual dysfunction following radical surgery. However, with improved surgical techniques these arguments no longer apply and, in my opinion, if young patients require an operation the procedure of choice is an ileal pouch-anal anastomosis. However, in older patients, an ileo-rectal anastomosis may be superior to a pelvic pouch provided there is minimal disease of the rectum and that the anal sphincters are competent.

Following ileo-rectal anastomosis, approximately 30%–35% of patients will require excision of their rectum at a later date. In the majority of patients this is due to recurrent proctitis but a few develop dysplasia or rarely a carcinoma. The average bowel frequency following ileo-rectal anastomosis is 4–6 motions per day. The majority of patients, however, require anti-diarrhoeal medication for 6–12 months following the operation. Stool consistency is usually semi-solid although some patients manage to pass a formed stool. Incontinence is uncommon but more than 50% of patients experience urgency particularly during the day or after a late evening meal.

Continent ileostomy (Kock pouch)

A continent ileostomy offers the advantages of a classical panproctocolectomy in that it eliminates the disease and the risk of malignancy and in addition provides the patient with a continent stoma. Although theoretically ideal, the adoption of this procedure has been limited, principally due to a high incidence of problems with the nipple valve. The patient has to intubate the reservoir to empty it and there is a high incidence of valve failure. As a result the procedure has largely been abandoned in favour of the pelvic pouch. However, patients who have had a classical panproctocolectomy and find the permanent stoma unacceptable can still opt for this procedure. It also provides an alternative in patients who have had a failed restorative proctocolectomy. If the failure is due to an unacceptably high defaecation frequency, then the pelvic pouch can be converted to a continent ileostomy. Patients who require pouch excision either for sepsis or pouchitis, and are determined to avoid an incontinent stoma should be offered a continent ileostomy.

At present most candidates for a continent ileostomy are: (1) those who wish to convert from a permanent end stoma; and (2) all patients who are unsuitable for sphincter-saving surgery. These patients include those with rectal cancer, poor sphincter function and patients whose jobs preclude frequent visits to the toilet. The results following continent ileostomy appear to be variable. This may simply reflect differences in the length of follow-up. Most series report results in the form of early experience and late experience. The early complication rates are reported to be around 8% (Gerber et al. 1983; Hulten and Svaninger 1984). The incidence of late complications has improved considerably. In particular, late complications requiring revisional surgery have decreased from more than 50% to between 10% and 25% (Hulten and Svaninger 1984, Barnett 1987, Vernava and Goldberg 1988). Operative mortality from this operation is almost down to zero now (Hulten 1984; Barnett 1987). However, the operation still carries significant morbidity in the form of nipple valve slippage seen in 30%–50% of patients (Hulten and Svaninger 1984; Kock et al. 1986), fistula formation, stomal stricturing due to either ischaemia or retraction of the terminal ileal segment (Olsson et al. 1987) and pouch ileitis.

Despite reasonably good results the Kock pouch has failed to gain widespread popularity and acceptance. The main reason for this is the complex nature of the operation and the high incidence of complication rates. The other important factor is the advent of sphincter-saving surgery. In my opinion, the Kock pouch is still a viable option in patients who want to convert from a permanent Brooke ileostomy and those who have failed after restorative proctocolectomy and still desire a continent stoma.

Restorative proctocolectomy

Restorative proctocolectomy has become the operation of choice for ulcerative colitis in the last 15 years. It offers most of the advantages of a panproctocolectomy in that the mucosal disease is eradicated. The initial operation consisted of a total colectomy, sub-total proctectomy and mucosal proctectomy, leaving behind a cuff of rectal muscle. However, more recently mucosectomy in the rectal cuff has been abandoned and the technique of pouch-anal anastomosis has been adopted. This may theoretically result in remnants of disease or colonic type mucosa which can either develop disease at a later date or even undergo malignant change. The main advantage of this operation is that it eliminates the need for a permanent ileostomy and gives the patient an acceptable bowel function. However, in approximately 5% of patients in most series the pouch has to be excised. Depending upon the condition of the patient, severity of disease and experience of the surgeon, the oper-

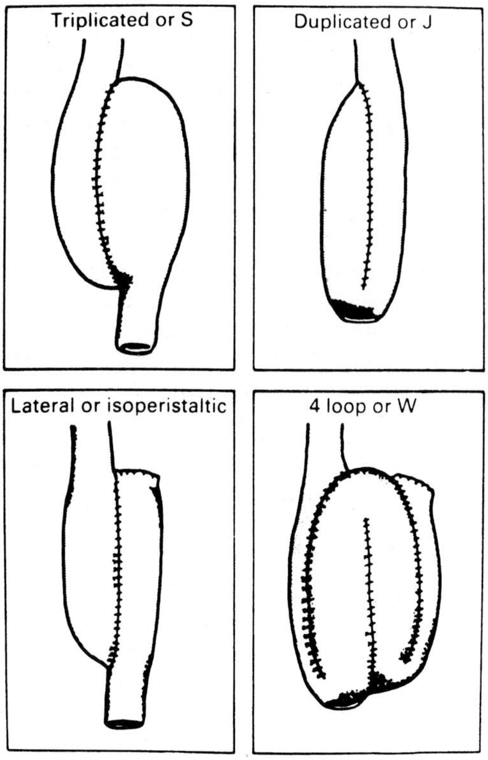

Fig. 21.1. The four commonly used pouch designs. (From Recent advances in gastroenterology, vol 6, by permission of Churchill Livingstone.)

ation is performed either as a one-stage, two-stage or even three-stage procedure. The main drawback of the three-stage operation is the prolonged hospital stay. However, it has advantages as well. I believe that minor degrees of sepsis do not become clinically evident in a three-stage operation. In the one-stage operation a total proctocolectomy is performed followed by the formation of an ileal pouch and a pouch-anal anastomosis. In a two-stage operation a sub-total colectomy with an ileostomy and mucus fistula is performed as the first stage followed by a proctectomy, formation of a pouch and pouch-anal anastomosis as a second-stage procedure. Alternatively in elective circumstances some people carry out a total proctocolectomy, formation of an ileal pouch, pouch-anal anastomosis, and a covering ileal stoma as the first stage followed by reversal of a loop ileostomy as a second-stage procedure. In a three-stage operation the first stage is sub-total colectomy with an ileostomy and mucus fistula. When the general condition of the patient has improved the second stage consists of the formation of the ileal pouch, its anastomosis to the anus and a covering loop ileostomy. The third stage is reversal of the loop ileostomy.

Restorative proctocolectomy is indicated in patients who need an elective resection for a definitive diagnosis of ulcerative colitis, whose general and nutritional status is satisfactory, with a strong dislike for permanent stomas and who are emotionally and psychologically stable. Old age was once considered a relative contraindication for this operation but now many surgeons perform this operation in patients in their 70s.

Since the first successful pouch-anal anastomosis in man by Parks and Nicholls (1978), a variety of pouch designs have emerged (Fig. 21.1).

There are 4 main pouch designs currently in use:

S pouch
J pouch
Lateral or isoperistaltic pouch
W pouch

S pouch

The S pouch or triplicated pouch was the initial pouch design described by Parks and Nicholls in 1978. The original triplicated pouch had an efferent limb which measured 5 cm and this resulted in ineffective or incomplete pouch emptying (Parks et al. 1980). A long efferent limb necessitated catheterisation of the pouch for emptying. Since then the efferent limb has been shortened and the need for catheterisation eliminated.

J pouch

The J pouch is the most commonly used pouch design (Utsunomiya et al. 1980). It is simple and empties well. The main problem with this pouch design is its small capacity and low compliance (Nasmyth et al. 1986). The J pouch can be modified by division of its apex so as to create a spout which simplifies the pouch and its anastomosis (Williams and Nasmyth 1988).

Lateral or isoperistaltic pouch

The lateral or isoperistaltic pouch design was described by Fonkalsrud (1981). It consists of a segment of ileum anastomosed to the terminal ileum in an isoperistaltic manner

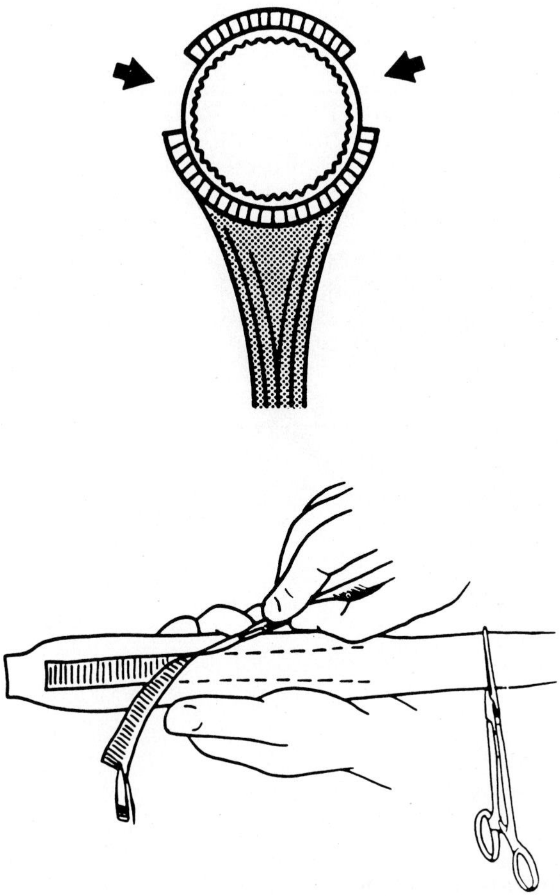

Fig. 21.2 Diagram of the technique of muscle stripping. Black arrows in the cross-sectional view mark the sites of the full-thickness dual myectomy. (From Strand and Yarbrough 1992 with permission.)

(Fig. 21.1). The isoperistaltic anastomosis is believed to be helpful in pouch emptying.

W pouch

This is the latest addition to pouch design. It utilises approximately 50 cm of the terminal ileum and provides a greater pouch capacity and compliance than the other two designs. Also it does not have any problems with spontaneous pouch emptying (Nicholls and Pezim 1985).

Alternatives to pelvic reservoir in restorative proctocolectomy

Ileal-mucosal transplantation in a rectal muscle tube has been attempted as an alternative to an ileal pelvic reservoir (Peck and Hallenbeck 1964). The results were unsatisfactory and therefore, the concept was abandoned. Ileal myotomy has also been performed with some success (Schmidt et al. 1984). In an experimental animal model, Strand and Yarbrough (1992) reported the results of strip myectomy. Two strips, 1 cm wide and 12–15 cm long, of full thickness muscle were removed from the antimesenteric side of the bowel (Fig. 21.2). In this series, there was no pelvic sepsis and all anastomoses healed without stricture. The myectomised animals were continent by three weeks. Necropsy examination at three months showed pelvic reservoirs in all the myectomised animals.

In another study, Sagar et al. (1990) reported the results of a similar operation (Fig. 21.3) in a dog model. Myectomy of single lumen ileum yielded similar results to those observed after a J pouch. Although the experience with these alternatives is very limited in the human, they may provide an easier option than the ileal pouch-anal anastomosis.

Which pouch?

The initial experience of most surgeons with pouch surgery was with the S pouch. The original S pouch has a long efferent limb which made spontaneous evacuation almost impossible. Since then several modifications in the S pouch design have come about and also other pouch designs have emerged. When we compare the functional results of one pouch design with another, there is considerable overlap. I favour the S pouch without a spout because it lies in the pelvis like a normal rectum and has no problems with spontaneous evacuation.

The type of pouch-anal anastomosis also varies. Some surgeons use a stapled anastomosis whereas others prefer a handsewn pouch-anal anastomosis. Again, there is very little to choose between the functional results of the two techniques. I believe that both techniques are useful and have a place in pouch surgery. The stapled anastomosis has the advantage that it puts minimal traction on the sphincter complex. How much of this relates to the functional result remains unclear.

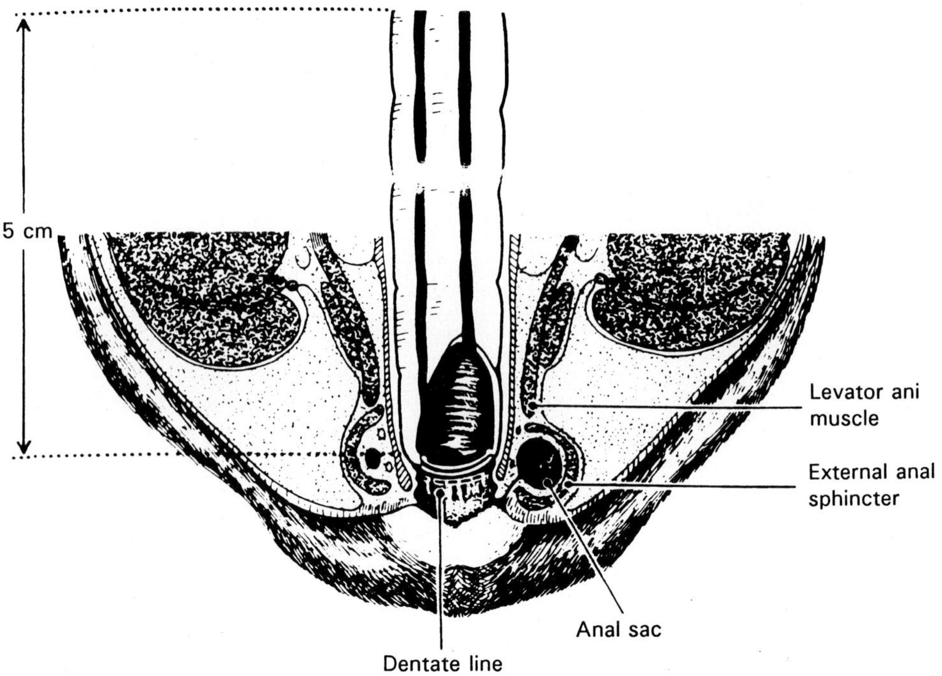

Fig. 21.3 A coronal section of the pelvis of the dog with double myectomy of single lumen ileum. The ileum is anastomosed to the top of the anal canal. (From Sagar et al. 1990 with permission.)

Reference

Barkel DC, Pemberton JH, Pezim ME, Phillips SF, Kelly KA, Brown ML (1988) Scintigraphic assessment of the anorectal angle in health and after ileal pouch-anal anastomosis. Ann Surg 208:42–49

Barnett WO (1987) New approaches for continent ostomy construction. J Miss State Med Assoc 28:1–3

Baudot P, Keighley MRB, Alexander-Williams J (1980) Perineal wound healing after proctectomy for carcinoma and inflammatory disease. Br J Surg 67:275–276

Berry AR, De Campos R, Lee ECG (1986) Perineal and pelvic morbidity following perimuscular excision of rectum for inflammatory bowel disease. Br J Surg 73:675–677

Fonkalsrud EW (1981) Endorectal pull through with lateral ileal reservoir for benign colorectal disease. Ann Surg 194:761–766

Fossard JBJ, Dixon MF (1989) Colonoscopic surveillance in ulcerative colitis – dysplasia through the looking glass. Gut 30:285–292

Gerber A, Apt MK, Craig PH (1983) The Kock continent ileostomy. Surg Gynecol Obstet 156:345–50

Greenstein AJ, Sachar DB, Gibas A et al. (1985) Outcome of toxic dilatation in ulcerative colitis and Crohn's colitis. J Clin Gastroenterol 7:137

Gruner OP, Flatmark A, Naas R et al. (1980) Ileorectal anastomosis in ulcerative colitis. Scand J Gastroenterol 15:123

Hawley PR (1988) Emergency surgery for ulcerative colitis. World J Surg 12:169–173

Hulten L, Svaninger G (1984) Facts about the continent ileostomy. Dis Colon Rectum 27:553–557

Jones HW, Grogono J, Hoare AM (1987) Acute colitis in a district general hospital. Br Med J 294:683–684

Kock NG, Brevinge H, Philipson BM, Ojerskog B (1986) Current ileostomy. The present technique and long-term results. Ann Chir Gynaecol 75:63–70

Kryt RH, Delemarre JBV, Doornbos J, Vogel HJ (1991) Normal anorectum dynamic MR imaging anatomy. Radiology 179:159–163

Morson BC (1985) Precancer and cancer in inflammatory bowel disease. Pathology 17:173–180

Nasmyth DG, Williams NS, Johnston D (1986) Comparison of the function of triplicated and duplicated pelvic ileal reservoirs after mucosal proctectomy and ileo-anal anastomosis for ulcerative colitis and adenomatous polyposis. Br J Surg 73:361–366

Nicholls RJ, Lubowski DZ (1987) Restorative proctocolectomy: the four loop (W) reservoir. Br J Surg 564–566

Nicholls RJ, Pezim ME (1985) Restorative proctocolectomy with ileal reservoir for ulcerative colitis and familial adenomatous polyposis: a comparison of three reservoir designs. Br J Surg 72:470–474

O'Connell PR, Kelly KA, Brown ML (1986) Scintigraphic assessment of neorectal motor function. J Nucl Med 27:460–464

O'Connell PR, Pemberton JH, Kelly KA. Motor function of the ileal J pouch and its relation to clinical outcome after ileal pouch-anal anastomosis. World J Surg 11:735–741

Oakley J, Jagelman DG, Fazio VW et al. (1985) Complications and quality of life after ileorectal anastomosis for ulcerative colitis. Am J Surg 149:108–114

Olsson SA, Fredlund P, Pettersson V, Petersson BG. (1987) Continent ileostomy. A follow-up study for 60 patients. Acta Chir Scand 153:119–122.

Parc R, Levy E, Frileux P, Loygue J (1985) Current results: ileorectal anastomosis after total abdominal colectomy for ulcerative colitis. In: Dozois RR (ed.) Alternatives to conventional ileostomy. Yearbook Medical, Chicago, pp 81–89

Parks AG, Nicholls RJ (1978) Proctocolectomy without ileostomy for ulcerative colitis. Br Med J ii:85–88

Parks AG, Nicholls RJ, Belliveau P (1980) Proctocolectomy with ileal reservoir and anal anastomosis. Br J Surg 67:533–538

Peck DA, Hallenbeck GA (1964) Fecal continence in the dog after replacement of rectal mucosa with ileal mucosa. Surg Gynecol Obstet 119:1312–1320

Sagar PM, Holdsworth PJ, King R, Salter G, Johnston D (1990) Single lumen ileum with myectomy: a possible alternative to the pelvic reservoir in restorative proctocolectomy. Br J Surg 77:1030–1035

Schmidt E, Imhof M, Spuler A, Rothhamer T, Henrich H, Wunsch P (1984) Ileoanal anastomosis, longitudinal myotomy to create an ileal reservoir. Coloproctology 6:353–356

Spence RAJ, Wilson W (1983) Surgically treated inflammatory bowel disease. J R Coll Surg Edinb 28:379–387

Strand JA, Yarbrough LW (1992) Straight ileoanal anastomosis after longitudinal strip myectomy in the swine model. Dis Colon Rectum 35:69–74

Turnbull RB, Hawk WA, Schofield P (1970) Choice of operation for the toxic megacolon phase of non-specific ulcerative colitis. Surg Clin North Am 50:1151

Utsunomiya T, Twama M et al. (1980) Total colectomy, mucosal proctectomy and ileoanal anastomosis. Dis Colon Rectum 23:459–466

Vasilevsky C, Rothenberger DA, Goldberg SM (1987) The S ileal pouch-anal anastomosis. World J Surg 11:742–750

Vernava AM III, Goldberg SM (1988) Is the Kock pouch still a viable option? Int J Colorect Dis 3:135–138

Williams NS, Nasmyth DG (1988) Ileostomy or ileal pouch for the surgical treatment of ulcerative colitis. Postgrad Med J 64:596–602

22 Pre-operative Assessment and Preparation

D. Kumar

Pre-operative assessment

Clinical

A careful clinical assessment of the patient is essential before operation. Different operations may be indicated for the same extent of disease depending on whether the patient is fit or sick, compromised or uncompromised. Signs of tachycardia, pyrexia and abdominal tenderness associated with a low haemoglobin, a high white cell count and a raised ESR and platelet count suggest a severe acute attack. Then the operation of choice is a subtotal colectomy, ileostomy and mucus fistula. A careful nutritional assessment is also essential. Patients who are hypoalbuminaemic and nutritionally compromised and those who have been on steroids for more than three months should not undergo definitive surgery such as a one-stage restorative proctocolectomy. Patients with signs of extra-intestinal manifestations such as arthritis, pyoderma gangrenosum, erythema nodosum and eye lesions should also be considered for a total colectomy with preservation of the rectum rather than a definitive procedure as the first choice operation.

Radiology

Before operation we always hold a careful review of all the past and present radiographs, including plain films as well as contrast studies, with a radiologist with a special interest in inflammatory bowel disease. This helps to exclude any features of Crohn's disease and if there is doubt about the diagnosis on any of the films then we review the choice of operation. In the presence of a doubtful radiological diagnosis, an initial colectomy is always a safer option than a restorative procedure.

Free gas under the diaphragm on plain abdominal radiography suggests colonic perforation and the presence of mucosal islands indicates severe extensive disease. If there is any doubt then we often use an instant air contrast study.

Histology

In the majority of patients a rectal biopsy reported on by a specialist gastrointestinal histopathologist is diagnostic and allows a clear distinction between ulcerative colitis and Crohn's disease. In patients referred from other centres our gastrointestinal histopathologist conducts a careful review of the biopsy slides from the referring hospital. If in doubt we perform a repeat rectal and/or colonic biopsy. Even with these precautions the diagnosis may change in approximately 10%–15% of patients after the colonic and/or rectal specimen is examined by the histopathologist.

Therefore, it is important that restorative surgery should not be undertaken in the presence of a doubtful histological diagnosis. When the pathological changes are non-specific, and the diagnosis is of indeterminate colitis, it is safest first to perform a colectomy with ileostomy and a mucus fistula. If examination of the colectomy specimen shows no features of Crohn's disease and no signs of Crohn's disease become apparent in the next 12 months then it is safe to perform a restorative proctectomy with pouch to anus anastomosis.

Physiological measurement

Because most patients with ulcerative colitis have a long history and a continuous challenge of the anal sphincter complex with liquid stool and because in many the rectum has become contracted and fibrotic, the majority suffer from urgency and some even incontinence. Therefore, it is important always to perform physiological measurements of the ano-rectum before restorative operations. A weak anal sphincter complex is likely to result in minor to moderate degrees of faecal incontinence, which may make the operation unacceptable to the patient. Abnormal rectal compliance in patients with longstanding disease, even in the presence of rectal sparing contraindicates ileo-rectal anastomosis, as this will result in persistent diarrhoea or frequent defaecation.

Anal endosonography can outline morphological changes in the anal sphincter complex and can detect minor fluid collections and oedema resulting in widening of the intersphincteric space; changes that suggest a diagnosis of Crohn's disease and may have an important bearing on the choice of operation.

On our unit we employ the following plan of physiological measurement prior to restorative operations for inflammatory bowel disease.

Ano-rectal manometry

Ano-rectal manometry is performed using a low-compliance pneumohydraulic perfusion system (Arndorfer et al. 1977). The perfusion ports are spaced 0.5 cm apart and are connected to pressure transducers and a multi-channel chart recorder. Assessment is performed in the left lateral position and we make a station pullthrough pressure profile of the anal canal. Both resting and squeeze pressures are recorded. The presence or absence of recto-anal inhibitory response is also documented using a rectal balloon attached to the end of the manometric assembly. Rectal compliance is measured by placing a large inflatable balloon in the rectum connected to a small tube into the rectal lumen.

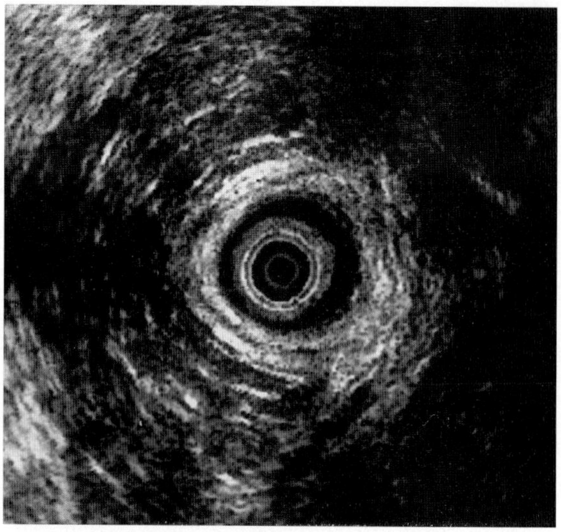

Fig. 22.1. Endo-anal ultrasound (EAU) showing normal morphology of the internal anal sphincter (IAS) and external anal sphincter (EAS).

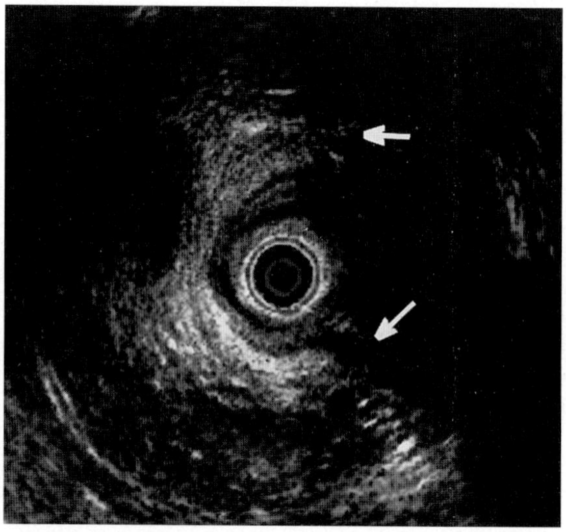

Fig. 22.2. EAU showing an anterior (A) defect in the internal anal sphincter (arrows) in a patient with chronic ulcerative colitis.

We also measure prolonged ambulant manometry for 24 hours in these patients to document the presence of spontaneous anal relaxation and rectal motor complexes.

Electromyography (EMG)

We make a concentric needle EMG of the external anal sphincter to assess spontaneous resting activity and motor unit potentials during voluntary squeeze. We have never recorded pudendal nerve terminal motor latencies before restorative proctocolectomy.

Endo-anal ultrasonography (EAU)

We always assess anal morphology by EAU before any anal anastomosis as it gives clear views of the morphology of the anal sphincter complex (Fig. 22.1). Also, it identifies deficiencies in the internal or external sphincter muscle (Fig. 22.2). These measurements are important because they identify patients who are likely to have problems with continence following restorative operations.

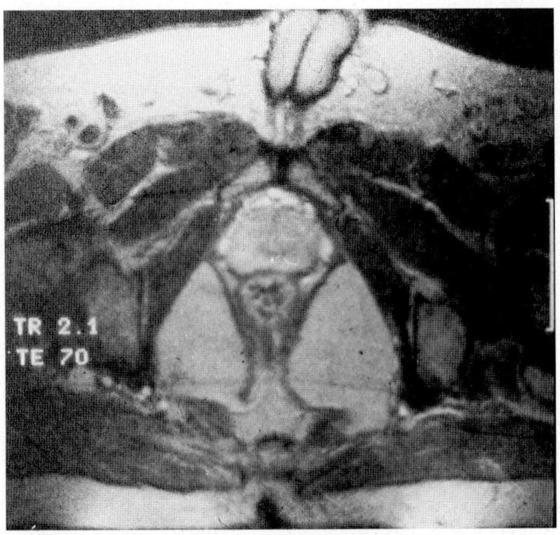

Fig. 22.3. Magnetic resonance (MR) image in the coronal plane showing a normal puborectal muscle and pelvic floor.

Cross-sectional imaging (MRI)

There is growing interest in magnetic resonance imaging of the pelvic floor to assess the morphology and measure various parameters such as the ano-rectal angle and perineal descent (Kruyt et al. 1991). Magnetic resonance imaging provides an accurate and clear picture of the pelvic floor morphology and its dynamics (Fig. 22.3, 22.4, 22.5). Magnetic resonance imaging is also able to depict the mobility of the posterior rectal wall and its descent during straining. Although our experience with this technique is limited I believe that MRI will prove useful in patient selection for restorative operations for inflammatory bowel disease.

Radioscintigraphic assessment

Ano-rectal function can also be measured using radioscintigraphy (O'Connell et al. 1987; Barkel et al. 1988). A Penrose drain connected to a catheter is used for this purpose. Technitium 99 is used as the radioisotope. The investigation is performed in the left lateral position. Isotope contrast is introduced into the Penrose drain via the connecting tube and gamma camera images obtained. The subject is asked to squeeze the drain, then to perform Valsalva manoeuvre without trying to defaecate the balloon and finally strain to expel the balloon. From the gamma camera images thus obtained an assessment of the ano-rectal angles is made. Others have also used scintigraphic assessment of rectal evacuation (O'Connell et al. 1986). In this investigation a known amount of a radioisotope is introduced into the rectum and the amount evacuated is

a

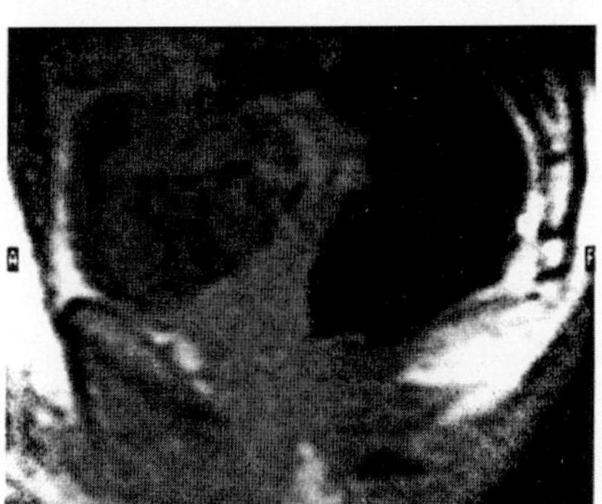

b

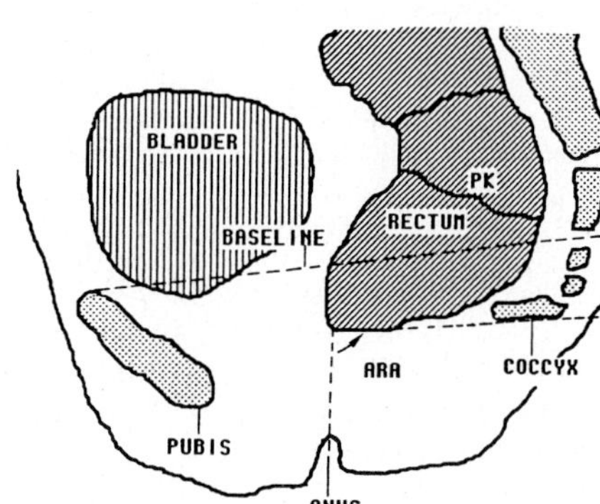

Fig. 22.4.a MR image obtained in the sagittal plane with gradient-echo pulse sequence with the patient at rest. A = anterior, P = posterior. **b** Schematic representation of a showing ano-rectal angle (ARA), baseline (junction line between cranial symphysis pubis and distal rectum) and plica of Kohlrausch (PK). (Reproduced from Kruyt et al. (1991) with permission.)

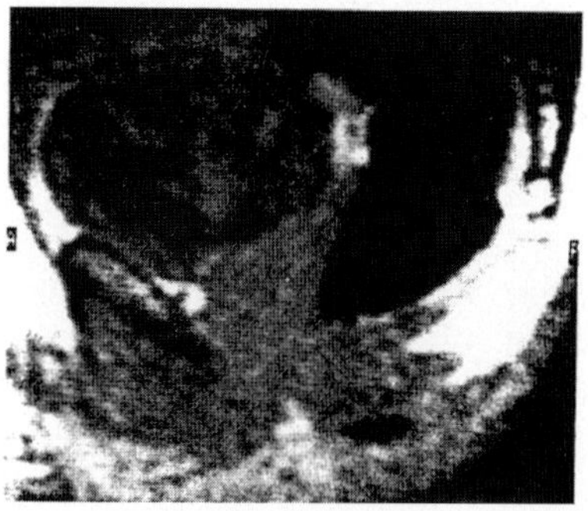

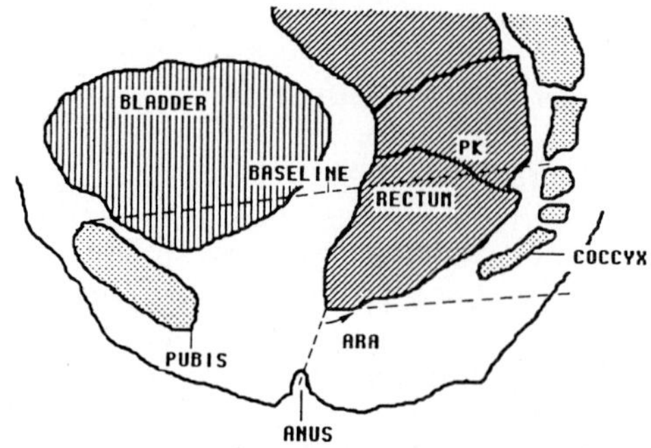

Fig. 22.5.a MR image of the same subject as in Fig. 22.4 during staining. **b** Schematic representation showing an increase in ARA and descent of the ano-rectal junction and plica of Kohlrausch (PK) in relation to the baseline. Note also the coccygeal descent during straining. (Reproduced from Kruyt et al. (1991) with permission.)

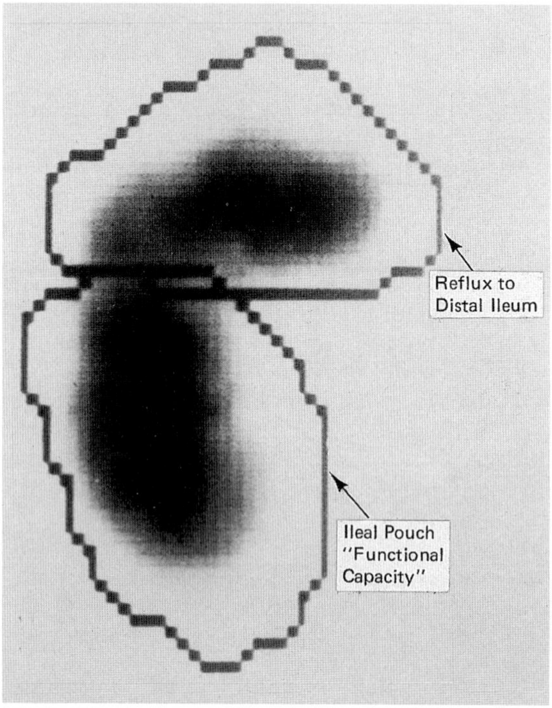

Fig. 22.6. Lateral scintigraphic scan of a patient with J pouch. Regions of interest outlined show ileal pouch "functional volume" and reflux into the distal ileum. (Reproduced from O'Connell et al. 1987 with permission.)

determined. The activity of the material evacuated is then compared with its activity before installation. Using this technique functional volumes of the rectum and the ileal pouch can also be obtained (Fig. 22.6).

Psychological assessment

A careful assessment of the patient's psychological status is extremely important. Only patients who are determined to avoid a stoma and are psychologically stable should be considered for restorative surgery. Similarly, adequate family support is vital in subsequent management of pouches. Patients who are emotionally unstable and psychologically disturbed are unsuitable for pouch surgery and should, therefore, be considered for panproctocolectomy and ileostomy. A detailed psychological assessment plan has been outlined in Chapter 4.

Preparation of the patient

Nutrition

During nutritional assessment (Chapter 3) particular attention is paid to hypoalbuminaemia, electrolyte imbalance and deficiency of minerals and folate. We always correct electrolyte imbalance and replenish the mineral deficiency before surgical intervention. If the patient is hypoalbuminaemic and malnourished nutritional supplements are given but total parenteral nutrition is rarely needed. The preferred route for enteral nutritional supplementation is via a fine-bore feeding tube. The patient may continue to require protein and calorie supplementation in the post-operative period, once the ileus has resolved.

Psychological

The psychological preparation of the patient is important and should include an open discussion with the patient and her/his family. A simple but detailed description of the disease and the treatment options should be given and the pros and cons of the different options explained and discussed. We always try to arrange for the patient to talk to someone who has undergone treatment for the same disease. This often helps them understand which procedure has been advised and why. It helps to alleviate anxieties about the operation. The patient should also be made aware of the impact of the operation on sexual function. We always counsel our female patients about pregnancy and advise them to have elective caesarian sections. For details of psychological preparation see Chapter 4.

Educational

Where possible patients should be given printed information, booklets, and/or videos explaining the procedure and possible complications and outcome of different surgical procedures. The help of illustrated material should be sought where possible to explain precisely what is involved in different operations. It helps to discuss various options after the patient has read booklets or printed material as it helps to dispel doubts that they might have about the operation.

Stoma marking

The involvement of the stoma therapy nurse specialist is invaluable. It is important that patients understand that they are to have either a temporary or permanent stoma. A visit by the stoma therapist is extremely helpful. We always ask the stoma therapist to visit the patient before operation. The stoma site should be clearly marked as badly sited stomas can lead to significant morbidity.

References

Arndorfer RC, Steff JJ, Dodds WJ, Linehan JH, Hogan WJ (1977) Improved infusion system for intraluminal oesophageal manometry. Gastroenterology 73:23–27

Barkel DC, Pemberton JH, Pezim ME, Phillips SF, Kelly KA, Brown ML (1988) Scintigraphic assessment of the anorectal angle in health and after ileal pouch-anal anastomosis. Ann Surg 208:42–49

Kruyt RH, Johannes BUM, Delemarre MD, Doornbos J, Vogel HJ (1991) Normal anorectum: : Dynamic MR imaging. Anat Radiol 179:153–163

O'Connell PR, Pemberton JH, Kelly KA (1987) Motor function of the ileal J pouch and its relation to clinical outcome after ileal pouch-anal anastomosis. World J Surg 11:735–741

O'Connell PR, Kelly KA, Brown ML (1986) Scintigraphic assessment of neorectal motor function. J Nucl Med 27:460–464

23 The Operation

D. Kumar

General consideration

Fluid and electrolyte balance are checked and corrected. If the patient is anaemic (haemoglobin less than 11 gm%) we usually transfuse at least 24 hours before operation. We cross match 2 units of blood unless we anticipate excessive losses such as in a difficult proctectomy.

Bowel preparation

We do not use any bowel preparation but the patients are advised to take a liquid only diet on the day before admission and continue on liquids until operation on the next day. In patients undergoing emergency surgery, no bowel preparation is used.

Antibiotics

We use intravenous metronidazole and a cephalosporin on induction and, if there is contamination, two further doses in the next 24 hours.

Position of the patient

Certain features are common to all operations for ulcerative colitis. The patient has a bladder catheter and a nasogastric tube. I prefer to perform these operations with the patient in the Lloyd Davis position, as it provides better access to the pelvis. Also an assistant can stand between the patient's legs to provide better retraction. Occasionally it is helpful for the assistant to push inward and upward with a fist in the perineum so that the abdominal surgeon can have better access to the pelvic floor.

Incision

A lower midline incision is made beginning at the symphysis pubis and extending above the umbilicus. Above the umbilicus I carry the incision slightly to the left towards the left subcostal margin as this provides optimum access to the splenic flexure. I incise the skin with a cutting diathermy which not only provides as neat a scar as opening by a scalpel incision, but also helps to minimise bleeding from the skin edges. The abdomen is opened in the midline along the entire length of the incision using a combination of cutting and coagulation diathermy and securing meticulous haemostasis of wound edges.

Total colectomy, ileostomy and mucus fistula

This is usually an urgent or emergency operation; it results in rapid improvement in the general health with minimal morbidity and it has the advantage that it leaves the options open for later restorative surgery.

Colectomy

After a full laparotomy, the colon is mobilised. The colon is usually friable and any rough

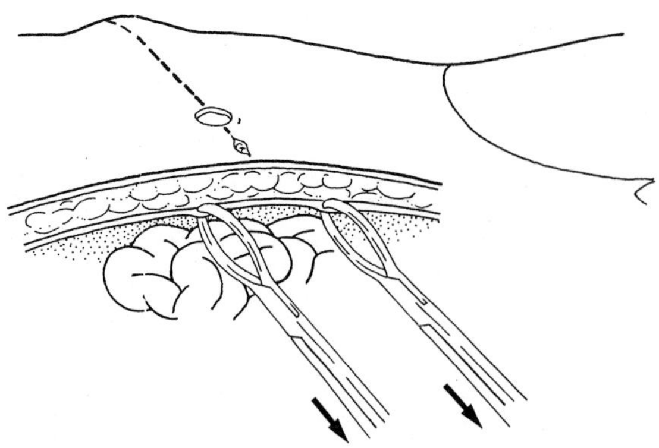

Fig. 23.1. Diagram showing that a disc of skin has been removed at the pre-marked stoma site. Note that the rectus sheath has been pulled medially by tissue forceps. (Repeat of Fig. 16.4)

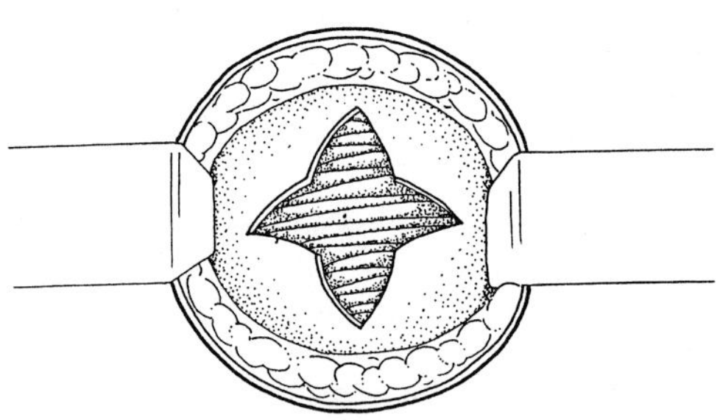

Fig. 23.2. A cruciate incision is made in the anterior rectus sheath. (Repeat of Fig. 16.5)

handling may perforate it and result in gross contamination. I use povidone-iodine-soaked gauze swabs to gently retract the colon and separate the tissue planes which are then cut by diathermy to minimise bleeding.

The splenic flexure is mobilised, preserving the spleen and the omentum. If the colon is entered inadvertently then every effort must be made to minimise contamination of the peritoneal cavity.

The colonic vessels are divided close to the bowel wall. The terminal ileum is divided between handle-less crushing clamps placed as close to the ileo-caecal valve as possible. The distal colon is divided between crushing clamps sufficiently proximal to the recto-sigmoid junction so that the end can be brought out as a mucus fistula. I take care not to devascularise the distal sigmoid and upper rectum as I have found this complication to be the commonest cause of collections in the left iliac fossa, because ischaemia leads to necrosis of the colon and/or rectum. I bring out the mucus fistula at the lower end of the main abdominal wound rather than as a separate stoma. I do not drain the peritoneal cavity unless there is faecal contamination during the procedure in which case I leave a suction drain in the left paracolic gutter.

Ileostomy

A 2 cm disc of skin is excised with cutting diathermy at the marked stoma site. The cylinder of subcutaneous fat is excised down to the anterior rectus sheath with cutting diathermy and maintaining meticulous haemostasis. Two retractors are placed to retract the skin and subcutaneous tissues to provide a clear view of the anterior rectus sheath (Fig. 23.1). A cruciate incision is made in the anterior rectus sheath with coagulation diathermy to expose the underlying rectus muscle (Fig. 23.2). The fibres of the rectus muscle are gently separated. The underlying peritoneum and posterior rectus sheath are pushed up with a large curved closed artery clip and held with a tissue forceps from above (Fig. 23.3). The peritoneum is

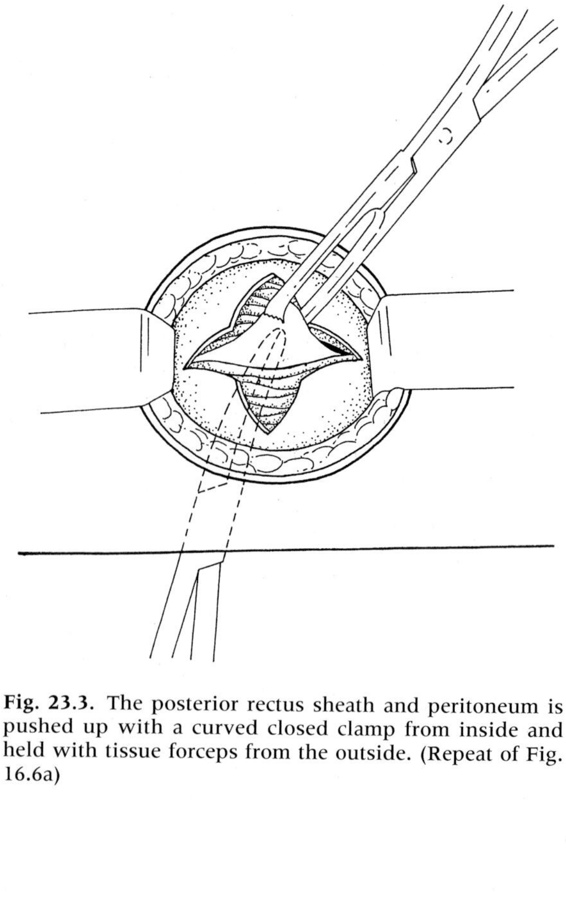

Fig. 23.3. The posterior rectus sheath and peritoneum is pushed up with a curved closed clamp from inside and held with tissue forceps from the outside. (Repeat of Fig. 16.6a)

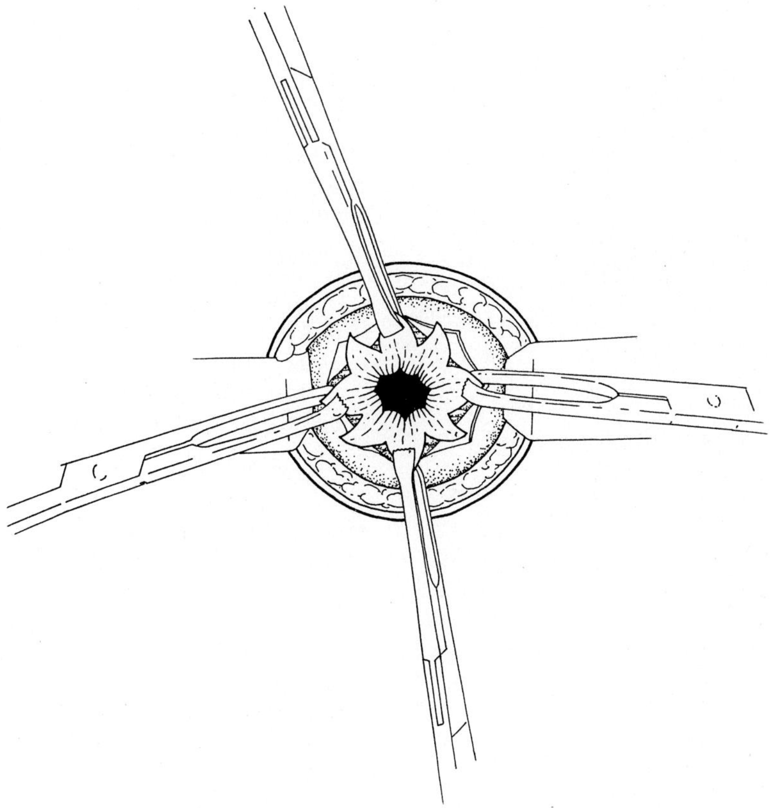

Fig. 23.4. The posterior rectus sheath is incised and the edges held by four tissue forceps. (Repeat of Fig. 16.7)

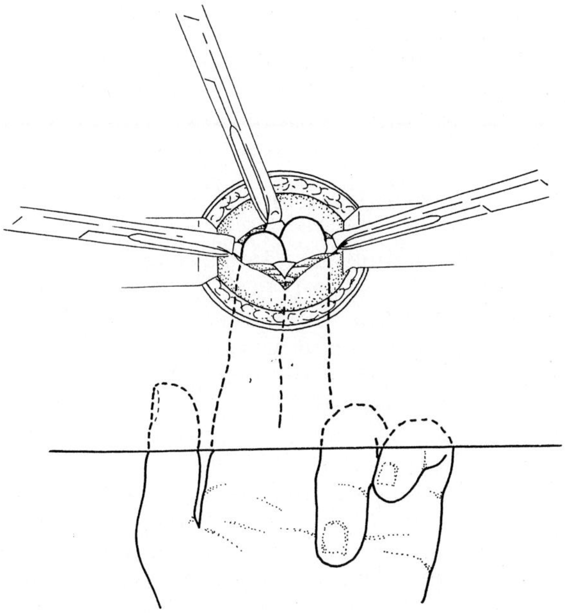

Fig. 23.5. The opening in the posterior rectus sheath admits two fingers. (Repeat of Fig. 16.8)

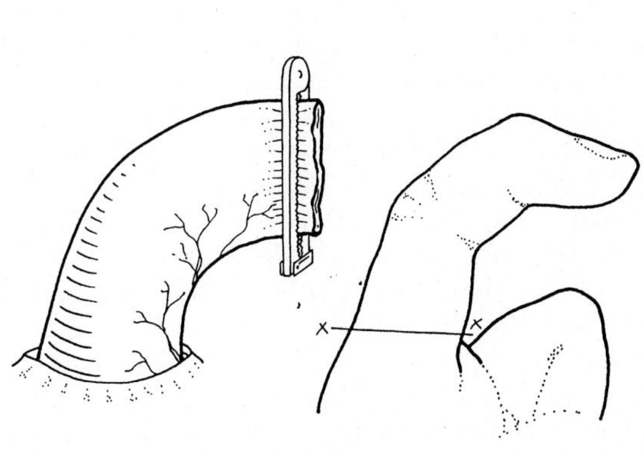

Fig. 23.6. The length of the ileum delivered through the abdominal wall roughly corresponds to the length of the index finger. (Repeat of Fig. 16.9)

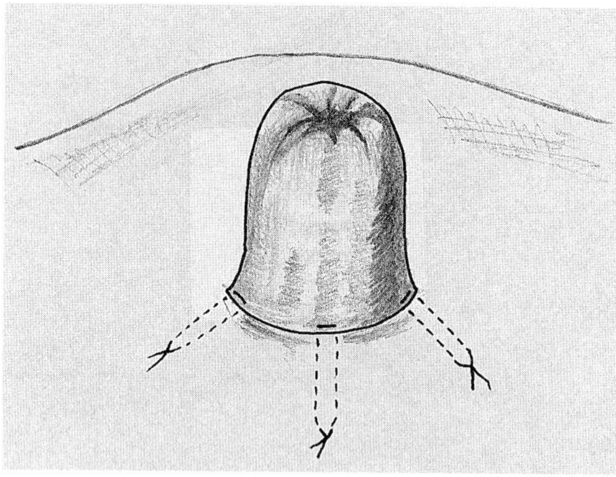

Fig. 23.7. An everted ileostomy stoma.

incised between two tissue forceps in a cruciate fashion (Fig. 23.4) and the edges held with four tissue forceps. The opening should not admit more than two fingers (Fig. 23.5). The ileal end is then delivered through the opening of the abdominal wall, making sure that approximately 5 cm of the distal end projects above the skin surface and is not under tension; a rough guide is the length of index finger of the operator (Fig. 23.6). The ileum is then anchored to the peritoneal edges, held by the tissue forceps, using 2/0 Polyglactin sutures between the peritoneal edge and seromuscular layer of the ileum. In my experience sutures placed in four quadrants are enough to anchor the ileum. The ileal end should be checked for viability, making sure that the blood supply has not been compromised during the anchoring procedure. To avoid contamination of the abdominal wound, the abdomen is closed before the ileostomy is everted and sutured to the skin.

I close the abdominal wound in a single layer using two lengths of number 1 Prolene on a large needle. I close the skin with 3/0 subcuticular Prolene and seal the wound with a plastic spray. The crushing clamp is now taken off the ileum and a tissue forceps is introduced through the lumen of the ileum and the end everted to form a spout measuring 2–3 cm (Fig. 23.7). The ileal mucosal edge is sutured to the cut edge of the skin using 5 to 6, 4/0 Prolene sutures placed circumferentially. A transparent stoma appliance should be then applied so that the stoma can be inspected to assess its viability.

Post-operative care

I usually continue nasograstic drainage and intravenous fluids until obvious intestinal contents appear in the ileostomy bag. This usually takes 48–72 hours. The presence of both gas and healthy ileal effluent suggests resolution of post-operative ileus and at this stage patients are commenced on oral intake. The passage of small amounts of liquid in the ileostomy bag may be misleading and should not be taken as evidence of a functioning stoma. Those on steroids before operation continue until satisfactory recovery when they are gradually reduced over 2–6 weeks.

Panproctocolectomy and ileostomy

The prefix "pan" implies the simultaneous removal of the colon, the rectum and the anal canal. This procedure is only performed in patients who are judged unsuitable for restorative proctocolectomy. The patient is positioned in the Lloyd Davis position and the buttocks are elevated on a sandbag to provide easy access to the anal canal. The anal margin is cleaned with povidone-iodine skin preparation and then the anal canal is occluded by a 2/0 silk purse-string suture. After preparing the abdominal skin the abdominal cavity is opened through a long lower midline incision as described previously.

Colonic mobilisation

The colon is mobilised in a similar manner to the operation of sub-total colectomy, ileostomy and mucus fistula. I make every effort to preserve the greater omentum and use it to fill the pelvic cavity at the end of the operation. The greater omentum is dissected free of the transverse colon and splenic flexure. Colonic blood vessels are divided close to the colonic wall. The splenic and hepatic flexures are mobilised taking care not to damage the spleen on the left side and the duodenum and the ureter on the right. I prefer to do the operation by sharp dissection using diathermy rather than finger mobilisation which tends to tear tissues. The ileum is divided between two crushing clamps as close to the ileo-caecal valve as possible.

Mobilisation of the rectum

I prefer to mobilise the rectum after the colon has been fully mobilised. The peritoneum on either side of the upper rectum is incised and this peritoneal incision is joined anteriorly in the recto-vesical or recto-vaginal pouch. At this stage it is important to identify the pelvic nerves as it is easy to enter the wrong plane and damage the nerve inadvertently. I ligate and divide the inferior mesenteric artery and vein away from its origin as I believe that it is at this stage the pelvic nerves are usually damaged. The plane between the pelvic nerves and the mesorectum is identified and followed in the pelvic cavity. The dissection is carried forwards around the mesorectum preserving the pelvic nerves all the time. I am aware of the arguments for staying close to the rectal wall but I believe that with care and attention damage to the pelvic nerves can be avoided in every case and the operation performed much more easily by staying in a relatively bloodless plane. The dissection is carried down in this plane to the pelvic floor. In my experience it is almost never necessary to ligate the lateral ligaments. I usually coagulate the vessels and divide them or simply divide them and pack with dry gauze whilst I do the same on the other side. The dissection is now carried into the intersphincteric plane from above by putting gentle traction on the rectum to open up the plane. At this stage it often helps if the perineal assistant pushes the perineum up with one hand and retracts the vagina and/or bladder with the other. I believe that most of this operation can be done from above, the advantage being that it leaves a small perineal wound which heals quickly without any problem. Using this technique I have never come across the problem of a non-healing or delayed healing perineal wound. After most of the dissection has been performed from above the perineal dissection is begun.

The perineal dissection

The skin is incised using cutting diathermy and staying close to the purse-string suture applied at the anal margin. The dissection is carried upwards in the intersphincteric plane avoiding damage to the external anal sphincter. As mentioned earlier, the perineal dissection often only involves incising the skin and carrying the dissection in the intersphincteric space for approximately 2 cm, when the plane of dissection from above can be met and the specimen removed from the abdominal end. After the specimen has been removed the levators are approximated with interrupted 0 chromic catgut sutures. The omentum is brought down by the abdominal operator to fill the pelvic cavity as much as possible so that loops of small bowel do not fall into the pelvis. The wound is washed with povidone-iodine solution before closing the skin. The skin is then closed with interrupted 3/0 Prolene sutures. I leave a suction drain in the pelvic cavity. An ileostomy is fashioned in the same way as described earlier and the abdominal wound closed with continuous Prolene in a single layer.

Post-operative care

The patient is maintained on intravenous fluids and nasogastric drainage until the ileostomy stoma starts to pass gas as well as ileal contents. Oral intake is commenced at this stage. The drain is left in place until the drainage is less than 25 ml in 24 hours. The patient is fully mobilised and then the urinary catheter is removed. I have seen bladder problems following this procedure. One patient needed re-catheterisation and transurethral resection of the prostate because of an enlarged prostate gland. I have not witnessed problems with a non-healing or delayed healing perineal wound. Some surgeons leave the perineal wound open, but I believe that this simply prolongs the hospital stay and has an adverse effect on the patient's psychology.

Ileo-rectal anastomosis

In patients whose rectum is relatively disease-free, an ileo-rectal anastomosis is performed. It must be emphasised at this stage that it is not simply the absence of ulceration or inflammation of the rectum that constitues an indication for ileo-rectal anastomosis. The rectum must also be free of the sequelae of previous chronic inflammation, such as fibrosis, strictures and impaired distensibility of the rectum. All these factors should be excluded by a careful pre-operative ano-rectal physiological assessment.

The abdomen is opened through a long lower midline incision and a full laparotomy performed.

Colectomy

The colon is mobilised as described previously. The colonic vessels are divided close to the bowel wall. The ileum is divided between two crushing clamps placed close to the ileocaecal valve to preserve as much of the terminal ileum as possible. The colon is divided at the recto-sigmoid junction near the sacral promontory. After clamping the colonic end to avoid spillage into the peritoneal cavity, the specimen is removed. The rectum is sucked empty of its contents. Any bleeding points at the cut edge of the rectum are controlled by coagulation diathermy.

The anastomosis

Inevitably there is a size discrepancy between the ileal lumen and the rectal lumen. For this reason many surgeons prefer to perform either an end-to-side anastomosis or a double-stapled ileo-rectal anastomosis. In my experience these techniques make subsequent follow-up more difficult and, therefore, I prefer to use an end-to-end hand sewn anastomosis as described below.

The ileal end is cleaned to excise the crushed tissue under the crushing clamp and any bleeding points controlled with coagulation diathermy. A soft clamp is placed approximately 15 cm away from the cut end to prevent spillage of ileal contents. Care should be taken not to obliterate the blood supply to the ileum by placing the clamp on the mesentry. Only the ileal lumen should be occluded. A 1–1.5 cm incision along the anti mesenteric border of the ileum helps to remove the size discrepancy between the ileum and the rectum. I prefer to perform a single layer extra-mucosal seromuscular anastomosis using 2/0 Polyglactin interrupted sutures anteriorly and a continuous seromuscular 2/0 Polyglactin stitch posteriorly. The mucosa is left unstitched. Two seromuscular stay stitches are placed at either end (Fig.23.8). The posterior layer is completed first, taking seromuscular bites approximately 5 mm apart making sure that there is no purse-stringing of the posterior layer. The posterior layer suture is tied when the second stay suture is reached. The anterior layer is now completed using interrupted 2/0 Polyglactin stitches taking seromuscular bites and leaving the mucosa unstitched (Fig. 23.9). The entire anastomosis can be performed using a continuous seromuscular stitch but I

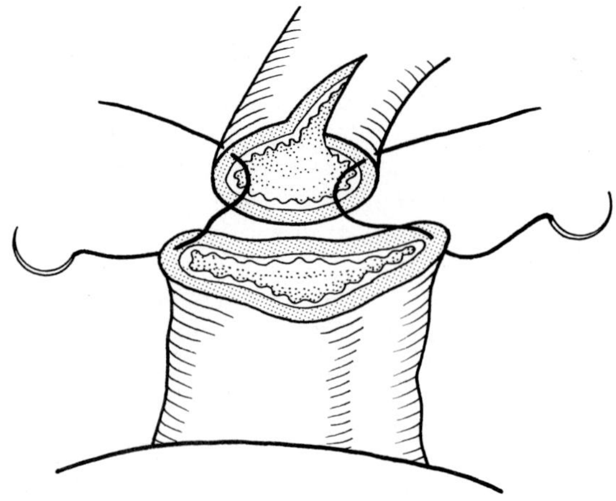

Fig. 23.8. Diagram showing an incision along the anti-mesenteric border to eliminate the discrepancy between the ileal and rectal lumen.

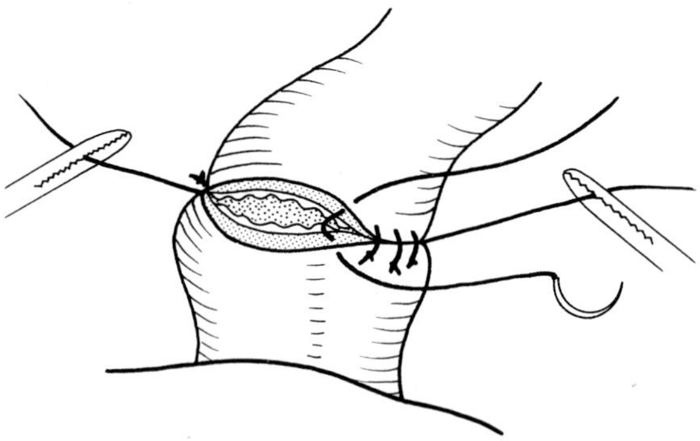

Fig. 23.9. Diagram showing a completed posterior continuous layer of ileo-rectal anastomosis and the beginning of an interrupted anterior layer.

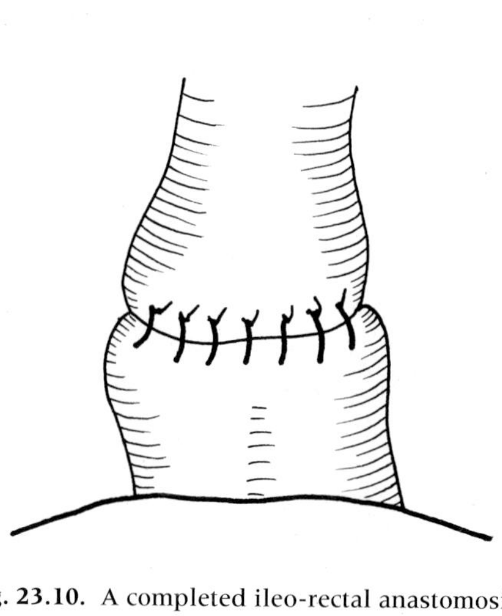

Fig. 23.10. A completed ileo-rectal anastomosis.

prefer to use an interrupted anterior layer as it prevents purse-stringing of the anastomosis. This is particularly important for the relatively inexperienced surgeon who is still in the learning phase. The interrupted stitches are placed approximately 5 mm apart (Fig. 23.10). I do not check the anastomosis with air insufflation at the end of the procedure because I believe it does not serve any useful purpose. I do not routinely cover an ileo-rectal anastomosis with an ileostomy.

Post-operative care

Intravenous fluids and electrolytes and continuous nasogastric drainage are maintained in the post-operative period. When signs of resolution of post-operative ileus are evident in the form of passage of flatus and stool, oral intake is commenced. Following an ileo-rectal anastomosis the patient often has diarrhoea in the early post-operative period and for this reason even if oral fluids are being taken, intravenous fluid and electrolyte therapy is maintained until the bowel frequency has settled to a more reasonable and acceptable level. Codeine phosphate or loperamide given orally often helps to reduce the stool frequency. Gradually the consistency of the stool starts to thicken and by about 10–14 days the patient starts to pass a semi-solid stool.

The continent ileostomy

In this operation a reservoir for storage of ileal contents is fashioned from the terminal ileum. At the outlet of the reservoir there is a nipple valve which ends in a flush stoma on the lower abdominal wall. The nipple valve prevents the escape of ileal contents and gas from the reservoir. The patient must intubate the reservoir three or four times a day to empty the contents. As mentioned previously the operation may be performed as a primary procedure or as a secondary procedure when the restorative proctocolectomy has failed, or when the patient wants a previous end ileostomy converted to a continent stoma. Patients who have had previous small bowel resections are unsuitable for this operation as are those who are emotionally and psychologically unstable.

No special pre-operative bowel preparation is needed. The patient is given prophylactic antibiotics intravenously in the form of metronidazole and cephalosporin. If the operation is carried out as a primary procedure the patient is placed in the Lloyd Davis position. When the operation is carried out as a second operation the procedure is performed in the supine position. A lower midline incision extending above the umbilicus is used. A previous ileostomy when present is taken down.

Formation of a reservoir

Approximately 12 cm of the distal ileum is left free for construction of the nipple valve and the stoma. In obese subjects a slightly longer length of the ileum may be needed for this purpose. A U loop of ileum is formed using 15 cm for each limb of the U. Two stay sutures are placed at the top and bottom end of the U loop to approximate the antimesenteric borders. The loop is opened along the antimesenteric border on both sides down to the mucosa using a cutting diathermy. A seromuscular continuous 3/0 Polyglactin suture forms the posterior suture line of the reservoir (Fig. 23.11). Now the mucosa is incised along the previous seromuscular incision. The cut

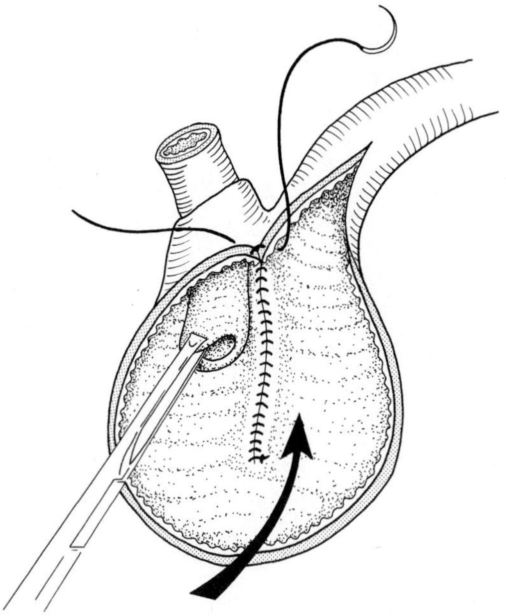

Fig. 23.11. Completed posterior layer of the pouch with invagination of the efferent loop as a nipple valve. Arrow shows how flap is folded over to complete pouch.

edge of the mucosa covers the posterior suture line and is left unstitched. A 1 cm wide strip of Prolene mesh soaked in povidone-iodine is brought through an opening in the mesentry close to the ileal wall at the base of the nipple valve limb. This is for later application around the base of the nipple valve.

Formation of the nipple valve

A Babcock forceps is passed up the valve limb and the bowel wall grasped to partially intussuscept the ileal segment into the lumen of the reservoir. The intussuscepted valve should be approximately 4–5 cm long and forms the future valve. The nipple is then fixed in position by applying a TA55 stapler. Alternatively a GIA stapler (without blade) may be used (Fig. 23.12). Four such applications are performed to maintain the nipple valve (Fig. 23.13). Long-term results with a hand-sewn nipple valve and stapled valve as described above compare favourably. The stapled valve does not run a higher risk of stenosis or slippage.

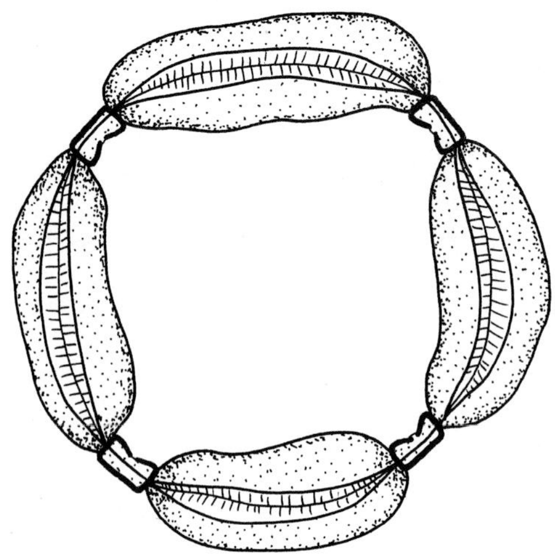

Fig. 23.13. Cross-section through the nipple valve showing four rows of staples.

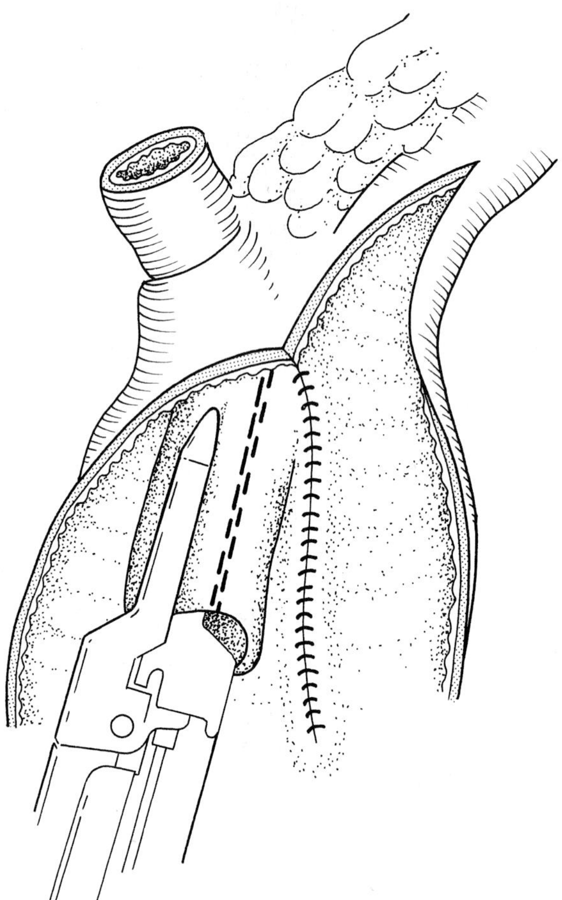

Fig. 23.12. Application of GIA stapler to prevent sliding of the nipple valve.

Completion of the reservoir

The opened reservoir is now folded and sutured with a continuous seromuscular 3/0 Polyglactin suture, similar to the formation of a reservoir in restorative proctocolectomy. The Prolene mesh is now positioned around the base of the outlet of the reservoir like a cylinder and the ends of the mesh are sutured together with non-absorbable sutures. Approximately half of the width of this cylinder is now embedded between the intussuscepted walls of the ileum forming the nipple valve.

Formation of the stoma

A trephine opening is made in the skin at a previously marked site for the ileostomy. The inner or peritoneal opening of the trephine hole should admit two fingers. The reservoir is placed underneath the trephine opening and the remaining visible part of the Prolene mesh is sutured to the rectus sheath using interrupted sutures. Care should be exercised at this stage to prevent obstruction to blood supply of the nipple. A stoma is now created flush with the skin level using mucocutaneous stitches. At the end of the procedure a tube drain is left in the reservoir for continuous drainage. The abdominal wound is closed with Prolene and the skin with a subcuticular running Prolene stitch.

Post-operative management

Intravenous fluids are administered until intestinal contents start draining through the drain in the reservoir. The reservoir itself is irrigated with 20 ml of saline three or four times a day until the flow of intestinal contents is well established. At this stage the catheter is removed and the patient is taught the technique of self-catheterisation approximately six to eight times a day initially and three or four times a day subsequently. The patients are instructed to irrigate the reservoir at least once a day. No special dietary instructions are required and the patients are followed-up jointly with a stoma nurse in the out-patient clinic.

Restorative proctocolectomy

The original operation as described by Parks and colleagues in 1980 was a triplicated or S-shaped reservoir with a long efferent limb. Since then, other pouch designs have been used, those commonly employed are a duplicated or J-shaped reservoir (Utsunomiya et al. 1980) and a 4-loop W pouch (Nicholls and Lubowski 1987). These pouches can be either hand sewn or stapled and use between 30 and 50 cm of terminal ileum. The operation of ileo-anal anastomosis is still under development. Initially the rectum was transected 10 cm above the pelvic floor and a trans-anal mucosectomy was performed by a complex and tedious dissection down to the dentate line (Parks and Nicholls 1978; Williams and Johnson 1985). More recently the rectum has been transected at the level of the pelvic floor leaving very little or no diseased mucosa to be removed (Nicholls and Lubowski 1987). The exact level of ileo-anal anastomosis is also controversial. Some authors argue that the anal transition zone just above the dentate line should be preserved to allow sensory discrimination (Martin et al. 1985; Keighley et al. 1987a). The functional results following different pouch designs show slight variations. It is generally believed that the bigger the pouch size the better the function. However, this remains controversial as people using pouch designs with a smaller capacity report equally good results.

The operation

As a matter of personal preference I use the triplicated or S reservoir without a spout. No pre-operative bowel cleansing is used. The patient is given prophylactic antibiotics in the form of intravenous metronidazole and a cephalosporin. Subcutaneous heparin 5000 units twice daily as anticoagulation prophylaxis is also given.

Position of the patient

The procedure is performed in the Lloyd Davis position with a foam wedge under the buttocks and a head-down tilt.

Incision

A long lower midline incision extending above the umbilicus is used. The skin incision above the umbilicus is directed towards the left subcostal margin. I believe that this facilitates the mobilisation of the splenic flexure. The peritoneal cavity is opened along the entire length of the incison. A complete laparotomy is performed. The mucus fistula, when present is taken down.

Proctocolectomy

The steps for colonic mobilisation are the same as described previously. The rectum is mobilised using the plane between the mesorectum and the pelvic nerves. Special care is taken not to damage the pelvic nerves which run posterior to the inferior mesenteric artery near its origin and then divide into two separate trunks just above the sacral promontory. These nerves are carefully preserved and the relatively bloodless plane anterior to these nerves is followed down to the pelvic floor. The rectum is mobilised along the lateral pelvic walls and anteriorly after incising the pelvic peritoneum. Care is taken not to damage the seminal vesicles and vas deferens in males and the vagina in females. The dissection is carried down to the pelvic floor until a supple tube of muscle is reached and then the

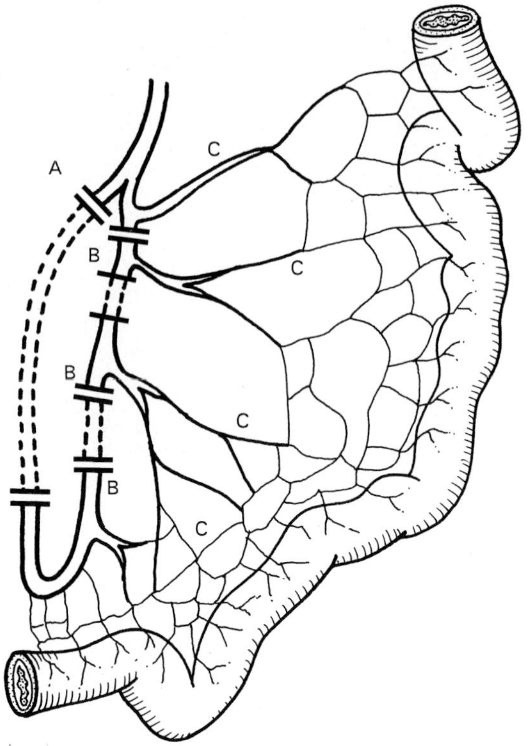

Fig. 23.14. Vascular mobilisation: A, ileo-colic artery divided; B, ileal artery divided; C, alternative route for blood.

dissection continued gently in the intersphincteric space. Using this technique the rectum and the upper anal canal can be mobilised from above. The lower end of the rectum is now clamped with a right-angled clamp and the anterior wall of the upper anal canal incised to place a purse-string suture for subsequent stapled anastomosis. The anal canal is incised as the purse-string suture is advanced and finally the specimen is removed and the purse-string completed. The pelvic cavity is now packed with gauze and attention diverted to formation of the reservoir.

Formation of the reservoir

An ileostomy when present is taken down and the mesenteric blood vessels are inspected against a bright light. The object is to obtain enough length on the blood vessels so that the reservoir can comfortably reach the upper anal canal without putting tension on blood vessels. Judicial division of blood vessels often achieves this objective (Fig. 23.14). I have never abandoned the procedure because of lack of length on the blood vessels. I prefer to use three 10 cm loops of ileum as shown in Fig. 23.15a. The loops are approximated by two stay sutures at the apex and bottom of the future reservoir. The antimesenteric bor- der of the S-shaped loop is now incised with cutting diathermy down to the mucosa (Fig. 23.15b). Beginning at the open end of the ileum a continuous seromuscular 3/0 Polyglactin stitch is applied to suture the posterior layer of the distal two limbs of the S reservoir (Fig. 23.15c). A similar continuous seromuscular stitch is applied to suture the posterior part of the proximal two limbs of the S up to the afferent limb (Fig. 23.15d). The mucosa is now incised and left unstitched to cover the seromuscular suture lines. The inside of the pouch is cleaned with povidone-iodine and any obvious bleeding points are cauterised.

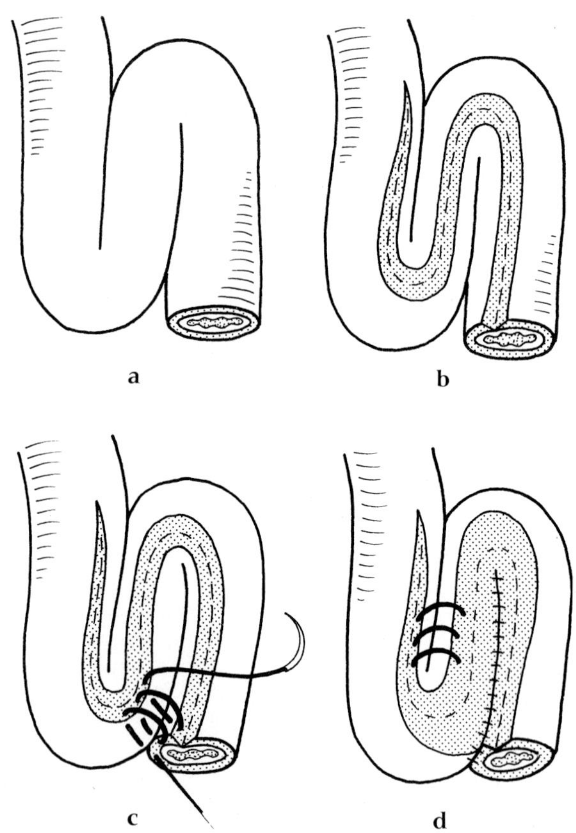

Fig. 23.15.a Diagram showing three loops of ileum (10 cm each) brought together in the shape of an S without a spout. **b** The antimesenteric border of the S loop has been incised down to the mucosa. **c** Beginning of the continuous suture of the layer of the distal two limbs. **d** The proximal limb suture line now begun.

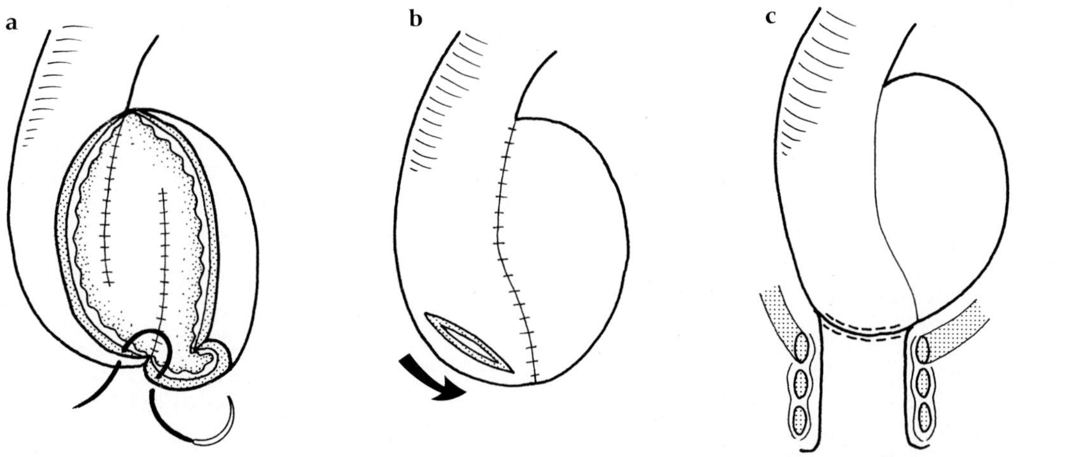

Fig. 23.16. **a** Diagram showing the beginning of the suture line for the anterior layer of the pouch. **b** A small hole, away from the suture line, is made in the proximal limb of the pouch. **c** Completed pouch-anal stapled anastomosis.

Once again beginning at the cut end of the ileum approximately seven or eight interrupted seromuscular 3/0 Polyglactin stitches are placed near the distal end of the pouch (Fig. 23.16a). The rest of the anterior layer of the reservoir is sutured using a 3/0 Polyglactin seromuscular stitch. When the anterior layer is half-complete the head of the staple gun is introduced into the pouch and positioned in the proximal limb of the reservoir away from the suture line through a small hole in the wall of the ileum (Fig. 23.16b). A purse-string suture is applied around this puncture hole to avoid tearing of ileal muscle during the anastomosis. The anterior suture line is now completed and the reservoir is ready to be brought down to the pelvis for ileo-anal anastomosis. The pelvic packs are removed and the pelvis is checked for haemostasis.

The anastomosis (Fig. 23.16c)

A size 31 EEA premier circular stapling gun without the head is now introduced through the anus and the purse-string stitch tied around the anvil. The head is now clicked into position making sure that the mesentry is not caught within the staple gun. The gun is now gradually approximated and fired when the green colour is visible through the window at the bottom of the gun handle. The gun head is opened by rotating the handle anticlockwise for two or three turns and the instrument is gently withdrawn through the anal canal. The assistant now checks the two tissue rings to make sure that they are complete. The abdominal operator gently checks the anastomosis for any invisible gaps. It is my practice not to check the anastomosis for air-tightness. A suction drain is positioned in the pelvis behind the pouch.

A double-staple anastomosis has been described in which the upper anal canal is stapled with a TA30 stapler (Fig. 23.17), the

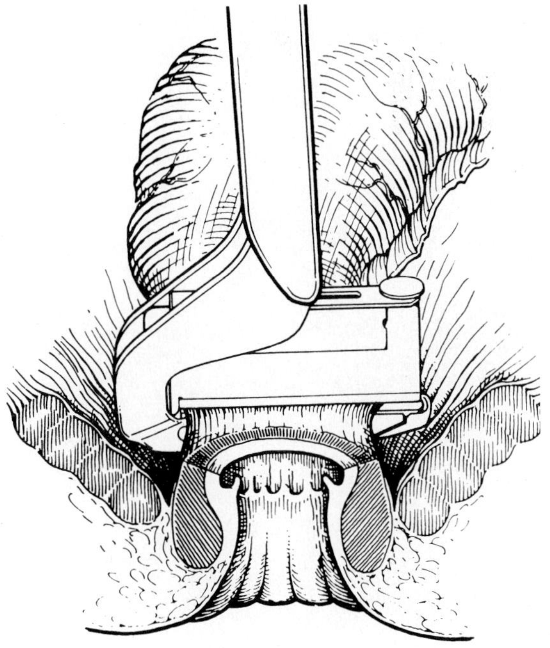

Fig. 23.17. Stapled transection of the upper anal canal using the TA30 stapler. (From Kmiot and Keighley 1989 with permission.)

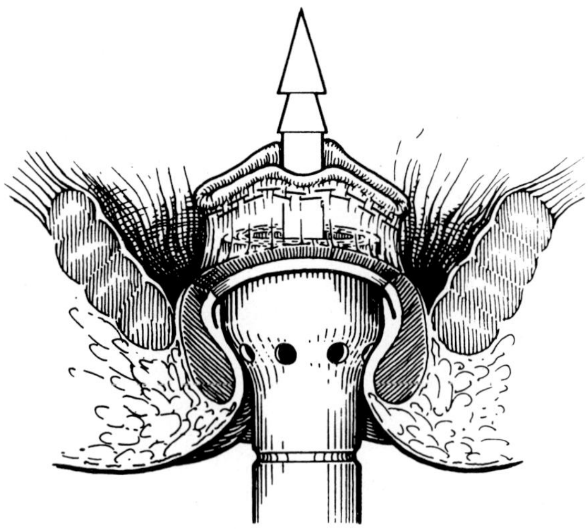

Fig. 23.18. Insertion of the central pin attached to the instrument head through the staple line of the previous transected anal canal. (From Kmiot and Keighley (1989) with permission.)

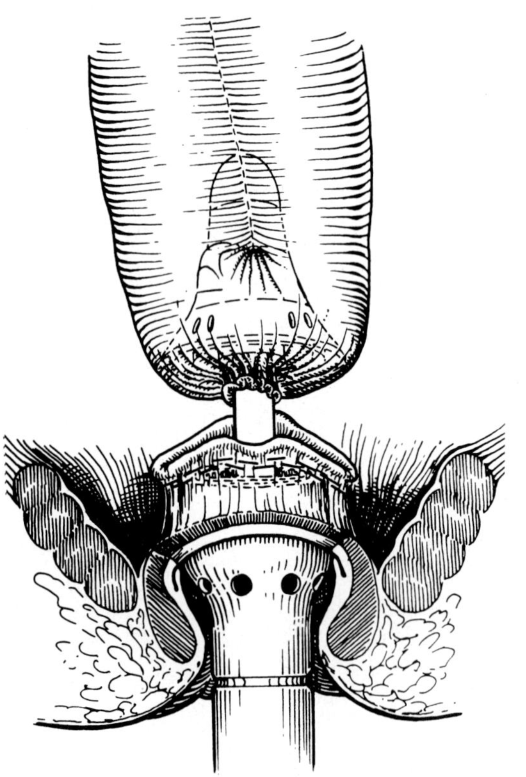

Fig. 23.19. Advancement of the anvil pin into the hollow end of the main instrument, thereby joining the pouch to the anal canal. (From Kmiot and Keighley (1989) with permission.)

central pin of a circular stapling instrument is introduced through the staple line (Fig. 23.18) and the anvil advanced into the hollow end of the main instrument to complete the anastomosis (Fig. 23.19). I believe that using this technique, there is greater risk of leaving diseased rectal mucosa behind.

Covering stoma

It is my practice to cover all ileal pouch-anal anastomoses with a loop ileostomy. The same hole used by the previous end ileostomy is used for the covering stoma. The stoma is raised as close to the pouch as possible. Occasionally because of the problems with length of blood vessels it is not possible to place a stoma close to the pouch. Under these circumstances the loop stoma is fashioned as close to the pouch as is practically feasible. A loop of ileum is brought through the trephine hole in the abdominal wall with a stitch to mark either the proximal or the distal limb (Fig. 23.20). The abdominal wound is now closed in single layer using a continuous Prolene stitch. The skin is closed with a subcuticular Prolene suture. The ileostomy is now opened with a diathermy and the proximal limb everted using a tissue-holding forceps (Fig. 23.21). Mucocutaneous sutures are applied using 4/0 Prolene and an ileostomy appliance is placed around the stoma at the end of the procedure.

Some authors have argued that it is not necessary to perform a covering ileostomy (Matikainen et al. 1990; Winslet et al. 1991). The reason usually advanced is that the covering loop ileostomy itself is a source of significant morbidity. Winslet et al. (1991) have reported a 41% and 30% complication rate with the formation and closure of loop ileostomy in a prospective series of 34 patients. In my experience most of the reported complications with covering stomata are technical and can be avoided by a meticulous surgical technique.

Post-operative management

The pelvic drain is left in situ until the drainage is less than 25 ml per day. The patients are given intravenous fluids and electrolytes until the covering stoma starts to function. Once the patient is taking nutrients orally, instructions are given regarding stoma care and change of stoma appliances. When

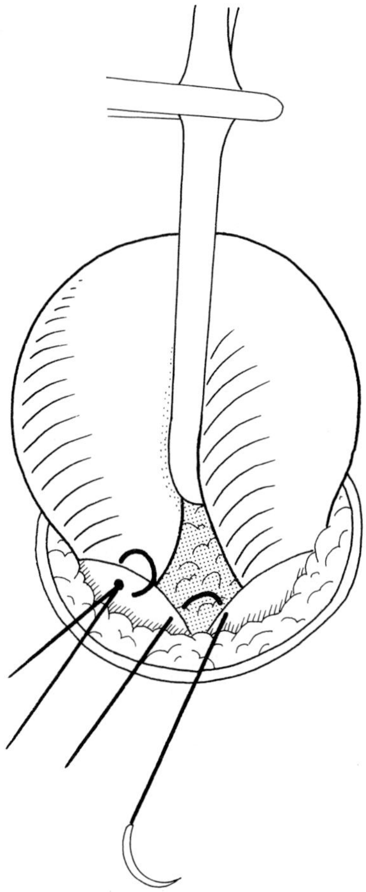

Fig. 23.20. A loop of ileum as close to the pouch as possible is pulled up through a trephine hole in the anterior abdominal wall. Note that the distal end is marked with a stitch.

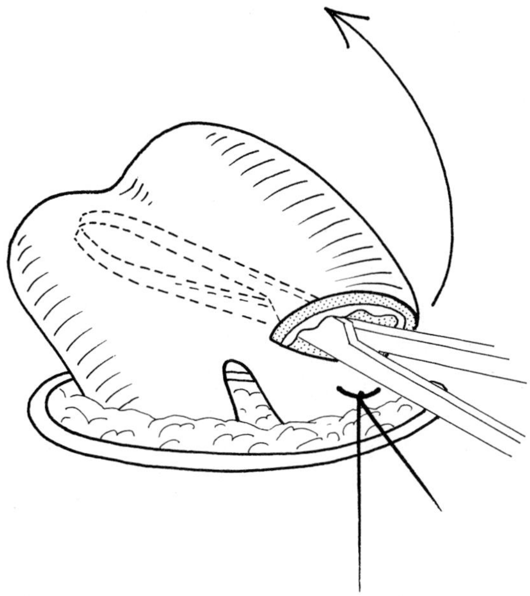

Fig. 23.21. The ileal loop is opened transversely with the diathermy and the proximal end everted with a tissue forceps to form a spout.

the patient is confident with the use and care of the stoma, he or she is allowed to leave hospital with arrangements to attend an out-patient clinic. It is my practice to perform a pouchogram (Fig. 23.22) at approximately six weeks post-operatively. The purpose is to check for minor leaks that may be present as small sinuses and also to see the position of the pouch in the pelvis. If the pouchogram is satisfactory then the ileostomy is closed at 8-10 weeks following the first operation.

Closure of ileostomy

The stoma is mobilised by cutting around the stoma at the mucocutaneous junction with a cutting diathermy. Now the loop is mobilised with a combination of blunt and sharp dissection down to the rectus sheath. Two

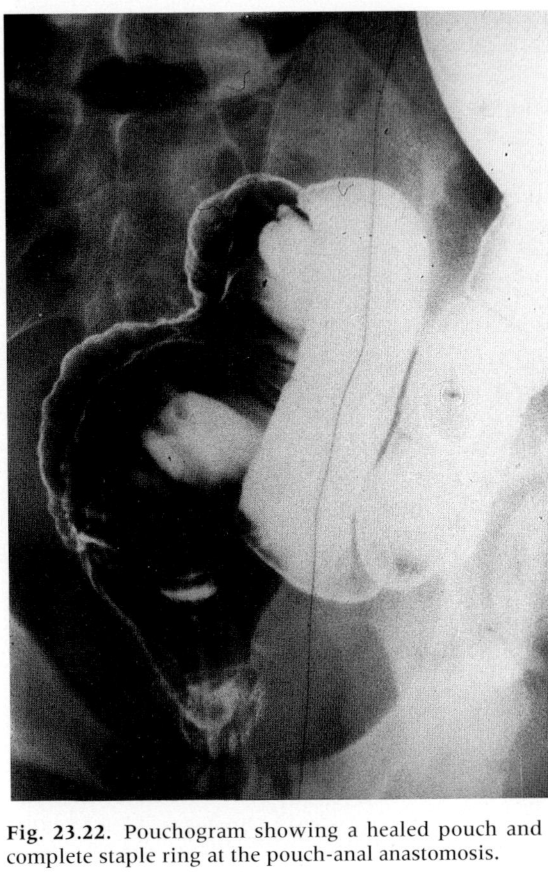

Fig. 23.22. Pouchogram showing a healed pouch and a complete staple ring at the pouch-anal anastomosis.

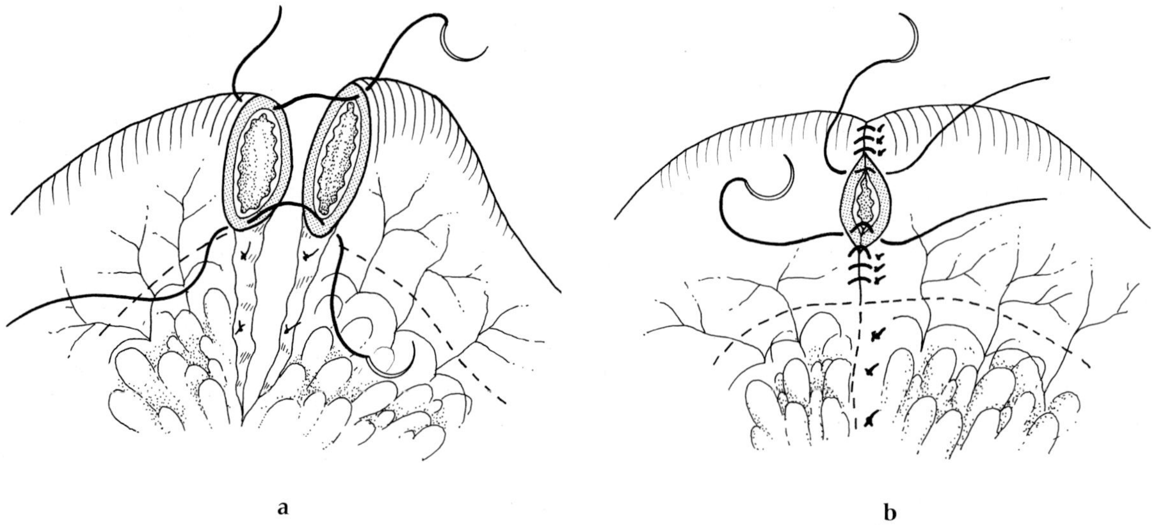

Fig. 23.23. a The edges of the ileum are cleaned and seromuscular stay-sutures inserted. **b** Extramucosal single layer seromuscular interrupted suture anastomosis.

Langenbeck retractors are now placed in position to retract the skin and subcutaneous tissues. The mobilisation is carried down to the peritoneal cavity staying close to the bowel wall. Once the peritoneal cavity is entered the ileal loop can be freed from inside by sweeping the index finger along the peritoneum. Care must be taken not to split the serosa during this manoeuvre. The loop is now pulled out and the edges trimmed until all the hard fibrous tissue is excised and healthy bleeding ends are reached. The ends are now anastomosed using 3:0 Polyglactin interrupted seromuscular stitches (Fig. 23.23). The ileal loop is reduced inside the peritoneal cavity. The rectus sheath is repaired with interrupted Prolene sutures. I wash the trephine wound with povidone-iodine and leave it open to granulate. This takes 4–6 weeks to heal completely but avoids an ugly scar.

Post-operative care

The patient is maintained on intravenous fluids and electrolytes until passage of flatus is resumed. Once the ileus has resolved, oral intake is commenced and the patient is allowed home.

References

Fasth S, Hulten L, Svaninger G (1987). The Kock continent ileostomy: influence of a defunctioning ileostomy and nipple valve stapling on early and late morbidity. Int J Colorect Dis 2:82–86

Keighley MRB, Winslet MC, Yoshioka K, Lightwood R (1987a) Discrimination is not impaired by excision of the anal transition zone after restorative proctocolectomy. Br J Surg 74:1118–1121

Keighley MRB, Winslet MC, Pringle W, Allan RN (1987b). The pouch as an alternative to permanent ileostomy. Br J Hosp Med 38: 286–293.

Kmiot WA, Keighley MRB (1989) Totally stapled abdominal restorative proctocolectomy. Br J Surg 76:961–964

Martin LW, Torres AM, Fischer JE, Alexander F (1985) The critical level for preservation of continence in the ileoanal anastomosis. J Pediatr Surg 20:664–667

Matikainen M, Santavirta J, Hiltunen KM (1990) Ileoanal anastomosis without covering ileostomy. Dis Colon Rectum 33:384–388

Nicholls RJ, Lubowski DZ (1987) Restorative proctocolectomy: the four loop (W) reservoir Br J Surg 74:564–566

Parks AG, Nicholls RJ (1978) Proctocolectomy without ileostomy for ulcerative colitis Br Med J ii:85–88

Utsunomiya J, Iwama T, Imajo M et al. (1980) Total colectomy, mucosal proctectomy and ileoanal anastomosis Dis colon Rectum 23:459–466

Williams NS, Johnston D (1985) The current status of mucosal proctectomy and ileoanal anastomosis in the surgical treatment of ulcerative colitis and adenomatous polyposis Br J Surg 72:159–168

Winslet MC, Barsoum G, Pringle W, Fox K, Keighley MRB (1991) Loop ileostomy after ileal pouchanal anastomosis – is it necessary? Dis Colon Rectum 34:267–270

24 Indeterminate Colitis

D. Kumar

In the majority of patients with inflammatory bowel disease the pathologist is able to make a confident diagnosis of either ulcerative colitis or Crohn's disease. However, in 10%–20% of patients it is not possible to make a confident histological diagnosis either of ulcerative colitis or Crohn's disease; even on the resected specimen.

The histological features suggestive of indeterminate colitis are:

Deep linear ulcers
Neural proliferation
Transmural inflammation
Retention of goblet cells
Absence of granulomas
Fissures
Unusual distribution of inflammation

Such pathology is described by the term "indeterminate colitis". In these patients not only the diagnosis but also the outcome remains uncertain. The pathological classification has crucial implications when considering subsequent surgery, particularly restorative proctocolectomy.

The incidence of indeterminate colitis has been reported as 10%–20% of all patients requiring operative treatment for ulcerative colitis (Hywell Jones et al. 1973; Price 1978; Lee et al. 1979; Pezim et al. 1989; Wells et al. 1991). The diagnostic difficulty is more common in those who have emergency or urgent operations (Morson and Dawson 1972). Wells et al. (1991) have shown that many cases considered to have indeterminate colitis in the operative specimen can be reassigned a diagnosis of Crohn's disease or ulcerative colitis with reasonable confidence when all the available features of the case are reviewed. They reported the outcome of 46 patients initially thought to have indeterminate colitis. Nineteen of 46 (40%) were reassigned as Crohn's disease, based on a pre-operative history of anal problems such as fissures, fistulas, abscesses or skin tags. Eleven patients were reassigned to the ulcerative colitis group because they had pre-operative radiological features typical of ulcerative colitis. In 16 patients it was still not possible to make a diagnosis of Crohn's disease or ulcerative colitis; even after reviewing the clinical presentation and the radiological investigations. However, only one of these 16 patients later was shown to have Crohn's disease on the basis of granulomata in a rectal biopsy.

In another series, Pezim et al. (1989) compared the outcome of 25 patients who were considered to have indeterminate colitis and underwent restorative proctocolectomy. With 489 patients who underwent restorative proctocolectomy for a definite diagnosis of chronic ulcerative colitis there was no significant difference between the groups in the complication rates, the stool frequency or incidence of incontinence or pouchitis. In another report Koltun et al. (1991) evaluated retrospectively 288 patients who had an ileal pouch-anal anastomosis, of whom 18 had indeterminate colitis. Half of those patients with indeterminate colitis experienced complications, the majority of which were perineal problems such as fistulae, abscesses and anastomotic dehiscence. Of the remaining 270 patients, only eight patients had experienced complications. Furthermore, the risk of a permanent ileostomy because of perineal complications of indeterminate colitis was 28% compared to 0.4% in patients with chronic ulcerative colitis.

With indeterminate colitis it is difficult to make a decision about the best operation. My personal preference is to postpone operation when a diagnosis of indeterminate colitis is made solely on the basis of the histological features of transmural inflammation, deep linear ulcers, neural proliferation, atypical distribution and fissures. A careful review of the presenting features, clinical signs and radiological investigations will make it possible to exclude the majority of patients with Crohn's disease. In my experience subsequent rectal biopsies taken during observations following the postponed operation are often helpful to eliminate the possibility of Crohn's proctitis. We believe, as do others (Pezim et al. 1989; Wells et al. 1991) that it is safe to carry out ileal pouch-anal anastomosis in patients who continue to show features of indeterminate colitis at the end of 12 months and cannot be assigned to either Crohn's disease or ulcerative colitis group. We can do so without putting the patient at an increased risk of developing complications.

True indeterminate colitis, seems to behave more like ulcerative colitis than it does like Crohn's colitis. However, there are still a number of unanswered questions such as the long-term outcome and the risk of developing dysplasia and cancer.

References

Hywell Jones J, Lennard-Jones JE, Morson BC et al. (1973) Numerical taxonomy and discriminant analysis to non-specific colitis. Q J Med 42:715–732

Koltun WA, Schoetz D, Roberts PL, Murray JJ, Coller JA, Veidenheimen MC (1991) Indeterminate colitis predisposes to perineal complications after ileal anal anastomosis. Dis Colon Rectum 34:857–860

Lee KS, Medline A, Shockey S (1979) Indeterminate colitis in the spectrum of inflammatory bowel disease. Arch Pathol Lab Med 103:173–176

Morson BC, Dawson IMP (eds) (1972) Gastrointestinal pathology. Blackwell Scientific, Oxford, p.467

Pezim ME, Pemberton JH, Beart RW Jr et al. (1989) Outcome of 'indeterminant' colitis following ileal pouch– anal anastomosis. Dis Colon Rectum 32:653–658

Price AB (1978) Overlap in the spectrum of non-specific inflammatory bowel disease – 'colitis indeterminate'. J Clin Pathol 31:567–577

Wells AD, McMillan I, Price AB, Ritchie JK, Nicholls RJ (1991) Natural history of indeterminate colitis. Br J Surg 78:179–181

25 Management of Cancer and Dysplasia in Ulcerative Colitis

D. Kumar

Patients who have had ulcerative colitis for 30 years have an approximately 20% risk of developing cancer or high grade dysplasia (Katzka et al. 1983; Lashner et al. 1989). The overall incidence of carcinoma in patients with ulcerative colitis is approximately 5% (McDougall 1964; Gozzetti et al. 1987). Patients with ulcerative colitis, when compared with those without colitis, develop colorectal cancer at a younger age, often at multiple sites in the colon and frequently present at sites other than the rectum or sigmoid colon (Greenstein et al. 1979; Vatn 1984). There appears to be a higher incidence of synchronous cancers in ulcerative colitis than in a control population, and also the cancers in ulcerative colitis tend to be less well differentiated.

The risk factors for the development of cancer in ulcerative colitis are total colitis, a chronic clinical course and onset of the disease at a young age (Cola 1989; Lashner et al. 1989). There is no unequivocal evidence to suggest that the risk of carcinoma increases with time (Kewenter 1978; Gozzetti et al. 1987).

The role of dysplasia in ulcerative colitis

The presence of dysplasia in ulcerative colitis is often regarded as an increased risk for the development of carcinoma. However, there are difficulties in assessing the significance of dysplasia in ulcerative colitis. Some believe that the evaluation of dysplasia is observer-dependent (Cola 1989). Discrepancy rates between expert histopathologists viewing the same slides vary from 4%–7.5%, with false positives being the commonest error (Dixon et al. 1988; Melville et al. 1988). Since dysplasia can develop in flat mucosa, sampling at the time of biopsy may be difficult and should not be confined to polypoidal areas, ulcer edges, stenotic areas and mucosal nodules. Biopsies must also be multiple and biopsy sites should be clearly recorded. Ransohoff et al. (1985) have shown that only 50% of specimens after colectomy for cancer show dysplasia distant from the cancer. Due to the patchy distribution of dysplasic lesions, even multiple biopsies may fail to identify them (Gyde 1990). Despite all these problems, dysplasia is still considered to be the most reliable marker of malignant transformation in ulcerative colitis.

Surveillance of patients at risk

Screening for dysplasia and for colorectal cancer in patients with ulcerative colitis has become routine practice. The aim of surveillance in ulcerative colitis is to identify patients with dysplasia and carcinoma, although it is uncertain whether it increases survival (Gyde

1990). However, it seems reasonable to suppose that early detection of colorectal cancer may lead to increased survival. There have been many reports of the number of cancers detected, their Duke's staging and the presence and grade of dysplasia. (Lennard-Jones et al. 1983; Nugent and Haggit 1984; Manning et al. 1987). The five-year survival with cancer complicating ulcerative colitis is poor (33%) without screening and that survival is dependent upon the stage at which the cancer is diagnosed (Gyde et al. 1984; Ritchie et al. 1981; Van Heerden et al. 1980). Survival for Dukes Class A cancer is in excess of 20 years whereas for Dukes Class B or C it tends to be poor. Colonoscopy is regarded as the most effective means of surveillance and should include multiple biopsies from at least ten sites between the caecum and rectum. Although this does not completely exclude the presence of dysplasia, it certainly reduces the chances of missing dysplasia or cancer in these patients. Patient compliance is an important factor in screening for cancer in ulcerative colitis – low compliance is the commonest reason for cancers being missed. Lennard-Jones et al. (1983) studied a group of 303 patients of which 43 discontinued follow-up and 20 of these refused screening. In another study (Jones et al. 1988) of 313 patients, 84 were lost to follow-up. Five of these were later found to have cancer. Khubchandani et al. (1982) recommend colonoscopy every six months but I feel that once yearly colonoscopy in patients who do not have evidence of dysplasia and six-monthly examinations in patients with features of dysplasia are adequate. Clearly surveillance is easier in patients who have had a colectomy and ileo-rectal anastomosis. The same surveillance strategy should be applied to this group of patients.

Surgical treatment of cancer in ulcerative colitis

Before the widespread adoption of the ileal pouch procedure the standard operations for carcinoma in ulcerative colitis were proctocolectomy, with permanent ileostomy or a colectomy with ileo-rectal anastomosis depending upon the site of cancer. The surgical option of restorative proctocolectomy and ileal pouch-anal anastomosis has made a great impact on the surgical management of dysplasia and cancer in ulcerative colitis. The proctocolectomy part of the operation eliminates the disease without sacrificing the anal sphincter mechanism. However, it does not seem to completely resolve the problem as there have been several reports of dysplasia, and carcinoma following an ileo-anal reservoir (Stern et al. 1990; Tsunoda et al. 1990; Lofberg et al. 1991). As discussed in an earlier chapter the radical operation of proctocolectomy with a permanent ileostomy carries all the morbidity associated with stomas and inherent problems with sexual and bladder function. These problems have largely been overcome by performing the rectal dissection as close to the rectal wall as possible. The indications for a conventional proctocolectomy, however, are becoming more and more limited with an increasing use of restorative proctocolectomy. The most common indication for a conventional proctocolectomy these days is a low rectal cancer where a restorative procedure cannot be performed. An alternative under these circumstances may be a continent stoma.

For a right-sided colonic cancer, a total colectomy and ileo-rectal anastomosis avoids a stoma but does not abolish the risk of cancer in the rectum. However, with meticulous monitoring and surveillance it may provide an easier alternative to restorative proctocolectomy. If subsequently the rectum does become diseased or dysplasic, rectal removal with an ileal reservoir is still an option. However, as yet our experience with restorative proctocolectomy in the treatment of cancer in ulcerative colitis is limited. Furthermore, the reports of dysplasia and cancer in the reservoir itself raise questions about the effectiveness of this operation. It is important to consider the location and the invasiveness of the tumour before deciding upon the surgical option. In case of doubt about tumour penetration, pan-proctocolectomy with a permanent stoma may be safer than restorative proctocolectomy. In patients with severe dysplasia the procedure of choice is proctocolectomy with an ileal reservoir and ileo-anal anastomosis. In cases with high grade dysplasia confined to the colon, an ileo-rectal anastomosis followed by meticulous follow-up of the rectum may be considered.

References

Cola B (1989) Inflammatory bowel disease and cancer. Int J Colorect Dis 4:128–133

Dixon MF, Brown LTR, Gilmour HM et al. (1988) Observer variation in the assessment of dysplasia ulcerative colitis. Histopathology 95:668–75

Gozzetti G, Cunsolo A, Grigioni WF, Vecchi R (1987) Coliti idiopatiche e cancro. Ciba-Geigy, Milano, pp 7–28

Greenstein AJ, Sachar DB, Smith H et al. (1979) Cancer in universal and left-sided ulcerative colitis: factors determining risk. Gastroenterology 77:290–294

Gyde SN (1990) Screening for colorectal cancer in ulcerative colitis: dubious benefits and high costs. Gut 31:1089–1092

Gyde SN, Prior P, Thompson H, Waterhouse JAH, Allan RN (1984) Survival of patients with colorectal cancer complicating ulcerative colitis. Gut 25:228–231

Hulten L, Kewenter J, Ahren C, Ojerskog B (1979) Clinical and morphological characteristics of colitis carcinoma and colorectal carcinoma in young people. Scand J Gastroenterol 14:673–678

Jones HW, Grogono J, Hoare AM (1988) Surveillance in ulcerative colitis: burdens and benefit. Gut 29:325–331

Katzka I, Brody RS, Morris E, Katz S (1983) Assessment of colorectal cancer risk in patients with ulcerative colitis: experience from a private practice. Gastroenterology 85:22–29

Kewenter J, Ahlman H, Hulten L (1978) Cancer risk in extensive colitis. Ann Surg 188:824–828

Khubchandani IT, Stasik JJ Jr, Nedwich A (1982) Prospective surveillance by rectal biopsy following ileorectal anastomosis for inflammatory bowel disease. Dis Col Rectum 25:343–347

Lashner BA, Silverstein MD, Hanauer SB (1989) Hazard rates for dysplasia and cancer in ulcerative colitis: results from a surveillance programme. Dig Dis Sci 34:1536–1544

Lashner BA, Turner BC, Bostwick DG, Frank PH, Hanauer SB (1990) Dysplasia and cancer complicating strictures in ulcerative colitis. Dig Dis Sci 33:349–352

Lennard–Jones JE, Morson BC, Ritchie JK, Williams CB (1983) Cancer surveillance in ulcerative colitis: experience over 15 years. Lancet ii:149–153

Lofberg R, Liljeqvist L, Lindquist K, Veress B, Reinholt, Tribukait B (1991) Dysplasia and DNA aneuploidy in a pelvic pouch. Dis Colon Rectum 34:280–284

McDougall IPM (1964) The risk of cancer in ulcerative colitis. Lancet ii:655–658

Manning AP, Bulgim OR, Dixon MF, Axon ATR (1987) Screening by colonoscopy for colonic epithelial dysplasia in inflammatory bowel disease. Gut 28:1489–1494

Melville DM, Jass JR, Shepherd NA et al. (1988) Dysplasia and deoxyribonucleic acid aneuploidy in the assessment of pre-cancerous changes in chronic ulcerative colitis: observer variation and correlations. Gastroenterology 95:668–675

Nugent FW, Haggit RC (1984) Results of a long-term prospective surveillance program for dysplasia in ulcerative colitis. Gastroenterology 86:1197

Ransohoff DF, Riddell RH, Levin B. (1985) Ulcerative colitis and colonic cancer: problems in assessing the diagnostic usefulness of mucosal dysplasia. Dis Colon Rectum 28:382–388

Ritchie JK, Hawley PR, Lennard-Jones JE (1981) Progress of carcinoma in ulcerative colitis. Gut 22:725–725

Stern H, Walfisch S, Mullen B, McLeod R, Cohen Z (1990) Cancer in an ileoanal reservoir: a new late complication? Gut 31:473–475

Tsunoda A, Talbot IC, Nicholls RJ (1990) Incidence of dysplasia in the anorectal mucosa in patients having restorative proctocolectomy. Br J Surg 77:506–508

Van Heerden JA, Beart RW (1980) Carcinoma of the colon. Section complicating chronic ulcerative colitis. Dis Colon Rectum 23:155–159

Vatn MH, Elgio K, Bergan A (1984) Distribution of dysplasia in ulcerative colitis. Scand J Gastroenterol 19:893–895

26 Pouch Function

D. Kumar

Clinical determinants of pouch function

Restorative proctocolectomy is now widely accepted as the optimum treatment for ulcerative colitis. However, despite improved surgical techniques and increasing experience the functional outcome is not always good. The four most commonly used determinants of clinical function are stool frequency, continence, ability to defaecate spontaneously and the ability to defer defaecation. However, all these parameters of pouch function are entirely subjective and, depending on their expectations, a good to excellent result for one patient may be a fair or even poor result to another. As a result clinicians have included physiological measurements to explain the variations in pouch function. These measurements have included anal manometry, pouch capacity, pouch compliance, motility and pouch scintigraphy. Pouch ecology has also been studied and attempts have been made to correlate pouch ecology with function.

Stool frequency

Large volume pouches are usually associated with lower stool frequency (Fig. 26.1). Therefore, the triplicated S and quadruplicated W pouches show the lowest stool frequencies. In this volume/frequency equation, often the length of ileum used is not considered. It is possible to make a large volume J pouch using a longer length of ileum than is used in the S or W pouch designs. The other important factor is the continuing improvement in stool frequency with the passage of time. Stool frequency also depends on the faecal output (Fig. 26.2): the greater the faecal output, the more the number of stools per day (Kelly 1992). The reported stool frequencies at 12 months vary between three and eight stools per day (Table 26.1). Some authors have compared clinical outcome in terms of stool frequency with different pouch designs. Hallgren et al. (1989) compared stool frequency between S and J pouches with 11 patients in each group. They found that the mean stool frequency with J pouch was six motions per 24 hours whereas with S pouches it was eight stools. Tuckson and Fazio (1991) in their series of 35 patients (J = 17, S = 18) found that the mean stool frequency per 24 hours was six in patients who had a J pouch whereas it was down to four in patients who had an S pouch. Others have compared pouch defaecation frequencies between S and W pouches and found that stool frequency per 24 hours in W pouches was significantly lower than S pouches (Sagar et al. 1992). In most series however, approximately 30% of patients were taking anti-diarrhoeal medication and it is not clear up to what extent the stool frequency was influenced by anti-diarrhoeal therapy. Nor is it known whether anti-diarrhoeals have different effects in different capacity pouches. It is conceivable that due to the different arrangement of ileal segments within the pouch, the motor effects of various segments may be different and therefore would respond differently to anti-diarrhoeals.

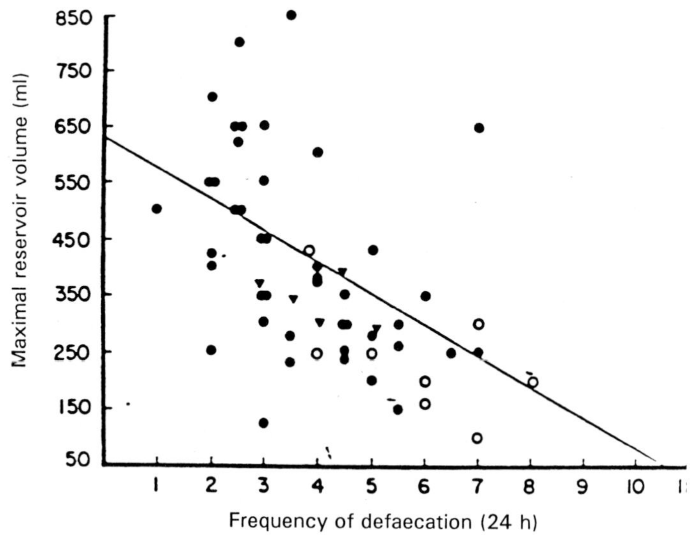

Fig. 26.1. The relationship between frequency of defaecation per 24 hours and maximal tolerated reservoir volume measured after closure of the ilestomy. Filled circles, S Pouch; open circles, J Pouch; filled triangles, W pouch ($r = 0.51$, $P < 0.05$). (From Nicholls and Pezim (1985) with permission.)

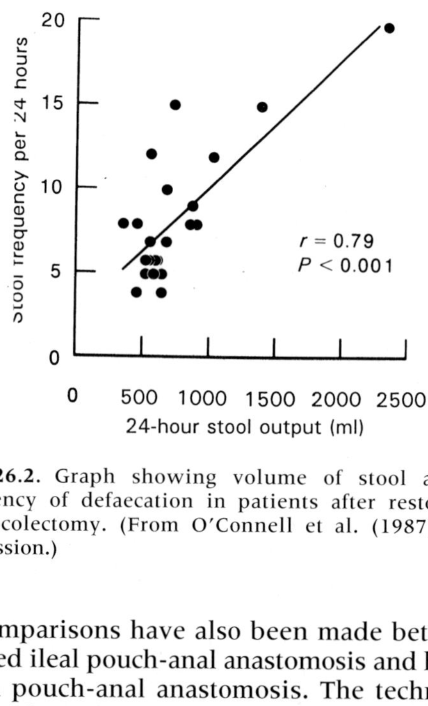

Fig. 26.2. Graph showing volume of stool against frequency of defaecation in patients after restorative proctocolectomy. (From O'Connell et al. (1987) with permission.)

Comparisons have also been made between stapled ileal pouch-anal anastomosis and hand-sewn pouch-anal anastomosis. The technique of pouch-anal anastomosis whether stapled or hand sewn does not appear to have any significant effect on stool frequency (Sugarman et al. 1990).

Nocturnal frequency seems to differ with different pouch designs. In a large series of J pouches from the Mayo Clinic, the mean nocturnal frequency is 1.2 whereas only 15% of patients with W pouches have night evacuation more than once a week (Dozois et al. 1986; Nicholls and Lubowsky 1987). The average reported nocturnal frequency seems to vary between zero and one.

Continence

This is an important marker on which the success of restorative proctocolectomy is judged. Normal continence has been reported in 50%–85% of patients with ileal pouches (Taylor et al. 1983; Williams and Johnston 1985; Rothenberger et al. 1985). However, the degree of continence is variable (Table 26.2). Major incontinence with solid or semi-solid stool is infrequent in all series. Approximately 2%–10% of patients experience major leaks and these episodes are more common at night (Williams and Johnston 1985; Nicholls 1987). Minor incontinence, on the other hand, is much more frequent and occurs in 10%–45% of patients (Table 26.2). Minor episodes of incontinence have been defined as leakage of faecal fluid or mucus that requires the use of a pad. Like stool frequency, continence also appears to improve with time. Episodes of minor faecal leakage continue to decrease for up to 12 months following surgery. This may be related to changes in the consistency of pouch contents over this time period.

Table 26.1 Stool frequency with different pouch designs

Author	Pouch design	Number	Frequency/24hrs	Nocturnal frequency
Hallgren et al. 1989	S J	11 11	8 6	4 2
Hatakeyama et al. 1989	W	16	3.8	NA
Williams et al. 1989	S	11 (stapled) 12 (trans-anal)	6 6	1 1
Sugarman et al. 1990	J	21 (stapled) 25	7.0 7.9	1.6 2.1
Chaussade et al. 1991	J	15	5.3	1.0
Wexner et al. 1991	J	15	5.6	0.6
Tuckson and Fazio 1991	S J	18 17	4 6	0 1.0
Sagar et al. 1992	S W	20 20	6.0 3.5	1.0 0
Fonkalsrud and Loar 1992	H	67	4.8	NA

Table 26.2. Incontinence following restorative proctocolectomy

Author	*n*	Pouch design	Incontinence/leakage day (%)	night (%)	Regularly take antidiarrhoeal medication (%)
Williams et al. 1989	23	S	18	51	73
Dozois et al. 1986	670	J	17	44	26
Tuckson and Fazio 1991	17 18	J S	29 22	53 29	71 29
Sagar et al. 1991	20	NS	0	10	35
Wexner et al. 1991	15	J	20	40	NS

Spontaneous evacuation

The majority of patients evacuate spontaneously following a restorative proctocolectomy. Catheter evacuation has only been reported in patients with S pouches and a few patients with isoperistaltic pouches. This was mainly a problem with pouch design and with experience the efferent limb of S pouches has been shortened and the need to catheterise eliminated (Nicholls and Pezim 1985; Rothenberger et al. 1985). Williams et al. (1989) reported incomplete pouch evacuation in 18% of their patients and the remaining 82% achieved spontaneous evacuation. Chaussade et al. (1991) have reported spontaneous evacuation in 94% of patients. We have had a similar experience with 23 patients. All our patients are able to evacuate spontaneously and have an evacuation frequency of three or four times per day and zero at night.

Deferment of defaecation

In our experience most patients are able to defer defaecation for at least 1–2 hours. Most published series report similar findings but urgency can be a feature in as many as 20% of patients (Hatakeyama 1989; Braun et al. 1991; Wexner et al. 1991; Fonkalsrud and Loar 1992). Like other clinical measures of pouch function, deferment of defaecation also improves with time.

Physiological determinants of pouch function

Manometry

Several authors have studied the effect of ileal pouch-anal anastomosis on anal canal manometry (Keighley et al. 1988b; O'Connell et al. 1988; Lindquist 1990; Miller et al. 1990). In most of these studies anal canal manometry employed a water-filled system with the patient lying in the left lateral position. Using this technique significant reductions in resting anal pressures have been reported after restorative proctocolectomy (Fig. 26.3). Also, this reduction in resting anal pressure has been found to correlate with poor function, particularly with continence. O'Connell et al. (1988) have studied 38 patients following restorative proctocolectomy and found that resting anal canal pressure was lower in patients than in controls. In their study the presence or absence of mucosal proctectomy did not have any effect on resting pressures. However, when they compared the continent patients with the incontinent group, there was a significant reduction in resting anal canal pressures in the incontinent group. In contrast, squeeze pressure was similar in patients and controls. Therefore, it appears that rectal mucosectomy had no effect on squeeze pressure, and once again squeeze pressures were lower in the incontinent group when compared with the continent group. Others have

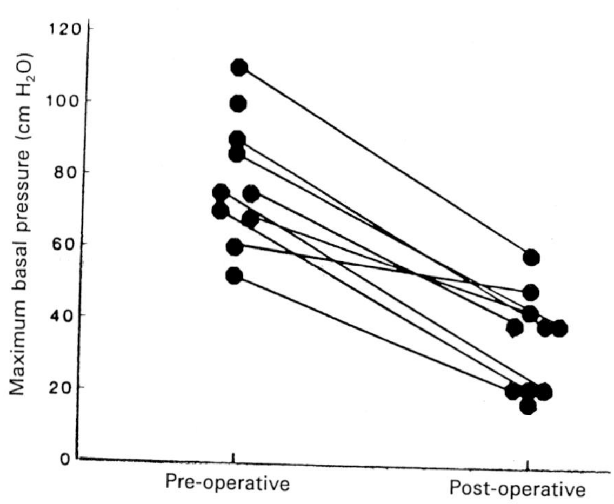

Fig. 26.3. Maximal basal anal canal pressure before and after pouch-anal anastomosis. The post-operative values are significantly different from the pre-operative values ($P < 0.01$). (From Williams et al. (1989) with permission.)

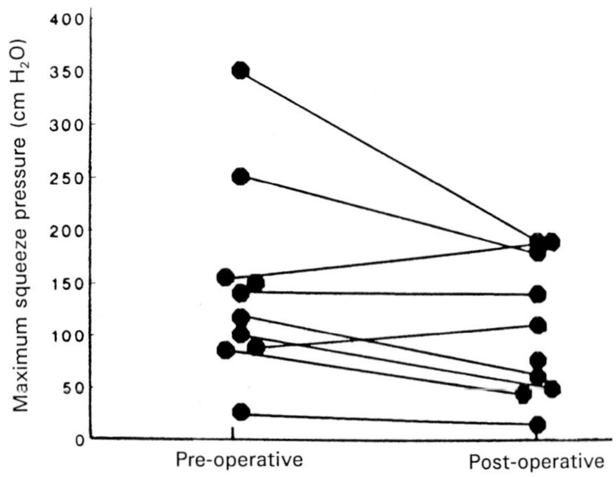

Fig. 26.4. Maximal squeeze anal canal pressure before and after pouch-anal anastomosis. (From Williams et al. (1989) with permission.)

also shown that maximal squeeze anal canal pressures before and after restorative proctocolectomy do not show any significant differences (Fig. 26.4) (Williams et al. 1989).

In another study, Johnston et al. (1987) compared anal canal manometry in 12 patients after a stapled pouch-anal anastomosis with 24 patients who underwent a handsewn ileal pouch-anal anastomosis. They found that the drop in resting anal canal pressures following a handsewn anastomosis was significantly greater compared to that observed after a stapled anastomosis (90 cm of water to 70 cm of water against 85 cm of water to 40 cm of water in the handsewn group). In this study there was no significant change in maximal squeeze pressure following restorative proctocolectomy. Others, however, have reported an increase in squeeze pressure after ileo-anal anastomosis in some patients (Becker 1984; Lindquist 1990). This increase in squeeze pressure following operation is said to be due to hypertrophy of the external sphincter.

The reasons for the change in internal anal sphincter function following restorative proctocolectomy are not clear. Heald and Allan (1986) believe that it was due to excessive stretching of the anal canal during a rectal mucosectomy. This view is supported by the findings of Johnston et al. (1987) who found a greater drop in resting anal pressures following a handsewn anastomosis than after a stapled anastomosis without mucosectomy. Others, however have failed to demonstrate a greater drop in resting tone following a handsewn ileo-anal anastomosis compared to a stapled anastomosis (Marzouk et al. 1989; Williams et al. 1989; O'Connell et al. 1988). There have been alternative explanations for the greater drop in resting anal tone following a mucosectomy. It has been suggested that some of the sphincter fibres may be stripped with the mucosa during this procedure resulting in poor function of the internal anal sphincter (Sharp et al. 1987). It has also been suggested that there may be fibrosis of the anal sphincters following a mucosectomy and ileo-anal anastomosis (Emblem et al. 1989). There is some evidence that the anal resting tone improves with time following restorative proctocolectomy. This would be consistent with the findings of improvement in continence function with time.

The length of the anal canal has been measured before and after restorative proctocolectomy. Most authors have found no change in anal canal length following an ileal pouch-anal anastomosis (Johnston et al. 1987; O'Connell et al. 1988).

Pouch capacity

It is generally believed that larger pouch volumes at the time of operation and subsequently are associated with better pouch function in terms of defaecation frequency. This hypothesis was originally tested in animal experimental studies and it was found that as pouch capacity increased post-operatively, stool frequency decreased (Rosemurgy 1983). These experimental studies are supported by observations in patients who have undergone restorative proctocolectomy. Nicholls and Pezim (1985) have reported improved function following W pouches. In their evaluation of reservoir volumes after following S, J and W configuration pouches after ileostomy closure, W pouches had the greatest capacity and this compared favourably with the functional results where W pouch design had a significantly lower evacuation frequency (Fig. 26.5). This inverse correlation between pouch capacity and evacuation frequency is also supported by the findings of Heppell et al. (1982), who found that pouch capacity was significantly greater in patients who had a good functional result compared to those who had a poor result. Similar results have been reported by Harms et al. (1990) who found better functional results after W pouches than after S pouches. However, others have failed to show a correlation between volume and function (Keighley et al. 1988a; Everett 1989). Pouch capacity is also related to the length of pouch segment at construction; the longer the pouch segment, the greater is the pouch volume (Fig. 26.6) (Oresland et al. 1990).

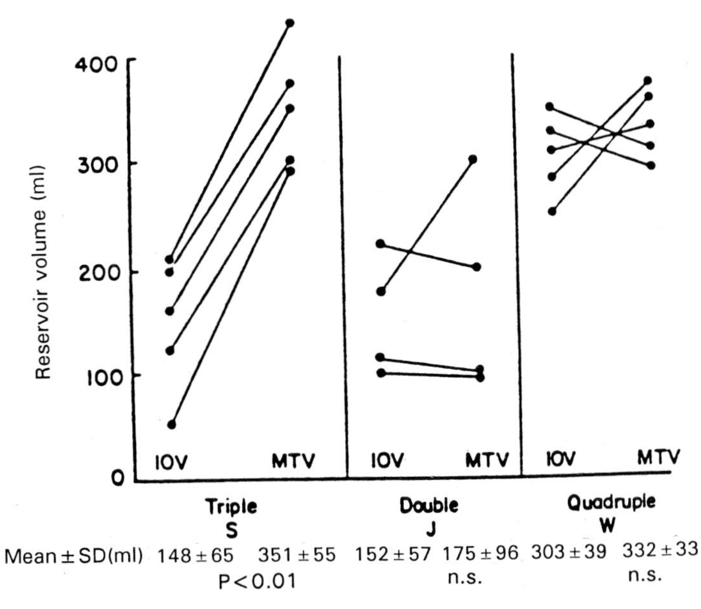

Fig. 26.5. Intra-operative reservoir volume (IOV) and maximal tolerated volume (MTV) after closure of the ileostomy. (From Nicholls and Pezim (1985) with permission.)

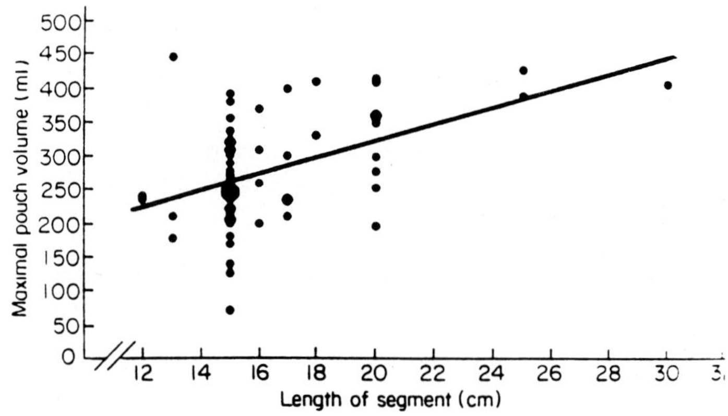

Fig. 26.6. Length of pouch segment at construction versus pouch volume 12 months after loop ileostomy closure. (From Oresland et al. (1990) with permission.)

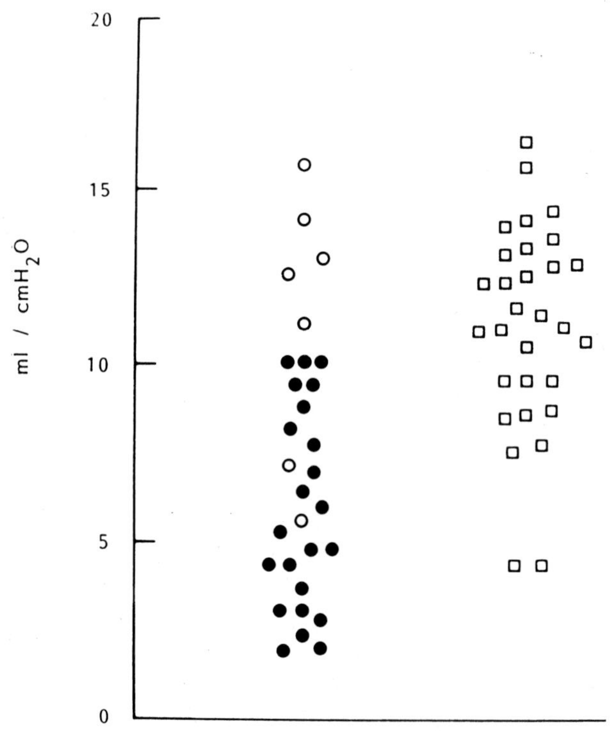

Fig. 26.7. Compliance (ml/cm H_2O) after restorative proctocolectomy compared with controls ($P < 0.05$). Filled circles, patients with good function; open circles, patients with poor function; open squares, controls. (From Keighley et al. (1988a) with permission.)

Compliance

Simultaneous measurement of pouch volume and intraluminal pressure enables calculation of pouch compliance. It is a measure of resistance to internal change in volume per unit change in pressure. It has been suggested that ileo-anal pouch compliance is an important determinant of function following restorative proctocolectomy (Taylor et al. 1983; Nasmyth et al. 1986; Harms et al. 1990). However, the validity of compliance measurements is doubtful and the technique of compliance determination has been criticised. Harms et al. (1990)

in their study of 50 patients who had a restorative proctocolectomy (S reservoirs = 12, W reservoirs = 38) found that reservoir compliance increased between two and 12 months for both S and W pouches. The mean compliance increased from 6.9 to 8.9 in the S pouches and from 7.8 to 10.6 in the W pouches. The W reservoirs always had a higher compliance at two and 12 months postoperatively. In another study of 23 patients two years following restorative proctocolectomy the capacity and compliance of ileal pouches was similar to that in the rectum of controls (O'Connell et al. 1987). In this study compliance of the pouch was not related to pouch function. Keighley et al. (1988a) have reported that pouch compliance in patients after restorative proctocolectomy is significantly lower than that in the rectum of healthy subjects (Fig. 26.7). In an experimental study Thayer et al. (1990) compared intrinsic and extrinsic compliance characteristics of three pouch designs (S, J and W) in 33 mongrel dogs. They found that in vivo and ex vivo compliance determinations do not correlate (Fig. 26.8). Although a useful experimental observation, it has little clinical application. However, this study shows that pouch compliance is dependent upon surrounding structures because compliance measurements taken ex vivo were more compliant than those taken in vivo.

Anal canal sensation

The sensory mechanisms in the anal canal allow discrimination of the nature of pouch content after pouch-anal anastomosis. Patients following restorative proctocolectomy are able to detect the need for evacuation of the pouch and can also discriminate between flatus an stool (Pemberton et al. 1987). Miller et al. (1990) studied 14 patients who had the anal transition zone preserved, eight who had the anal transition zone removed and 20 controls, measuring anal sensation, manometry and functional results. They found improved sensation in those patients with a preserved anal transition zone although functional results were not significantly improved. Nevertheless, there was a non-significant trend towards improved continence and discrimination in those with the anal transition zone preserved.

Holdsworth and Johnston (1988a) studied anal sensation in 16 patients who had an end-to-end ileo-anal anastomosis without a mucosectomy and 13 patients after endo-anal anastomosis. They found that patients who

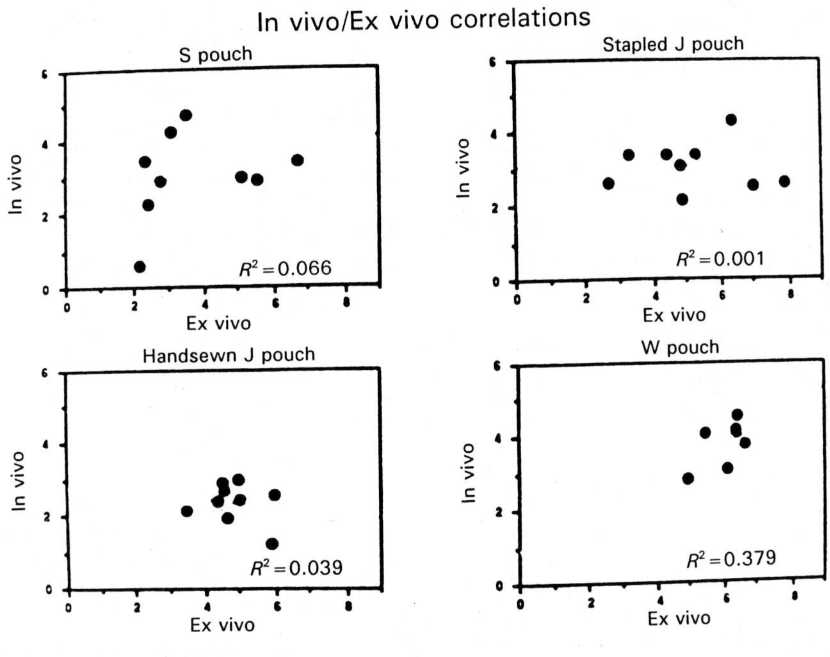

Fig. 26.8. Correlation of in vivo and ex vivo compliance for S, J and W pouches. (From Thayer et al. (1991) with permission.)

had undergone mucosectomy had a significantly higher sensory threshold in the upper anal canal compared with those who had an end-to-end anastomosis and control patients. There was no significant difference in electrosensitivity thresholds in the mid- and lower anal canal amongst the three groups. In addition, all patients in the end-to-end anastomosis group were able to discriminate between flatus and faeces whereas only 77% of those with endo-anal anastomosis were able to do so. Keighley et al. (1987) assessed anal sensation in 21 patients after restorative proctocolectomy. Fifteen of these patients had excision of anal transition zone whereas six had the operation with the anal transition zone preserved. In their series the median threshold values for electrosensitivity in the upper, mid- and lower anal canals were greater than 15 mA in the upper and mid-anal canal and 6.8 mA in the lower anal canal. When compared to controls the mid- and upper zone threshold anal sensation was significantly lower when the transition zone had not been removed. Despite changes in electrosensitivity post-operatively they could not detect any clinical benefit in patients who had the anal transition zone preserved. Discrimination was normal in all except one of their patients. They concluded that excision of the anal transition zone does not eliminate the ability to discriminate and does not increase the risk of impaired continence after ileal pouch-anal anastomosis. In a subsequent study by the same authors (Keighley et al. 1988b), 30 patients who had undergone restorative proctocolectomy were compared with a group of age- and sex-matched controls. In this study they reported loss of sensation in mid-anal canal in 25 (76%) of their pouch patients. The remaining five (15%) patients with normal sensation had an intact anal transition zone.

It appears that although abnormalities of anal sensation following restorative proctocolectomy can be detected by electrosensitivity measurements, they have very little impact on the clinical outcome.

Recto-anal inhibitory reflex

Acute rectal distension produces relaxation of the internal anal sphincter and contraction of the external anal sphincter. This response is called the recto-anal inhibitory reflex and can be elicited in all healthy subjects.

It is generally believed that the recto-anal inhibitory reflex allows the rectal contents to come in contact with the sensitive anal transition zone mucosa while the external sphincter contracts to prevent leakage. The preservation of recto-anal inhibitory reflex following restorative proctocolectomy remains controversial. In reported series the incidence of recto-anal inhibitory reflex in pouch patients varies from 4% to 75% (Pescatori and Parks 1984; Holdsworth and Johnston 1988b; O'Connell et al. 1988; Oresland et al. 1990). O'Connell et al. (1988) showed that neorectal (pouch) anal inhibitory reflex could be elicited in only 4% of their patients whereas Holdsworth and Johnston (1988b) reported that the reflex was present in 75% of their patients. The explanation for the difference is that Holdsworth and Johnston's patients all had an end-to-end anastomosis without mucosectomy whereas the patients reported by O'Connell et al. (1988) had long rectal cuffs. In another study (Oresland et al. 1990), sphincter inhibition on pouch distension could be detected in 25% of patients. They found that the distension pressures required to elicit the in-

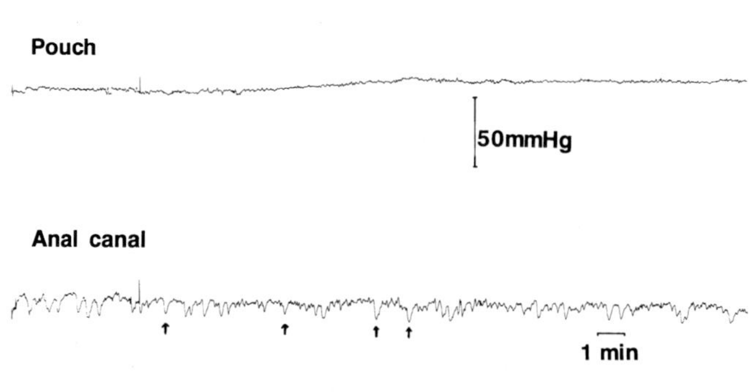

Fig. 26.9. Prolonged and ambulant pressure recordings showing neo-recto-anal inhibitory reflexes (arrows).

hibition in pouch patients were higher than those in control subjects. However, the functional result was similar irrespective of whether sphincter inhibition was present or absent. In our experience, using prolonged manometry for 24 hours, recto-anal inhibitory reflex occurs in all patients who have had restorative proctocolectomy (Fig. 26.9).

It appears that the preservation of neorectal-anal inhibitory reflex has no beneficial effect on the functional outcome of restorative proctocolectomy.

Pouch and anal canal motility

Pouch motility

Ileal pouches exhibit a significantly different pattern of contractile activity from that seen in the normal rectum. The rectum exhibits periodic activity in the form of rectal motor complexes and in addition has isolated prolonged contractions and clustered contractions (Kumar et al. 1989). In contrast, the pouch exhibits two types of motor activity. The predominant activity is in the form of large amplitude (giant) contractions (more than 50 mmHg which last for approximately 30 seconds (Fig. 26.10)). These contractions do not appear to be related to pouch filling. Also, these giant contraction waves are more frequent in pouches with a capacity of 300 ml or less. There is no difference in the frequency of giant contraction waves during wakefulness and sleep. When three or more giant contraction waves appear over five minutes the patient feels an urge to defaecate. The second type of motor activity seen in ileal pouches occurs with a frequency of 6–8 per minute and is seen predominantly after feeding (Fig. 26.10). Giant contraction waves are also seen in association with the 6–8 per minute activity. This postprandial response in the pouch lasts for 2–3 hours and once again the predominant activity is giant contraction waves (Kumar et al. 1989). Similar motor activity has been described by others who also showed that the pattern of motility in J pouches is similar to that seen in Kock pouches (O'Connell et al. 1987).

Although frequent giant contraction waves produce the urge to defaecate, pouch evacuation appears to occur with raised intra-abdominal pressure (Fig. 26.11). We measured simultaneously duodenojejunal motility and pouch motility using a fine bore solid state catheter. As can be seen from Fig. 26.11 the patient showed frequent giant contraction waves which were associated with an urge to defaecate. The act of pouch evacuation was accomplished by a rise in intra-abdominal

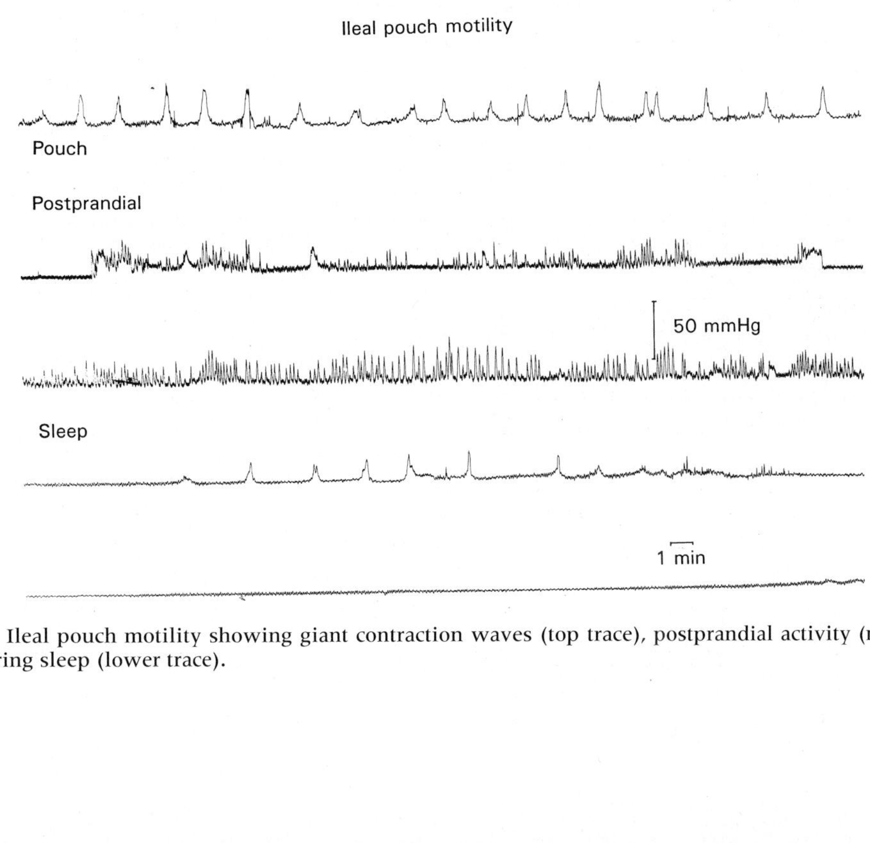

Fig. 26.10. Ileal pouch motility showing giant contraction waves (top trace), postprandial activity (middle trace) and activity during sleep (lower trace).

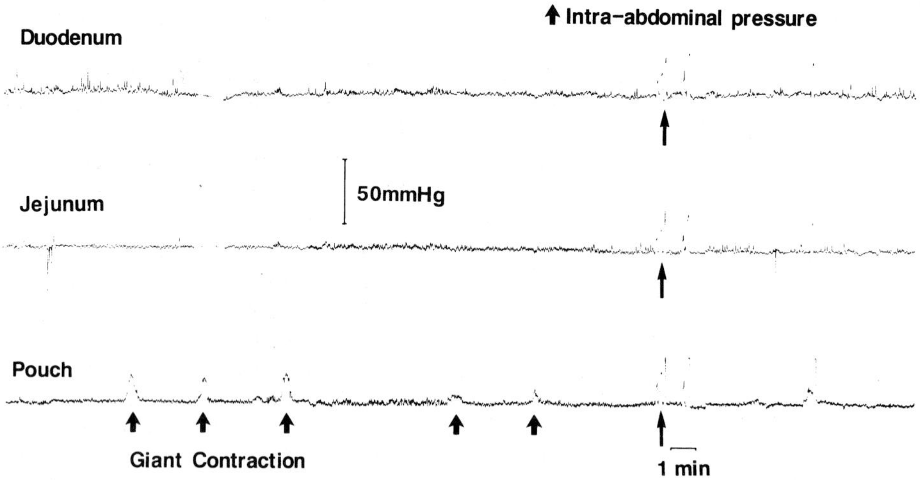

Fig. 26.11. Trace showing simultaneous measurement of duodenojejunal and pouch motility. The urge to defaecate is initiated by frequent giant contraction waves whereas defaecation is achieved by a rise in intra-abdominal pressure recorded by all the transducers simultaneously (arrows).

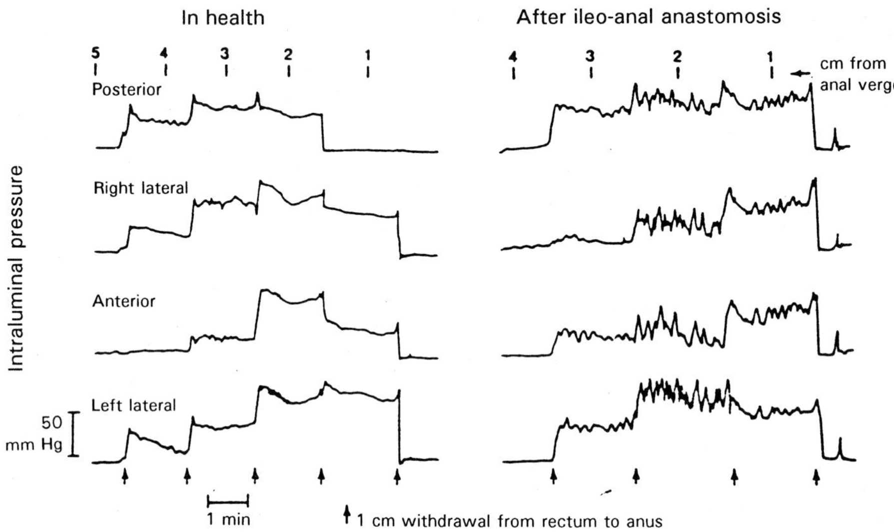

Fig. 26.12. Pressure recordings from the anal canal of a healthy volunteer and a patient after restorative proctocolectomy. Note the phasic fluctuations in the anal canal tone after restorative proctocolectomy. (From O'Connell et al. (1988) with permission.)

pressure which was registered simultaneously at all three recording sites. Stryker et al. (1986) have reported that these giant contraction waves are abolished by evacuation of stool. In our study we did not observe abolition of giant pressure waves on pouch evacuation.

Anal canal motility

The resting tone in the anal canal shows phasic fluctuations in all patients following ileal pouch-anal anastomosis and approximately 80% of healthy subjects (Fig. 26.12) (O'Connell et al. 1988). However, the slow wave frequency was less in the patient group (8.4 ± 0.4 per minute) compared with that in controls (13.8 ± 0.5 per minute). Slow wave amplitude was greater in the patient group when compared with the control group (Fig. 26.13).

Giant slow waves were not seen in any of the controls but were present in 23 of the 50 patients studied. The giant slow waves were not associated with differences in

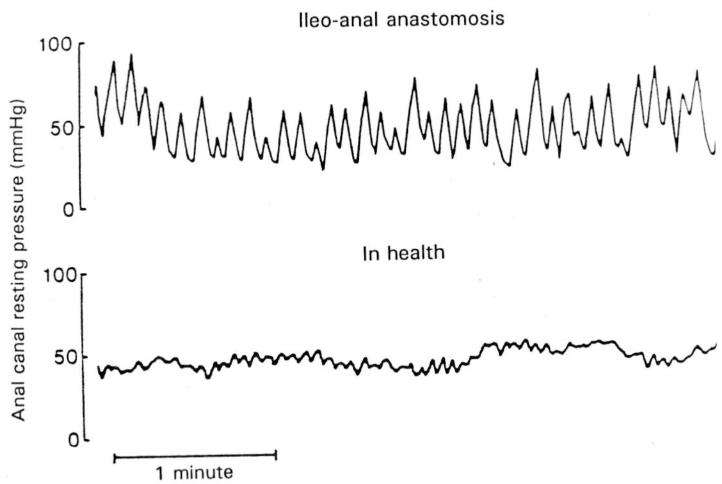

Fig 26.13. Pattern of anal canal motility and after ileo-anal anastomosis and in health as demonstrated by pressure recordings. Note the greater amplitude of slow waves in patients after ileo-anal anastomosis. (From O'Connell et al. (1988) with permission.)

sphincter length, resting anal pressure and maximal squeeze pressure. These variations in motility patterns, however, were not related to continence.

Radiology and scintigraphy

Assessments of pouch function have been made radiologically both by static films (Pescatori et al. 1983; Hillard et al. 1985; Brown et al. 1990) and videoproctography (pouchography) (Kmiot et al. 1990). Pouchograms were performed to assess healing and anatomical integrity of the pouch and to evaluate pouch emptying. Pescatori et al. (1983) in their study assessed 34 patients radiologically after an S pouch restorative proctocolectomy. Patients were studied in two groups, those who could evacuate spontaneously and those who had to catheterise the pouch. Barium was introduced into the pouch and the patients were sat upright on a commode. A lateral film was taken at rest and then the patients were asked to evacuate. A second film was taken at the end of pouch evacuation. From these films they attempted to evaluate parameters such as pelvic floor descent, filling of the efferent limb and the angle between the efferent limb and the pouch. They concluded that patients with short efferent limbs were able to evacuate better than those who had a long efferent limb. Pouch configuration, angle between the efferent limb and the pouch and pelvic floor descent were unimportant in pouch evacuation. Kmiot et al. (1990) used videoproctographic assessments after restorative proctocolectomy. They studied 40 patients to evaluate pouch emptying, ano-pouch angle and pelvic floor movements. They also compared two pouch designs. Using this technique, they found no difference between pouch designs and also emptying did not influence either the frequency of defaecation or faecal soiling rate. The only positive finding in their study was that the presence of an anal stricture was associated with poor emptying. Levit et al. (1991) made similar assessments to compare patients who had good pouch function and spontaneous defaecation with patients who had disordered pouch evacuation. They also found that a pouch-anal stricture resulted in poor pouch evacuation.

Scintigraphy

O'Connell et al. (1986) developed a Technitium 99 sulphurcolloid radio-labelled artificial stool which was used to assess pouch function after restorative proctocolectomy. They studied 23 patients and seven controls. The labelled stool was introduced into the pouch until the maximal tolerable volume was reached. This was previously assessed using balloon manometry. Following a pre-evacuation scan, dynamic images were recorded during defaecation. The total activity of the excreted stool and activity per gram weight were also obtained. They found that the patients emptied approximately 61% of the labelled stool. Three patients who took more than 90 seconds to evacuate were only able to empty 37% of the labelled stool. The evacuation efficiency in controls was similar to that in patients. In controls the sigmoid colon first emptied into the rectum which became distended and then evacuated. In pouch patients the ileum and the pouch emptied as one single unit. Similar techniques have been used to study ano-pouch angle (Barkel et al. 1988).

Ecology of ileal pouches

Bacteriology

The normal terminal ileum is relatively sterile whereas a permanent ileostomy has bacterial flora which is qualitatively and quantitatively intermediate between normal ileal content and normal stool (Gorbach et al. 1976). The flora of ileal reservoirs closely resembles that of the normal colon and rectum (Kelly et al. 1983; Nasmyth et al. 1989a).

Sager et al. (1992) studied faecal bacteriology in 20 patients with a triplicated S pouch and 20 patients with a W pouch. They found that the number of bacteroides was significantly greater in the effluent from S reservoirs than that from W reservoirs ($P < 0.05$). However, there was no significant difference in the numbers of streptococci, staphylococci, enterobacter, clostridia, lactobacilli, bifidobacteria or coliforms. Similarly, the ratios of anaerobes to aerobes was not significantly different between the two designs of reservoir. There was no significant correlation between the numbers of bacteria and the efficiency of pouch emptying. In a previous study, Nasmyth et al. (1989a) assessed 11 patients after restorative proctocolectomy and compared these to 12 patients who had conventional ileostomy. They found that the ratio of anaerobes to aerobes in pouch effluent was significantly greater than in faeces from ileostomies. Also, the median number of bifidobacteria and bacteriodes was greater in the ileal pouch patients. When they compared bacteriology of pouch effluent between J and S pouches there were no significant differences.

Volatile fatty acids

Volatile fatty acids in the faeces are the metabolites of anaerobic fermentation of carbohydrates by intestinal microflora. The most commonly measured short chain (2–5 carbon atoms) fatty acids are acetic, propionic, butyric and valeric acids. In the human ileum they are present in low concentrations. It has been shown that median concentrations of propionic and butyric acid are significantly greater in the faeces of pouch patients than in the effluent fluid from a conventional ileostomy (Nasmyth et al. 1989). When the same authors compared short chain fatty acids in pouch faeces with those in normal controls' faeces, they found no difference except for a higher concentration of acetic acid in pouch effluent. Sagar et al. (1992) measured the concentration of short chain fatty acids in 20 patients with S pouches and 20 patients with W pouches. They found that the concentrations of acetic and propionic acids were significantly greater in the S pouch effluent than in that from W pouches (acetic: S, 231.7 μmol/g; W, 95.0 μmol/g; $P < 0.05$); (propionic acid: S, 60.1 μmol/g; W, 16.7 μmol/g; $P < 0.05$). They did not observe any differences in the other short chain fatty acids in the two pouch designs.

The greater concentration of volatile fatty acids may have some beneficial effect. Increased production of volatile fatty acids in animals suppresses enteropathic bacteria (Hentges 1983). Greater concentrations of butyrate appear to have a protective effect against villous atrophy whereas acetic and propionic acid concentrations have a significant correlation with the degree of mucosal inflammation.

Mucosal morphology

It is well recognised that compared with normal ileal mucosa the pouch mucosa shows histopathological abnormalities such as shortening of villi, submucosal inflammation and colonic metaplasia (Fiorentini et al. 1987; Lerch et al. 1989; Santavirta et al. 1991b). It has also been found that in about 50% of patients the pouch mucin changes from small bowel type sulphomucin to colorectal type sulphomucin (Shepherd et al. 1987). In a recent study de Silva et al. (1991b) investigated mucosal characteristics of ileal pouches to determine the degree of colonic metaplasia by histochemical and immunohistochemical techniques. They studied biopsies from 25 patients with ileal pouches, eight of whom had pouchitis at the time of biopsy. The biopsies were studied using routine histology, mucosal morphometry, mucin histochemistry and immunoperoxidase staining with monoclonal antibodies. They found that the index of villous atrophy (villous height : total mucosal thickness) was significantly lower in pouches with pouchitis than in those without pouchitis and the index was lower in pouches without pouchitis when compared with normal ileal controls. Mean villous height was significantly lower and crypt depth significantly greater in patients with pouchitis compared with those without pouchitis. They did not detect any significant differences in total mucosal thickness amongst pouches with pouchitis, without pouchitis and normal controls. Thirteen of the 25 pouch biopsies showed sub-total or total villous atrophy and crypt hyperplasia histologically resembling colonic mucosa. Of these 25 pouches, the mucosa of nine had colorectal type sulphomucin. These changes were not seen in patients with less severe villous abnormalities. The conclusion from this study was that ileal pouches acquire certain colonic characteristics but complete colonic metaplasia does not occur.

De Silva et al. (1991c) in another study investigated the effect of faecal stream and stasis on pouch mucosa. They studied nine patients in whom two pouch biopsies were obtained at the time of pouch formation, ileostomy closure, and at three, six and 12 months after operation. Biopsies were assessed for the degree of acute and chronic inflammation, mucin type, villous atrophy index and crypt cell proliferation. They found that at three months the scores for acute and chronic inflammation, the degree of sulphomucin and crypt cell proliferation were significantly higher and the villous atrophy index significantly lower than at pouch formation or at ileostomy closure. The changes seen at six and 12 months were not significantly different from those at three months. They concluded that exposure to the faecal stream is necessary for changes to take place in the pouch mucosa and that mucosal changes occur soon after ileostomy closure and then remain stable. There was no significant correlation between the efficiency of pouch evacuation and any of the mucosal changes reported.

Sagar et al. (1992) have also studied mucosal morphology and found blunting of ileal villi, chronic inflammatory infiltration of lamina propria and crypt hyperplasia in pouches. They did not see fibrosis of the lamina propria. The degree of mucosal inflammation in their study was similar for S and W pouch designs. De Silva et al. (1991a) have also to studied biopsies from pouch patients to characterise the mucosal cellular infiltrate in ileal reservoirs with and without pouchitis. T lymphocyte and macrophage subpopulations were characterised immunohistochemically in pouch biopsies using monoclonal antibodies. Lymphocyte density in pouches with and without pouchitis was significantly less than in normal ileum. There was no significant difference between pouches with and without pouchitis. Low intra-epithelial lymphocyte counts may suggest an adaptive response to the new luminal environment.

Bile acid absorption

The entero-hepatic circulation of primary conjugated bile acids is dependent upon active transport in the terminal ileum. Only a small proportion of bile acids are passively absorbed from the proximal small intestine or colon. Approximately 95% of conjugated bile acids are absorbed through the specialised system of active transport in the ileum. Of the small residuum entering the large intestine, some is passively reabsorbed and the rest is deconjugated by anaerobic bacteria and excreted as secondary bile acids. Although increased hepatic synthesis can compensate for small increases in bile acid excretion, larger losses may result in depletion of the pool of bile acids. Therefore, resection or disease of the terminal ileum may result in an increased loss of bile acids from the entero-hepatic circulation. It is conceivable that after an ileal pouch-anal anastomosis changes in ileal mucosal morphology may have an adverse effect on the absorptive capacity of the ileum. Nasmyth et al. (1989b) studied 15 patients with a conventional ileostomy, 13 patients with a pouch and 10 healthy controls to establish whether absorption of bile acids after total colectomy was significantly impaired in patients who had undergone ileal pouch formation. Samples of ileal and pouch effluent were collected and bile acids were extracted from the effluent using gas-liquid chromatography. Lithocholate was present in all samples. Deoxycholate was found in 18% of samples from ileostomies but 88% of samples from ileal pouches. The percentage of secondary bile acids exceeded the percentage of primary bile acids in 50% of pouch samples but in only 9% of ileostomy samples. Hojlund et al. (1985) compared S pouch effluent with normal stool. Normal stool had a predominance of secondary bile acids whereas the pouch effluent excreted mainly primary bile acids. Also, the overall bile acid excretion was greater in the pouch effluent.

Most of the published studies suggest that the bile acid metabolism following restorative proctocolectomy is abnormal. The most significant abnormality is the presence of high levels of lithocholic acid in the pouch. It remains to be seen whether this will produce abnormalities of liver function in the long term.

Water and electrolyte balance

The normal colon absorbs approximately 1 litre of water and 100 mmol of sodium chloride daily (Phillips and Giller 1973). Following proctocolectomy, a conventional ileostomy is associated with chronic water and salt depletion resulting in renal conservation of water and sodium (Clarke et al. 1967, Kennedy et al. 1983). There are very few reports of water and electrolyte balance after ileal pouch-anal anastomosis. Santavirta et al. (1991a) investigated 30 patients with J pouches and ten patients with conventional ileostomies with nine patients with quiescent ulcerative colitis serving as controls. In all the patients, they measured daily urine volumes, serum electrolyte concentrations and losses of sodium, potassium and chloride. They found that the serum chloride in patients with ileal pouches was significantly lower than in those with conventional ileostomies or in unoperated patients. Daily urinary loss of sodium in non-operated patients was significantly higher than in patients with ileal pouches or conventional ileostomies. Similarly, daily loss of potassium in patients with ileal pouches was significantly higher than in those with conventional ileostomies. From this study it appeared that changes in water and sodium balance after ileal pouches were similar to those after conventional ileostomies, but chloride balance was more altered after ileal pouch-anal anastomosis. Christie et al. (1990) investigated 14 patients with conventional ileostomies and 20 patients with J pouches where the extra cellular water volume was measured by bromide dilution method. Patients and controls had a 48-hour collection of urine for volume and sodium and potassium estimation. Similarly, a 48-hour collections of effluent were also made for analysis of volume and sodium and potassium. Total body weight, total body fat and fat-free mass were also measured. They showed that the body content of water and extra-cellular fluid in ileostomy patients and pouch patients is normal. Also, the effluent volume and chemistry was similar in both groups resulting in a similar and significant degree of urinary sodium retention.

Rectal, bladder and sexual function after restorative proctocolectomy

Proctocolectomy with a permanent ileostomy has been reported as associated with a high incidence of sexual dysfunction in men (Watts et al. 1966; Burnham et al. 1977). Bladder dysfunction has also been reported in some patients after proctectomy (Neal et al. 1982a). These complications have been thought to be related to damage to pelvic autonomic nerves during dissection around the rectum. Neal et al. (1982b) studied prospectively 33 patients who underwent a mucosal proctectomy, most for ulcerative colitis. Each patient had sexual and bladder function assessed before and after operation. Sixty-seven per cent of patients underwent filling and voiding pressure-flow cystometry before and after operation. In this study there was no detectable impairment of bladder or sexual function after mucosal proctectomy and ileal pouch-anal anastomosis. None of the patients reported impotence or failure of ejaculation. Similarly none of the patients reported bladder dysfunction following the pouch procedure. It is now known that damage to the autonomic nerves supplying the urinary bladder and those responsible for sexual function can be preserved either by a dissection close to the rectum or carefully dissecting in the plane between the mesorectum and the pelvic nerves. In my personal series none of the 23 patients who have had restorative proctocolectomy using the technique of total mesorectal excision have had bladder or sexual problems.

References

Barkel DC, Pemberton JH, Pexim ME et al. (1988) Scintigraphic assessment of the anorectal angle in health and after ileal pouch-anal anastomosis. Ann Surg 208:42–49

Becker JM (1984) Anal sphincter function after colectomy mucosal proctectomy and endorectal ileoanal pull-through. Arch Surg 119:526–531

Braun J, Treutner KH, Harder M, Lerch MM, Tons C, Schumpelick V (1991) Anal sphincter function after intersphincteric resection and stapled ileal pouch-anal anastomosis. Dis Colon Rectum 34:8–16

Brown JJ, Balfe DM, Heiken JP et al. (1990) Ileal J-pouch: radiologic evaluation in patients with and without postoperative infectious complications. Radiology 174:115–120

Burnham WR, Lennard-Jones JE, Brooke BN (1977) Sexual problems among married ileostomists. Gut 18:673–677

Chaussade S, Michopoulos S, Hautefeuille M, Valleur P, Hautefeuille P, Guerre J, Couturier D. Clinical and physiological study of anal sphincter and ileal J pouch before perileostomy closure and 6–12 months after closure of loop ileostomy. Dig Dis Sci 36:161–167

Christie PM, Knight GS, Hill GL (1990) Metabolism of body water and electrolytes after surgery for ulcerative colitis: conventional ileostomy versus J pouch. Br J Surg 77:149–151

Clarke AM, Chirnside A, Hill GL et al. (1967) Chronic dehydration and sodium depletion in patients with established ileotomies. Lancet ii:740–743

de Silva HJ, Jones M, Prince C, Kettlewell M, Mortensen NJ, Jewell DP (1991a) Lymphocyte and macrophage subpopulations in pelvic ileal pouches. Gut 32:1160–1165

de Silva HJ, Millard PR, Kettlewell M, Mortensen NJ, Prince C, Jewell DP (1991b) Mucosal characteristics of pelvic ileal pouches. Gut 32:61–65

de Silva HJ, Millard PR, Soper N, Kettlewell M, Mortensen NJ, Jewell DP (1991c) Effects of the faecal stream and stadid on the ileal pouch mucosa. Gut 32:1166–1169

Dozois RR, Goldberg SM, Rothenberger DA et al. (1986) Symposium on restorative proctocolectomy with ileal reservoir. Int J Colorectal Dis 1:2–19

Emblem R, Erichsen AA, Morkrid L et al. (1989) Failed ileoanal anastomosis: correlations between clinical function and anal canal neurophysiologic and histologic examinations. Scand J Gastroenterol 24:623–631

Everett WG (1989) Experience of restorative proctocolectomy with ileal reservoir. Br J Surg 76:77–81

Fiorentini MT, Locatelli L, Ceccopieri B et al. (1987) Physiology of ileoanal anastomosis with ileal reservoir for ulcerative colitis and adenomatosis coli. Dis Colon Rectum 30:267–272

Fonkalsrud EW, Loar N (1992) Long-term results after colectomy and endorectal ileal pullthrough procedure in children. Ann Surg 215:57–62

Gorbach SL, Nakas L, Weinstein L (1976) Studies of intestinal microflora. IV. The microflora of ileostomy effluent: a unique microbial ecology. Gastroenterology 53:874–877

Hallgren T, Fasth S, Nordgren, Oresland T, Hallsberg L, Hulten L (1989) Manovolumetric characteristics and functional results in three different pelvic pouch designs. Int J Colorect Dis 4:156–160

Harms BA, Pahl AC, Starling JR (1990) Comparison of clinical and compliance characteristics between S and W ileal reservoirs. Am J Surg 159:34–40

Hatakeyama K, Yamai K, Muto T (1989) Evaluation of ileal W pouch-anal anastomosis for restorative proctocolectomy. Int J Colorect Dis 4:150–155

Heald RJ, Allen DR (1986) Stapled ileoanal anastomosis: a technique to avoid mucosal proctectomy in the ileal pouch operation. Br J Surg 73:571–572

Hentges DJ (1983) Role of intestinal microflora in host defences against infection. In: Hentges DJ (ed) Human intestinal microflora in health and disease. Academic Press, New York, pp 311–331

Heppell J, Kelly KA, Phillips SF et al. (1982) Physiologic aspects of continence after colectomy mucosal proctectomy and endorectal ileoanal anastomosis. Ann Surg 195:435–443

Hillard AE, Mann FA, Becker JM, Nelson JA. The ileoanal J pouch: radiographic evaluation. Radiology 155:591–594

Hojlund PB, Simonsen L, Hansen LK et al. (1985) Bile acid malabsorption in patients with an ileal reservoir with a long efferent leg to an anal anastomosis. Scand J Gastroenterol 20:995–1000

Holdsworth PJ, Johnston D (1988a) Anal sensation after restorative proctectomy for ulcerative colitis. Br J Surg 75:993–996

Holdsworth JP, Johnston D (1988b) Use of the end-to-end anastomosis without mucosal stripping diminishes morbidity and time in hospital after restorative proctocolectomy. Br J Surg 75:1232

Johnston D, Holdsworth PJ, Nasmyth DG et al. (1987) Preservation of the entire anal canal in conservative proctocolectomy for ulcerative colitis: a pilot study comparing end-to-end ileoanal without mucosal resection with mucosal proctectomy and endo-anal anastomosis. Br J Surg 74:940–944

Kawarasaki H, Fujiwara T, Fonkalsrud EW (1985) Electric activity and motility in the side-to-side isoperistaltic ileal reservoir. Arch Surg 120:1045–1047

Keighley MRB, Kmiot W (1990) Surgical options in ulcerative colitis: role of ileo-anal anastomosis. Aust NZ Surg 60:835–845

Keighley MRB, Winslet MC, Yoshioka K, Lightwood R (1987) Discrimination is not impaired by excision of the anal transition zone after restorative proctocolectomy. Br J Surg 74:1118–1121

Keighley MRB, Yoshioka K, Kmiot W (1988a) Prospective randomised trial to compare the stapled double lumen pouch and the sutured quadruple pouch for restorative proctocolectomy. Br J Surg 75:1008–1011

Keighley MRB, Yoshioka K, Kmiot W, Heyen F (1988b) Physiological parameters influencing function in restorative proctocolectomy and ileal pouch-anal anastomosis. Br J Surg 75:997–1002

Kelly DG, Phillips SF, Kelly KA et al. (1983) Dysfunction of the continent ileostomy: clinical features and bacteriology. Gut 24:193–201

Kelly KA (1992) Anal sphincter saving operations for chronic ulcerative colitis. Am J Surg 163:5–11

Kennedy HJ, Al-Dujaili EAS, Edwards CRW et al. (1983) Water and electrolyte balance in subjects with a permanent ileostomy. Gut 24:702–705

Kmiot WA, Yoshioka K, Pinho M, Keighley MRB (1990) Videoproctographic assessment after restorative proctocolectomy. Dis Colon Rectum 33:566–572

Kumar D, Waldron D, Nicholls RJ, Williams NS (1989) Motor functon of the ileal reservoir following restorative proctocolectomy. Gastroenterology 96:A276

Lerch MM, Braun J, Harder M et al. (1989) Postoperative adaptation of the small intestine after total colectomy and J pouch-anal anastomosis. Dis Colon Rectum 32:600–608

Levitt MD, Kamm MA, Nicholls RJ (1991) Pouch dynamics – a simple test of ileoanal pouch evacuation. 6:158–160

Lindquist K (1990) Anal manometry with microtransducer technique before and after restorative proctocolectomy. Sphincter function and clinical correlations. Dis Colon Rectum 33:91–98

Marzouk D, Williams NS, Hallan RI (1989) Function after stapled ileal pouch-anal anastomosis for ulcerative colitis. Br J Surg 76:A627

Miller R, Orrom WJ, Duthie et al. (1990) Ambulatory anorectal physiology in patients following restorative proctocolectomy for ulcerative colitis: comparison with normal controls. Br J Surg 77:895–897

Mortensen N (1988) Progress with pouch-restorative proctocolectomy for ulcerative colitis. Gut 29:561–565

Nasmyth DG, Williams NS, Johnston D (1986) Comparison of the function of triplicated and duplicated pelvic ileal reservoirs after mucosal proctectomy and ileoanal anastomosis for ulcerative colitis and adenomatous polyposis. Br J Surg 73:361–366

Nasmyth DGN, Godwin PGR, Dixon MF, Williams NS, Johnstone D (1989a) Ileal ecology after pouch-anal anastomosis or ileostomy. Gastroenterology 96:817–824

Nasmyth DG, Johnston D, Williams NS, King RFG, Burkinshaw L, Brooks K (1989b) Changes in the absorption of bile acids after total colectomy in patients with an ileostomy or pouch-anal anastomosis. Dis Colon Rectum 32:230–234

Neal DE, Parker AJ, Williams NS et al. (1982a) The long-term effects of proctectomy on bladder function in patients with inflammatory bowel disease. Br J Surg 69:349–352

Neal DE, Williams NS, Johnston D (1982b) Rectal, bladder and sexual function after mucosal proctectomy with and without a pelvic reservoir for colitis and polyposis. Br J Surg 69:599–604

Nicholls RJ (1987) Restorative proctocolectomy with various types of reservoir. World J Surg 11:751–762

Nicholls RJ, Lubowski DZ (1987) Restorative proctocolectomy: the four loop (W) reservoir. Br J Surg 74:564–566

Nicholls RJ, Pezim ME (1985) Restorative proctocolectomy with ileal reservoir for ulcerative colitis and familial adenomatous polyposis: a comparison of three reservoir designs. Br J Surg 72:470–474

O'Connell PR, Rankin DR, Weiland LH, Kelly KA (1986) Enteric bacteriology, absorption, morphology and emptying after ileal pouch-anal anastomosis. Br J Surg 73:909–914

O'Connell PR, Pemberton JH, Brown ML et al. (1987) Determinants of stool frequency after ileal pouch-anal anastomosis. Am J Surg 153:157–163

O'Connell PR, Stryker SJ, Metcalf AM et al. (1988) Anal canal pressure and motility after ileoanal anastomosis. Surg Gynecol Obstet 166:47–54

Oresland T, Fasth S, Nordgren S, Akervall S, Hulten L (1990) Pouch size: the important functional determinant after restorative proctocolectomy. Br J Surg 77:265–269

Pemberton JH, Kelly KA, Beast RW et al. (1987) Ileal pouch-anal anastomosis for chronic ulcerative colitis: long-term results. Ann Surg 206:504–513

Pescatori M, Parks AG (1984) The sphincteric and sensory components of preserved continence after ileoanal reservoir. Surg Gynecol Obstet 158:517–521

Pescatori M, Manhire A, Bartram CI Evacuation pouchography in the evaluation of ileoanal reservoir function. Dis Colon Rectum 26:365–368

Phillips SF, Giller J (1973) The contribution of the colon to electrolyte and water conservation in man. J Lab Clin Med 81:733–746

Rosemurgy AS, Schraut WH, Block GE (1983) The physiological effects of ileal reservoirs and efferent conduits complementing ileoanal anastomosis: an experimental study in dogs. Surgery 94:697–703

Rothenberger DA, Wong WD, Buls JG, Goldberg SM (1985) In: Dozois RR (ed) Alternatives to conventional ileostomy. Yearbook Medical, Chicago, pp 345–362

Sagar PM, Holdsworth PJ, Godwin GR, Quirke P, Smith AN, Johnstone D (1992) Comparison of triplicated (S) and quadruplicated (W) pelvic ileal reservoirs: studies on manovolumetry, fecal bacteriology, fecal volatile fatty acids, mucosal morphology, and function results. Gastroenterology 102:520–528

Santavirta J, Harmoninen A, Karvonen AL, Matikainen M (1991a) Water and electrolyte balance after ileoanal anastomosis. Dis Colon Rectum 34:115–118

Santavirta J, Mattila J, Kokki M, Matikainen M (1991b) Mucosal morphology and faecal bacteriology after ileoanal anastomosis. Int J Colorec Dis 6:38–41

Sharp FR, Bell GA, Seal AM, Atkinson KG (1987) Investigations of the anal sphincter before and after restorative proctocolectomy. Am J Surg 153:496–472

Shepherd NA, Jass JR, Duval I, Moskowitz RL, Nicholls RJ, Morson BC (1987) Restorative proctocolectomy with ileal reservoir: pathological and histochemical study of mucosal biopsy specimens. J Clin Pathol 40:601–607

Shepherd NA, Jass JR, Duval I et al. (1989) Restorative proctocolectomy with ileal reservoir: a pathological and histochemical study of mucosal biopsy specimens. J Clin Pathol 40:601–607

Stryker SJ, Kelly KA, Phillips SF et al. (1986) Anal and neorectal function after proctocolectomy and ileal pouch-anal anastomosis. Ann Surg 203:55–61

Sugarman HJ, Newsome HH, Decosta G, Zfass AM (1991) Stapled ileoanal anastomosis for ulcerative colitis and familial polyposis without a temporary diverting ileostomy. Ann Surg 213:606–619

Taylor BM, Beart RW, Dozois RR, Kelly KA, Phillips SF (1983) Straight ileoanal anastomosis v. ileal pouch-anal anastomosis after colectomy and mucosal proctectomy. Arch Surg 118:696–701

Thayer ML, Madoff RD, Jacobs DM, Bubrick MP (1990) Comparative intrinsic and extrinsic compliance characteristics of S, J and W ileoanal pouches. Dis Colon Rectum 33:86

Tuckson WB, Fazio VW (1991) Functional comparison between double and triple ileal loop pouches. Dis Colon Rectum 34:17–21

Watts J McK, de Dombal FT, Goligher JC (1966) Long-term complications and prognosis following major surgery for ulcerative colitis. Br J Surg 53:1014–1023

Wexner SD, James K, Jagelman DG (1991) The double-spaced ileal reservoir and ileoanal anastomosis: a prospective review of sphincter function and clinical outcome. Dis Colon Rectum 34:487–494

Williams NS, Johnston D (1985) The current status of mucosal proctectomy and ileoanal anastomosis in the surgical treatment of ulcerative colitis and adenomatous polyposis. Br J Surg 72:159–168

Williams NS, Marzouk DEMM, Hallan RI, Waldron DJ (1989) Function after ileal pouch and stapled pouch-anal anastomosis for ulcerative colitis. Br J Surg 76:1168–1171

27 Complications of Restorative Proctocolectomy

D. Kumar

The concept of an ileal pouch-anal anastomosis is attractive to the patient because it eliminates the need for a permanent ileostomy and is also attractive to the surgeon because it cures the patient of ulcerative colitis. Although the mortality from this complex procedure is remarkably low, there is a substantial morbidity. Approximately a third of all patients will develop complications (Hulten 1986; Vasilevsky et al. 1987; Beart 1988). The commonest complications following restorative proctocolectomy are:

1. Haemorrhage from the pouch
2. Leak from the pouch suture line
3. Pouch necrosis
4. Pouch-anal anastomotic stenosis
5. Pelvic sepsis
6. Intestinal obstruction
7. Pouchitis
8. Pouch-anal or pouch-vaginal fistulae
9. Pouch failure

The incidence of the complications mentioned above is variable and to a large extent depends upon the experience of the surgeon and patient selection.

Early complication

Haemorrhage from the pouch

Haemorrhage from the pouch is an uncommon complication. I have never seen an example. However, most of the reported cases have required re-laparotomy to stop the bleeding. Some surgeons leave a tube drain in the pouch to drain any blood or collections from within the pouch. I have used this in the past but remain sceptical of its value.

Leak from the pouch suture line

The reported incidence of suture line leakage from the pouch itself is around 5%. Such leaks either present early as pelvic sepsis, or at a later stage as pouch-cutaneous fistulas. If this does occur, a defunctioning loop ileostomy with adequate drainage of sepsis may help in salvaging the pouch. These are serious complications and often result in pouch excision.

Pouch necrosis

Necrosis is usually the result of ischaemia either due to undue tension on mesenteric vessels or an inadvertent twist in the mesentry at the apex of the pouch. Although Pescatori et al. (1988) have reported a 4% incidence of pouch necrosis in their series, it is fortunately a rare complication. When it does occur it requires pouch excision.

Pouch-anal anastomotic stenosis

The incidence of anastomotic stenosis after pouch-anal anastomosis varies between 1% and 8% (Skarsgard et al. 1989; Wexner et al. 1990). A minor degree of anastomotic stenosis is common, particularly during the time when the pouch is defunctioned by a temporary loop ileostomy. Most of the anastomotic strictures will respond to simple once only dilatation. Less than 5% of patients will require intermittent dilatation for recurrent stenotic problems. In the few patients with recurrent stenotic problems a biopsy should be taken from close to the strictured anastomosis to exclude histological evidence of Crohn's disease.

Pelvic sepsis

The incidence of pelvic sepsis following ileal pouch-anal anastomosis varies between 10% and 30% (Nicholls 1987) (Table 27.1). The commonest cause of pelvic sepsis following ileal pouch-anal anastomosis is an infected pelvic haematoma but occasionally this is due to an anastomotic dehiscence or disruption of the pouch suture or staple line. When surgeons used to leave a rectal muscular cuff through which the pouch was pulled and anastomosed to the dentate line, cuff abscess was the commonest form of pelvic sepsis. Since the introduction of a stapled ileal pouch-anal anastomosis, which does not involve a rectal cuff this complication has been eliminated because there is no residual space between the rectal muscular wall and the pouch. Cuff abscess usually resulted in partial dehiscence of the ileo-anal anastomosis and subsequent drainage of the collection into the pelvis, causing an abscess or peritonitis. Disruption of the pouch suture or staple line, although uncommon, may also cause spillage of pouch contents into the pelvis and result in pelvic sepsis (Taylor et al. 1983; Freshman et al. 1988).

Table 27.1. Pelvic sepsis following restorative proctocolectomy

Author	*n* (Pouch type)	sepsis *n*	%
Becker and Raymond 1986	100 (J)	0	0
Beart 1988	188 (J)	21	11
Scott et al. 1988	500	30	6
Keighley et al. 1988	18 (J) 15 (W)	2 1	11 6.7
Hatakeyama et al. 1989	16 (W)	2	12.5
Nicholls et al. 1989	152	26	17
Pemberton et al. 1987	390 (J)	20	5
Sugarman et al. 1991	46 (J) 18 (S)	6 4	13 22

Pelvic sepsis is the commonest cause of pouch failure and results in pouch excision in approximately 5%–10% of all ileal pouch-anal anastomoses. The treatment is adequate surgical drainage of the collection per abdomen and defunctioning of the pouch with a loop ileostomy. Intestinal continuity should not be restored until sepsis has settled completely. Occasionally pelvic abscesses can drain spontaneously into the pouch (Schoetz et al. 1986) but may still require pouch excision (Fonkalsrud 1985).

There is evidence that the incidence of pelvic sepsis, like other complications following ileal pouch-anal anastomosis, improves with increasing experience. Scott et al. (1988) reported a 6% overall incidence of postoperative sepsis; it was 11% for the first 100 procedures and it decreased to 5% in the next 300 patients and was 4% in the last 100 patients.

Females appear to be more prone to pelvic sepsis following restorative proctocolectomy as do those who are underweight, or have a carcinoma or systemic toxicity complicating their colitis (Scott et al. 1988). The use of prophylactic antibiotics or pre-operative corticosteroids does not seem to influence the incidence of pelvic sepsis (Higgens et al. 1980). Scott et al. (1988) also found that patients who had had a previous sub-total colectomy and Brooke ileostomy were not protected after complications against restorative surgery. However, their findings contradict a previous report (Martin et al. 1977) which suggested that a preceding ileostomy and sub-total colectomy may protect an ileal pouch-anal anastomosis from complications.

If laparotomy is required to deal with sepsis, the pouch usually has to be removed. However, in those patients in whom pelvic sepsis had been treated successfully and conservatively with pouch preservation, the com-

Table 27.2 Intestinal obstruction following ileal pouch-anal anastomosis

Author	*n*	Pouch	Obstruction conservative management (%)	Laparotomy (%)
Becker and Raymond 1986	100	J	8	7
Pemberton et al. 1987	390	J	3	10
Fleshman et al. 1988	NA	S,J	10	9
Nicholls et al. 1989	152	S,J,W	NA	13
Keighley et al. 1989	65	S,J,W	6	8

plication has no adverse influence on stool frequency or continence (Pemberton et al. 1987).

Intestinal obstruction

Obstruction is the commonest early complication and is usually due to adhesions (Table 27.2). Approximately 15%–20% of patients undergoing ileal pouch-anal anastomosis experience episodes of obstruction and about half of these will require a further laparotomy. The majority of episodes of small bowel obstruction following restorative proctocolectomy have been related to the temporary ileostomy. The incidence of small bowel obstruction is higher in patients who have had a previous subtotal colectomy than in those who have not undergone a previous colectomy (Francois et al. 1989). In a series of 188 patients from the Mayo Clinic (Beart 1988) 23% of patients showed clinical evidence of small bowel obstruction. In a third of these patients the obstruction was related to ileostomy closure. In this series laparotomy was required in approximately 30% of the patients with small bowel obstruction. It is not invariably such a dismal picture; in my experience with 23 patients having restorative proctocolectomy, episodes of intestinal obstruction occurred in only four patients and all of these settled with conservative management.

Pouchitis

Some degree of mucosal inflammation is seen frequently in ileal pouches. This is often transient and asymptomatic and does not justify the designation "pouchitis". However, as experience with this procedure grows it is evident that recurrent pouchitis or severe mucosal inflammation of the reservoir has become a major long-term problem. The reported incidence of pouchitis is between 7% and 42% of patients (Dozois 1985; Dozois et al. 1986; Moskovitz et al. 1986; Tytgat and Van Deventer 1988). It seems likely that the variation in incidence of pouchitis is due to different authors having different definitions and diagnostic criteria. However, some patients, present with an obvious clinical syndrome which is associated with endoscopic and histopathological inflammation of a severe degree (Nicholls 1987).

The symptoms of pouchitis include frequency of defaecation which correlates with the histological grade of inflammation (Fig. 27.1), loose watery stools, malaise, fatigue and occasionally reactivation of extra-intestinal manifestations such as arthropathy (Nicholls 1987). Using these diagnostic criteria a prevalence of 11% has been reported from St Mark's Hospital (Shepherd et al. 1989). They recommended that pouchitis should be diagnosed by a combination of clinical, endoscopic and histopathological criteria; particularly the severity of mucosal inflammation. It is only acute, not chronic, inflammation that is diagnostic of pouchitis. In another series of 90 patients from St Mark's Hospital, 87% showed some degree of chronic inflammation and only 30% acute and it was only those with acute changes who had symptoms (Nicholls 1989).

The aetiology of pouchitis is unknown. It is believed that acute pouchitis is found exclusively in patients who suffered with ulcerative colitis before colectomy. Also

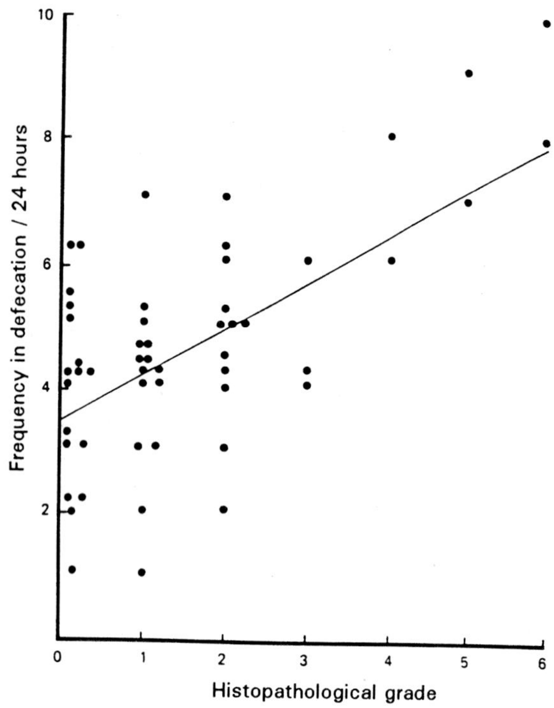

Fig. 27.1. Frequency of defaecation and histological grade of inflammation (correlation coefficient of linear regression $r = 0.65$; $P < 0.001$). (From Moskowitz et al. (1986) with permission.)

patients who had total colitis are more likely to develop pouchitis than are those who had their protocolectomy for predominantly distal disease (Madden et al. 1990). The association of pouchitis and total colitis led to the belief that pre-operative backwash ileitis may be responsible. However, Gustavsson et al. (1987), in their series of 131 patients, only found backwash ileitis in 15. Twenty of their 131 patients developed pouchitis and only two of these had had backwash ileitis.

Since pouchitis responds favourably to antimicrobial treatment it was postulated that it may be bacterial in origin and this has led to the study of bacterial flora within the pouches. Quantitative anaerobe counts are greater in the luminal contents of pouch patients than in those with an end ileostomy. More importantly, neither total counts nor particular concentrations of pathogens appear to be associated with the presence of acute pouchitis (Luukkonen et al. 1988). Others have measured crypt cell production rates in patients with and without pouchitis. In these studies crypt cell production rates correlated well with the degree of villous atrophy but not with pouch bacteriology (Kmiot et al. 1989; Keighley et al. 1990). Therefore, it seems unlikely that a known intestinal pathogen is the cause of pouchitis. It has been postulated that the disease may be caused by a yet unidentified abnormality in the microbacteriological profile or in the immune response to that profile.

Faecal bile acids have been studied in patients with pouchitis to determine whether the diarrhoea and severe inflammation in pouchitis could be due to an abnormally high intestinal bile acid concentration. Owen et al. (1984) studied faecal steroids in 20 healthy pouch patients who had restorative proctocolectomy for chronic ulcerative colitis, six ileal pouches for ulcerative colitis with pouchitis and seven pouch patients who had familial adenomatous polyposis (FAP). They compared faecal steroids of pouch patients treated for FAP with those treated for ulcerative colitis. The faecal steroids were mainly deconjugated in 68% of pouch patients and 81% of pouch patients who had FAP. Similarly, in 23% of the pouch patients (FAP and ulcerative colitis) free bile acids had undergone dehydroxilation. This study did not reveal a high faecal bile acid concentration in pouchitis. Pouchitis patients tended to have a slightly lower bile acid concentration compared to those with healthy pouches.

O'Connell et al. (1986) investigated 20 patients following ileal pouch-anal anastomosis to test the hypothesis that stasis within an ileal reservoir is a prerequisite for the development of pouchitis. They correlated with the clinical outcome the ileal and jejunal bacterial count and the efficiency of ileal pouch evacuation. Enteric bacterial counts and the efficiency of ileal pouch evacuation were no different in patients with recurrent pouchitis than in those with a good clinical outcome. However, they did identify jejunal bacterial overgrowth in patients with a poor clinical outcome. Similar observations have been reported by Moskowitz et al. (1986) and Heppel et al. (1987). Therefore, it seems that quantitative bacterial overgrowth within the pouch is not responsible for acute pouchitis but it is uncertain whether a qualitative change in ileal pouch flora is responsible (O'Connell et al. 1986).

The long-term effects of pouchitis in pouch patients is unknown. Most patients show an immediate favourable response to metronidazole (Dozois et al. 1986). Occasionally patients with severe pouchitis have been treated successfully with corticosteroids and 5-aminosalicylic acid (Tytgat and van Deventer 1988). However, experience is limited and randomised controlled trials are needed to validate the efficacy of treatment. It is rarely necessary to excise the pouch and convert to a permanent end ileostomy for pouchitis although it may be required in those who find unacceptable symptoms of recurrent pouchitis.

Pouch-anal or pouch-vaginal fistulas

This is a well-recognised yet uncommon complication of ileal pouch-anal anastomosis. In a multi-centre study, reported from North America, 304 pouch operations were performed in female patients, 21 developed pouch-vaginal fistulas; an overall incidence of 6.9%. Of patients in this series, 85% had a covering loop ileostomy and 88% had their pelvis drained at operation. Contrary to what might be expected, 30% of the pouch-vaginal fistulas presented before ileostomy closure and only 12% of the patients were found to have Crohn's disease (Wexner et al. 1989). In this series also, sepsis was the most common associated complication. Thirteen different forms of treatment were used and the majority of them underwent more than one procedure. Five of the 21 had local treatment and another five had more aggressive treatment. Five patients ultimately required pouch excision. The most successful local treatments of the fistula were sphincteroplasty and an advancement flap. Closure via the trans-anal or trans-vaginal route were the next most successful forms of treatment while debridement and fistulectomy was the least successful. Some have reported Seton fistulotomy for the treatment of pouch-vaginal fistula (Keighley et al. 1988) and others trans-vaginal advancement flaps and anoplasties.

Based on the varied experiences of many authors of pouch-vaginal and pouch-anal fistulas it can be concluded that:

1. Sepsis is an important aetiological factor
2. It is important to exclude Crohn's disease
3. Sepsis, when present, should be adequately drained
4. A defunctioning loop ileostomy stoma may have to be performed
5. In approximately 50% of patients local procedures such as a mucosal advancement flap will successfully treat this complication; others may require more aggressive forms of intervention

Re-operation for complications of restorative proctocolectomy

With long-term follow-up, an increasing number of patients are presenting for treatment of specific pouch-related complications. Reoperation may be necessary when these complications are refractory to conservative treatment. However, the safety, efficacy and function results of salvage operations is not known.

Galandiuk et al. (1990) retrospectively reviewed the results of 114 patients who had reoperation for pouch-related complications. Patients with small bowel obstruction were excluded from this analysis. Pouch-related complications were divided into four groups:

1. Anastomotic stricture (42 patients)
2. Perianal abscess, fistula or sinus (30 patients)
3. Intra-abdominal fistula or abscess (29 patients)
4. Functional problems including impaired pouch emptying and incontinence (13 patients)

Eighty-two percent of patients had J pouches, 9% S and the remaining 9% had other types of pouches. Thirty-six percent of patients still had a diverting loop ileostomy before reoperation. The salvage operations included anal dilatation under general anaesthesia, Seton fistulotomy, deroofing of sinuses, simple drainage of abscesses, drainage of intra-abdominal sepsis and partial or complete reconstruction of reservoirs in patients who had inadequate pouch emptying.

After reoperation, further complications occured in 70 patients (61%) requiring subsequent operations. After a mean follow-up of three years, 22 patients had their pouches excised, 15 had ileostomies with intact pouches and 77 had functioning pouches; of these 77

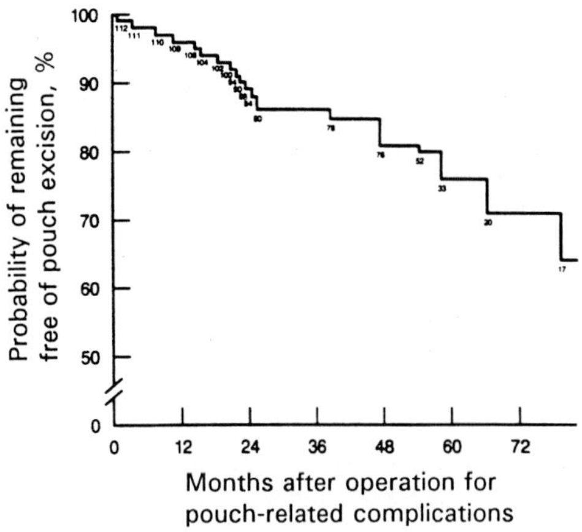

Fig. 27.2 Probability of pouch excision against time among all patients with pouch-related complications requiring operation after ileal pouch-anal anastomosis. (From Galandiuk et al. (1990) with permission.)

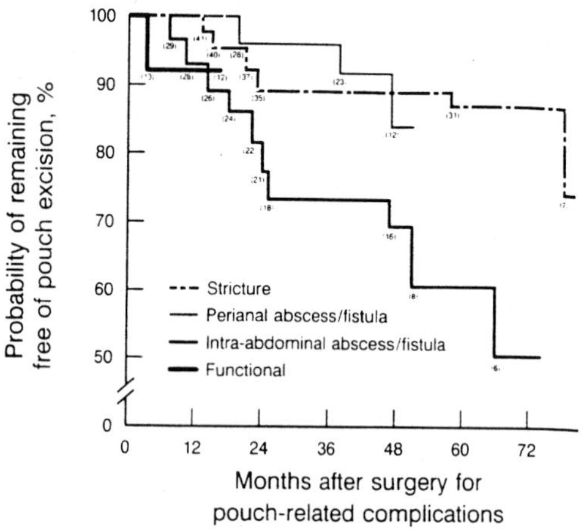

Fig. 27.3. Probability of pouch excision against time among groups of patients with pouch-related complications requiring reoperation after ileal pouch-anal anastomosis. (From Galandiuk et al. (1990) with permission.)

patients, 54 (70%) had a satisfactory functional result. The probability of pouch excision against time is greater amongst patients who have pouch-related complications and require reoperation (Fig. 27.2, 27.3). In this series, 69% of patients requiring more than one operation for pouch-related complications had their pouch excised compared to 14% who had only one operation for pouch-related complications.

Salvage operations for pouch-related complications can be done safely and restore good pouch function in approximately two thirds of patients. Complications after reoperation will, however, lead to pouch excision in about 20% of patients. In patients who have pelvic sepsis pouch excision is common.

Quality of life after ileal pouch-anal anastomosis

It is generally believed that patients undergoing ileal pouch-anal anastomosis experience a better quality of life than those undergoing proctocolectomy and conventional ileostomy. The quality of life following a permanent ileostomy is generally regarded as satisfactory (Becker and Raymond 1986; Pemberton et al. 1987; Cohen and McCloud 1988). Nevertheless, it has been reported that following conversion to a continent ileostomy there is an improvement in the patient's quality of life (Kock et al. 1980, 1981; Gerber et al. 1984, McCloud and Fazio 1984). Pemberton et al. (1989) have shown that patients with ileal pouch-anal anastomosis are better able to perform their daily activities compared with those with a conventional ileostomy. It is not clear, however, whether the good quality of life after pouch operations is due to the avoidance of a permanent stoma or due to achieving faecal continence. To try to answer this question a recent study (Cola et al. 1991) investigated 796 patients. They compared function and performance in patients with a conventional ileostomy with those with a continent ileostomy and those with ileal pouch-anal anastomosis. Patients were surveyed by a questionnaire or telephone and the follow-up was continued until 300 consecutive patients had responded. Dietary restrictions were reported by 46% of continent ileostomy patients compared to 28% conventional ileostomy and 22% ileal pouch-anal anastomosis patients. There were no detectable differences in overall satisfaction among patients with any of the three operations. However, amongst patients who were informed of the possibility of alternative procedures, more patients with conventional ileostomies and continent ileostomies desired a change than did those with ileal pouch-anal anastomosis. Patients with continent ileostomies had greater travel restrictions than those with permanent ileostomies.

Most reported series on quality of life after ileal pouch-anal anastomosis are limited by the fact that patients in the continent ileostomy and conventional ileostomy groups have had the procedure performed for a much longer period of time than those who have had the newer restorative proctocolectomy. The other factor that makes comparison invalid is that patients with psychological and emotional instability are regarded as a relative contraindication for a restorative proctocolectomy. The standard proctocolectomy with conventional end-ileostomy is offered to all comers including the unstable and disturbed. This is likely to bias the results in favour of ileal pouch-anal anastomosis selected as they are on the basis of stable personalities.

References

Beart RW (1988) Proctocolectomy and ileoanal anastomosis. World J Surg 12:160–163

Becker JM, Raymond JL (1986) Ileal pouch-anal anastomosis: a single surgeons experience with 100 consecutive cases. Ann Surg 204:375–383

Cohen Z, McCloud RS Proctocolectomy and ileoanal anastomosis with J shaped or S shaped ileal pouch. World J Surg 12:164–168

Dozois RR (1985) Ileal J pouch-anal anastomosis. Br J Surg 72:580–582

Dozois RR, Goldberg SM, Rothenberger DA et al. (1986) Symposium: restorative proctocolectomy with ileal reservoir. Int J Colorect Dis 1:2–19.

Fleshman JW, Cohen Z, McCleod RS, Stern H, Blair J (1988) The ileal reservoir and ileoanal anastomosis procedure: factors affecting technical and functional outcome. Dis Colon Rectum 31:10–16

Fonkalsrud EW (1985) Endorectal ileal pullthrough with isoperistaltic ileal reservoir for colitis and polyposis. Ann Surg 202:145–152

Francois Y, Dozois RR, Kelly KA et al. (1989) Small intestinal obstruction complicating ileal pouch-anal anastomosis. Ann Surg 209:46–50

Galandiuk S, Scott NA, Dozois R et al. (1990) Ileal pouch-anal anastomosis: re-operation for pouch-related complications. Ann Surg 212:446–454

Gerber A, Apt MK, Craig PH (1984) The improved quality of life with the Kock continent ileostomy. J Clin Gastroenterol 6:513–517

Gustavsson S, Weiland LH, Kelly KA (1987) Relationship of backwash ileitis to ileal pouchitis after ileal pouch-anal anastomosis. Dis Colon Rectum 30:25–28

Hatakeyama K, Yamai K, Muto T (1989) Evaluation of ileal W pouch-anal anastomosis for restorative proctocolectomy. Int J Colon Dis 4:150–155

Heppell J, Belliveau P, Taillefer R et al. (1987) Quantitative assessment of pelvic ileal reservoir emptying with a semisolid radionuclide enema: a correlation with clinical outcome. Dis Colon Rectum 30:81–85

Higgens C, Allan RN, Keighley MRB, Arabi Y, Alexander-Williams J (1980) Sepsis following operation for inflammatory intestinal disease. Dis Colon Rectum 23:102–105

Hulten L (1986) In:Symposium: restorative protocolectomy with ileal reservoir. Int J Colorect Dis 1:2–19

Keighley MRB, Yoshioka K, Kmiot W (1988) Prospective randomised trial to compare the stapled double lumen pouch and the sutured quadruple pouch for restorative proctocolectomy. Br J Surg 75:1008–1011

Keighley MRB, Winslet MC, Flinn R, Kmiot W (1989) Multivariate analysis of factors influencing the results of restorative proctocolectomy. Br J Surg 76:740–743

Keighley MRB, Kmiot WA, Youngs DJ (1990) Recovery from pouchitis: the mechanism of adaptive ileal villous regrowth. Dis Colon Rectum 33:33

Kmiot WA, Youngs DJ, Keighley MRB (1989) Recovery from pouchitis: the mechanism of adaptive ileal villous regrowth. Br J Surg 76:1338

Kock Ng, Myrvoid HE, Nilsson LO (1980) Progress report on the continent ileostomy. World J Surg 4:143–148

Kock NG, Myrvoid HE, Nilsson LO, Philipson BM (1981) Continent ileostomy. An account of 314 patients. Acta Chir Scand 147:67–72

Kohler LW, Pemberton JH, Zinsmeister AR, Kelly KA (1991) Quality of life after proctocolectomy. A comparison of Brooke ileostomy, Kock pouch, and ileal pouch-anal anastomosis. Gastroenterology 101:679–684

Luukkonen P, Valtonen V, Sivoren A et al. (1988) Faecal bacteriology and reservoir ileitis in patients operated on for ulcerative colitis. Dis Colon Rectum 31:864–867

Madden MV, Farthing MJG, Nicholls RJ (1990) Inflammation in ileal reservoirs: 'pouchitis'. Gut 31:247–249

Martin LW, LeCoultre C, Schubert WK (1977) Total colectomy and mucosal proctectomy with preservation of continence in ulcerative colitis. Ann Surg 186:477–480

McCloud RS, Fazio VW (1984) Quality of life with the continent ileostomy. World J Surg 8:90–95

Moskowitz RL, Shepherd NA, Nicholls RJ (1986) An assessment of inflammation in the reservoir after restorative proctocolectomy with ileoanal ileal reservoir. Int J Colorect Dis 1:167–174

Nicholls RJ (1987) Restorative proctocolectomy with various types of reservoir. World J Surg 11:751–762

Nicholls RJ, Holt SDH, Lubowski DZ (1989) Restorative proctocolectomy with ileal reservoir: comparison of two-stage vs. three-stage procedures and analysis of factors that might affect outcome. Dis Colon Rectum 32:323–326

O'Connell PR, Rankin DR, Weiland LH, Kelly KA (1986) Enteric bacteriology, absorption, morphology and emptying after pouch-anal anastomosis. Br J Surg 73:909–914

Owen RW, Thompson MH, Hill MJ (1984) Analysis of metabolic profiles of steroids in faeces of healthy subjects undergoing chemodeoxycholic acid treatment by liquid-gel chromatography and gas-liquid chromatography-mass spectrometry. J Steroid Biochem 5:593–600

Pemberton JH, Kelly KA, Beart RW Jr, Dozois RR, Wolff BG, Ilstrup D (1987) Ileal pouch-anal anastomosis for chronic ulcerative colitis: long-term results. Ann Surg 206:540–513

Pemberton JH, Phillips SF, Ready RR, Zinmeister AR, Beahrs OH (1989) Quality of life after Brooke ileostomy and ileal pouch-anal anastomosis. Ann Surg 209:620–628

Pescatori M, Mattana C, Castagneto M (1988) Clinical and functional results after restorative proctocolectomy. Br J Surg 75:321–324

Schoetz DJ Jr, Coller JA, Veidenheimer MC (1986) Ileoanal reservoir for ulcerative colitis and familial polyposis. Arch Surg 121:404–409

Scott NA, Dozois RR, Beart RW Jr, Pemberton JH, Wolff BG, Ilstrup DM (1988) Postoperative intra-abdominal and pelvic sepsis complicating ileal pouch-anal anastomosis. Int J Colorect Dis 1988, 3:149–152

Shepherd NA, Hulten L, Tytgat GNJ, Nasmyth DG, Hill MJ, Fernandez F, Gertner DJ, Rampton DS, Hill MJ, Owen RW, Kmiot WA, Keighley MRB, O'Connell PR, Kumar D, Williams NS (1989) Workshop. Int J Colorect Dis 4:205–229

Skarsgard ED, Atkinson KG, Bell GA et al. (1989) Function and quality of life results after ileal pouch surgery for chronic ulcerative colitis and familial polyposis. Am J Surg 157:467–471

Sugarman HJ, Newsome HH, Decosta G, Zfass AM (1991) Stapled ileoanal anastomosis for ulcerative colitis and familial polyposis without a temporary diverting ileostomy. Ann Surg 213:606–619

Taylor BM, Cranley B, Kelly KA, Phillips SF, Beart RW, Dozois RR (1983) A clinico-physiological comparison of ileal pouch-anal and straight ileoanal anastomosis. Ann Surg 198:462–468

Tytgat GNJ, van Deventer SJH (1988) Pouchitis. Int J Colorect Dis 3:226–228

Vasilevsky CA, Rothenberger BA, Goldberg SM. The S ileal pouch-anal anastomosis. World J Surg 11:742-750

Wexner SD, Rothenberger DA, Jensen L et al. (1989) Ileal pouch vaginal fistulas: incidence etiology and management. Dis Colon Rectum 32:460–465

Wexner SD, Wong WD, Rothenberger DA, Goldberg SM (1990) The ileoanal reservoir. Am J Surg 159:178–18

Section IV

28 Management of Stomas

D. Kumar

The most commonly employed stoma in the surgical management of inflammatory bowel disease is an ileostomy. Occasionally, in the management of Crohn's disease some surgeons employ a colostomy. Despite the fact that several hundreds of thousands of permanent ileostomies have been constructed throughout the world in patients with inflammatory bowel disease, the prospect of living with a permanent stoma continues to cause patients to have a significant psychological morbidity. It is to reduce this morbidity that technical developments in the surgical management of inflammatory bowel disease have taken place over the last two to three decades. Although operations such as ileo-rectal anastomosis, continent ileostomy and restorative proctocolectomy have significantly reduced the need for a permanent conventional ileostomy, a panproctocolectomy and ileostomy still remains one of the best options in the surgical management of inflammatory bowel disease. Although stomas function well, there is a significant complication rate (Goldblactt et al. 1977; Weaver et al. 1988). The common complications of stomas include parastomal hernia (1%–5%), stenosis (5%–10%), retraction (5%–10%), sepsis and fistula (1%–4%), and prolapse (1%–6%) (Ritchie 1971). Furthermore, patients developing complications from their ileostomy often require operative revisions. Some of the problems related to stomas can be avoided by careful stoma marking and patient counselling before operation.

Stoma siting

Siting is one of the most important aspects of formation of a stoma. A stoma site should be marked precisely and carefully by the operating surgeon or stoma therapist on the patient's skin with a permanent ink marker. Care must be taken that the stoma site does not lie on the waistline in an area where patients may fasten their clothes. Care must also be exercised in obese people as the site of the stoma may change when they stand up. What looks like an appropriate site in the lying down position may end 15 cm lower in the standing position. Therefore, in such subjects an assessment of stoma site should be made in the upright position. Similarly, skin creases can cause leakage of ileostomy effluent and therefore patients should be assessed in the sitting position so that skin creases can be identified. Attention must also be paid to the suitability of the skin for appliance application. If the patient has scars close to the standard site for an ileostomy stoma they may interfere with the application of the appliance, resulting in leakage and skin problems. The patient should be able to see the stoma to be able to manage it well.

Patient counselling

It is important to prepare the patient mentally for life with a stoma. The majority of patients who agree to have a permanent stoma performed do not understand fully the implications. They must be made aware of the common problems and also they must be well trained in the art of looking after a stoma. The patients should be seen by a stoma care nurse who can explain to them the various changes they may have to make in their work or social environment. Written and verbal information about the operation and stoma management is helpful. Similarly, the family members should be counselled as the quality of life assessment with a stoma does not just apply to the patient but to the whole family as a unit.

Operative technique

For a permanent ileostomy, a 2 cm disc of skin is excised with electrocautery at the preselected stoma site. The subcutaneous fat is excised in the shape of a cylinder down to the anterior rectus sheath, again with the help of cutting diathermy and maintaining meticulous haemostasis. A cruciate incision is made in the anterior rectus sheath and the underlying fibres of the rectus muscle are gently teased apart making sure that the opening does not admit more than 2 fingers. The underlying peritoneum and posterior rectus sheath is incised and the peritoneal edges held with a tissue-holding forceps. The cut end of the ileum with a handleless clamp is then delivered through the opening in the abdominal wall making sure that approximately 5 cm of the ileal end projects above the skin surface and is not under tension. The ileum is then anchored to the peritoneal edges held by tissue forceps. In my experience 2/0 Polyglactin sutures between the peritoneal edge and seromuscular layer of the ileum placed in four quadrants are sufficient for this purpose. At this stage the ileal end should be checked for viability making sure that the blood supply has not been compromised during the anchoring procedure. A tissue-holding forceps is then introduced through the lumen of the ileum and the end everted to form a spout measuring 2–3 cm. The ileal mucosal edge is sutured to the cut edge of the skin using 5 or 6 4/0 Prolene sutures placed circumferentially. A transparent stoma appliance is applied so that the stoma can be inspected post-operatively to assess the viability of the stoma.

Ileostomy effluent

In patients who have a well-functioning and well-matured ileostomy the volume of ileal effluent varies between 200 and 700 ml per 24 hours (Kramer 1966). In the first week after operation the ileal effluent is usually thin and green in colour and the volumes are small until the patient is eating. By about the tenth day the effluent starts to become thicker and the output maintained at around 600 to 700 mls per day. In patients with Crohn's disease the ileostomy output is usually higher. In health, the effluent volume shows little variation despite changes in diet. Sudden increases in ileostomy output may indicate small intestinal obstruction or recurrence of Crohn's disease. Biochemically, the sodium content of ileal effluent is three times greater than that of normal stool. However, the body compensates by increased renal conservation of salt and water and as a result patients with ileostomies do not show signs of salt depletion (Gallagher et al. 1962; Hill 1990). Occasionally patients with a high output ileostomy show evidence of magnesium depletion.

Ileostomy effluent is rich in pancreatic proteolytic enzymes. Therefore, if the ileal effluent is allowed to come in prolonged contact with the skin as a result of an ill-fitting appliance skin excoriation will occur. Due to disturbed entero-hepatic circulation in patients with ileostomies some people have reported a higher incidence of asymptomatic gall stones compared with the general population (Kurchin et al. 1984).

Complications of stomas

Approximately 20%–25% of patients with stomas will experience a stoma-related complication and of these nearly 50% will require surgical intervention (Ritchie 1971; Carlstedt et al. 1987). Complications following the formation of stomas can be broadly divided into those due to technical problems and those due to functional problems. The majority of complications described below are common to both ileostomies and colostomies.

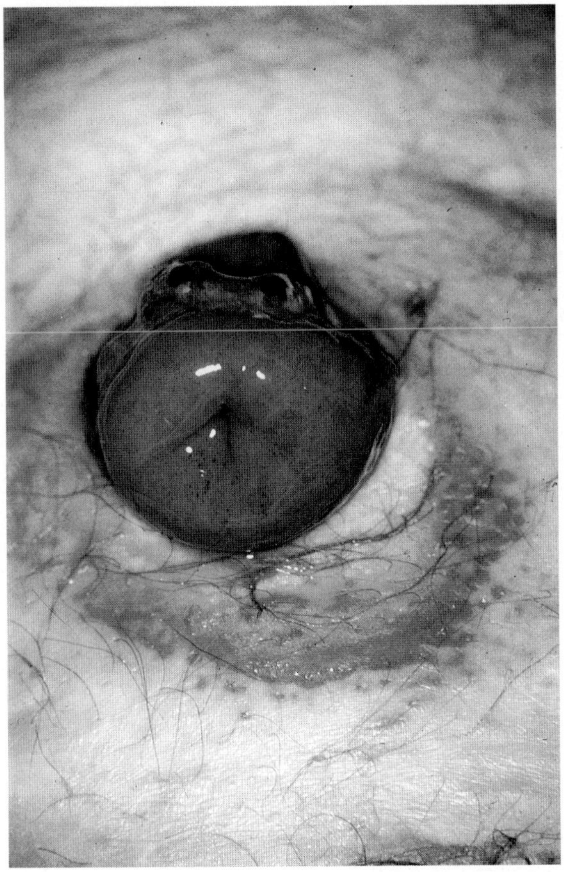

Fig. 28.1. An ileostomy with ulceration due to an ill-fitting appliance.

Early complications

Ill-fitting appliance

In the majority of patients this is due to stomal oedema in the immediate post-operative period. This usually settles down within 48 to 72 hours when a better fitting stoma appliance can be applied and the problem is resolved. Patients who continue to have problems with ill-fitting appliances (Fig. 28.1), usually because of a badly sited stoma, invariably require revision of their stoma.

Parastomal sepsis or abscess

This is usually due to the separation of the mucosa-skin interface. It commonly occurs between the seventh and the tenth day. If it is a small infected area then it is left alone to resolve. If there is an established abscess cavity (Fig. 28.2) then a formal drainage of the abscess may be necessary.

Ischaemia

If stomal ischaemia develops it will be obvious within 24 to 48 hours. If the necrosis is superficial and confined to part of the mucosa it can be left alone to slough and re-epithelialise; a stomal stricture almost invariably develops as the tissues heal. If the

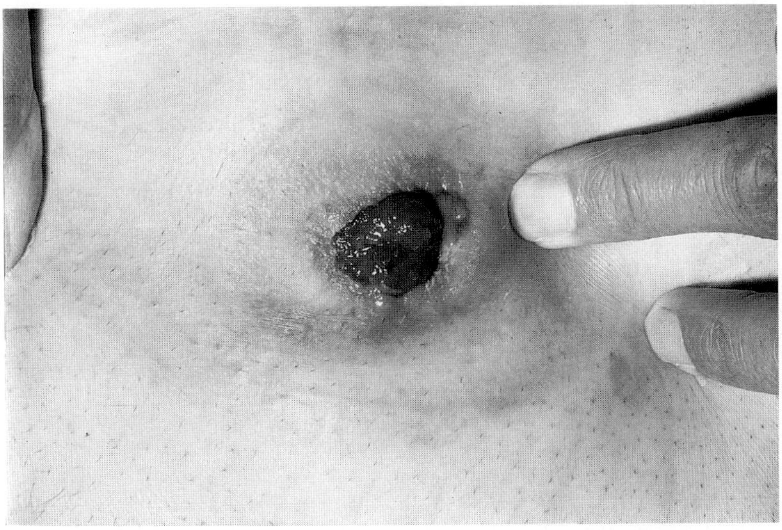

Fig. 28.2. A parastomal abscess.

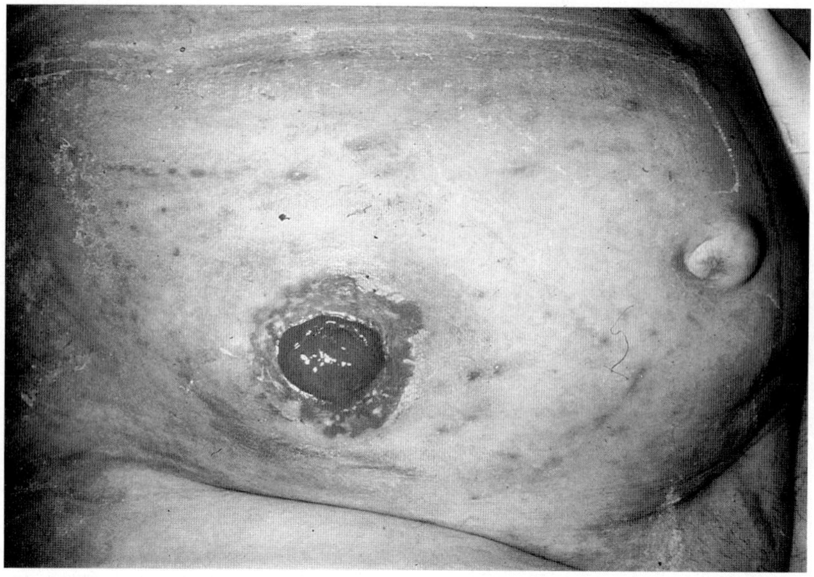

Fig. 28.3. A retracted ileostomy. Note that the position of the ileostomy is lateral to the right rectus muscle.

ischaemic necrosis extends below the fascia then re-laparotomy and re-fashioning of the stoma is required. Occasionally, a gentle examination with a flexible endoscope may help in diagnosing extensive ischaemic necrosis.

Skin excoriation

The effluent from the ileostomy contains pancreatic proteolytic enzymes that can digest the skin. If the stoma is badly constructed or if the appliance is not well fitting there will be leakage of ileal effluent resulting in excoriation of parastomal skin. Initial treatment is by the stoma therapist using a better fitting appliance, if this is not effective usually the stoma will need re-fashioning or re-siting. Occasionally patients develop contact dermatitis either to adhesives or other components of the appliance. In these cases a skin patch test should be performed and the appliance or the adhesive changed.

Stoma retraction

This is often due to inadequate fixation of ileal serosa to the rectus sheath. The principal factor fixing the length of the ileostomy stoma is the contact of the serosa with the fibres of the rectus muscle. Stomas that are brought out lateral to the rectus sheath often retract (Fig. 28.3). Some surgeons suture the ileal serosa to the posterior rectus sheath; others do not. Most fix the ileal mesentery to the posterior rectus sheath. Retraction also occurs if an inadequate length of ileum has been used to fashion the stoma, or if the patient gains a large amount of weight post-operatively. In my experience, local mobilisation and re-fashioning of stomas is often inadequate and usually a formal laparotomy, mobilisation of bowel and re-fashioning of ileostomy is necessary.

Intermediate and late complications

Obstruction

Most patients with stomas experience transit episodes of obstruction. Often this is the result of a high-fibre food bolus obstruction; the patient usually presenting with colicky abdominal pain, distension, sometimes vomiting and cessation of ileostomy output. Occasionally the obstruction may be secondary to intestinal adhesions and can then be a closed loop obstruction. I believe that all patients with a stoma presenting with signs and symptoms of intestinal obstruction should be admitted to hospital. They should be managed with nasogastric suction and intravenous fluids. A bolus obstruction can sometimes be differentiated from adhesive proximal obstruction by irrigating the stoma with 25–50 ml of normal saline. If the irrigating fluid comes back mixed with food particles then a bolus obstruction should be suspected. However, if the irrigation fluid is clear then it suggests proximal obstruction. In such cases a retrograde ileogram is the investigation of choice to

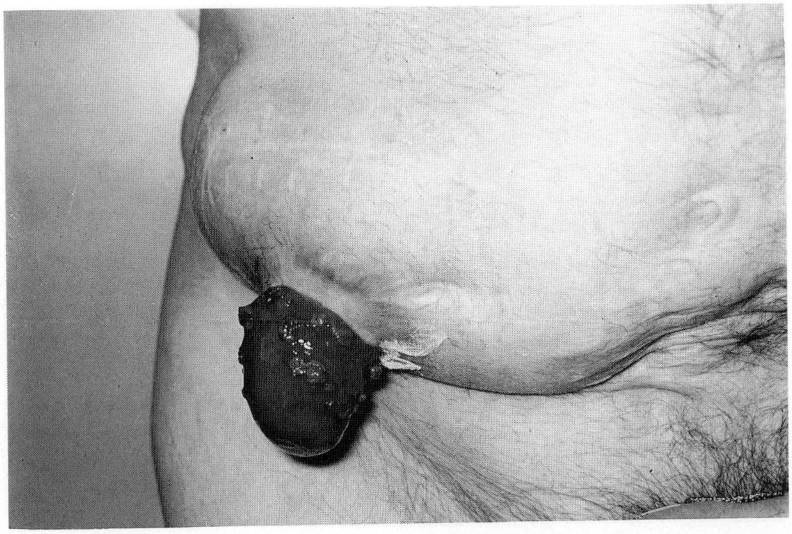

Fig. 28.4. A recurrent paraileostomy hernia. The scar from a previous repair can be seen. Note that the stoma has been sited in the right iliac fossa over a skin crease and lateral to the rectus muscle.

identify the site and nature of obstruction. In cases of bolus obstruction, continuous irrigation will often relieve the obstruction and its associated signs and symptoms. Simple adhesive obstructions occasionally settle on conservative measures whereas band adhesions will require a laparotomy and division of the band. The danger of closed loop obstruction should always be considered and an unnecessary laparotomy is better than an ischaemic length of gut from neglected strangulation.

Parastomal hernias

This is a common complication of both ileostomies and colostomies. The commonest cause is a large fascial defect or a stoma which has been sited lateral to the rectus sheath (Fig. 28.4). If such hernias are asymptomatic they do not require surgical treatment. Whereas if the patient complains of persistent pain around the stoma or presents with symptoms of intestinal obstruction due to entrapped small bowel then the best treatment is relocation of the stoma to the other side of the abdomen and closing the hernial defect.

Prolapse

Prolapse (Fig. 28.5) is another common complication of stomas (both ileostomies and colostomies). It is usually due to intussusception of the bowel which may be a result of too large a fascial defect as with parastomal hernia above. Usually conservative management or local refashioning with amputation of the prolapsed gut is unsuccessful. Re-siting the stoma to the opposite side of the abdomen

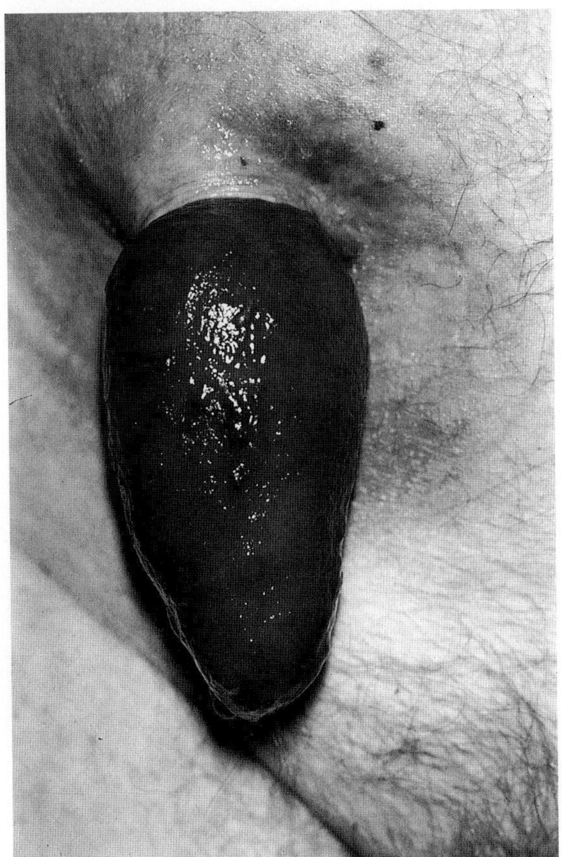

Fig. 28.5. Prolapse of an ileostomy stoma.

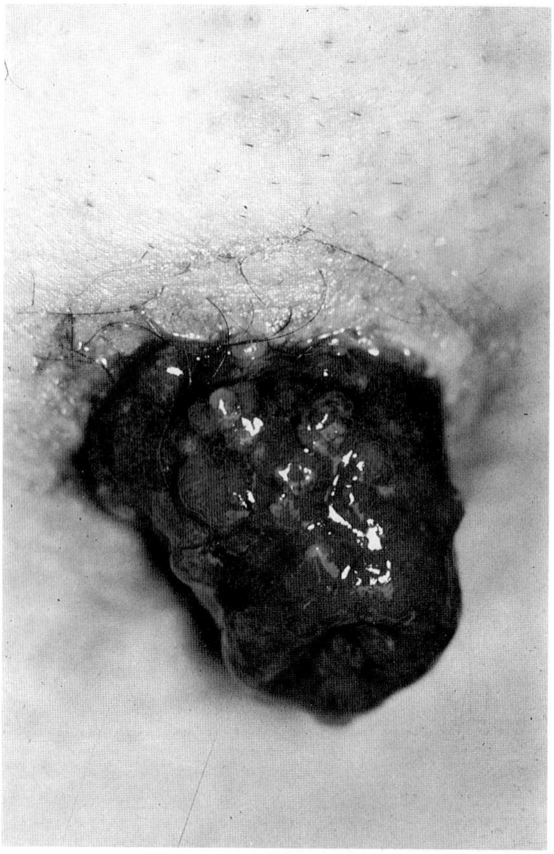

Fig. 28.6. Ileostomy granulomas seen as small polypoid lesions on the mucosal surface.

and bringing it out through the muscle fibres of the rectus sheath is the best management.

Stenosis

Stricture of the stoma occurs in approximately 5%–10% of patients with a colostomy. The stenoses of colostomies and ileostomies have different aetiologies: in colostomies it is due to improper maturation of the stoma with healing by granulation; in ileostomies it is due to chronic ulceration due to too high or too rigid a face plate. Local refashioning is not often effective and once again re-siting the best treatment. Dilatation with balloon or finger gives only transient relief and is not recommended.

Ileostomy granulomas

These are often small polypoid lesions on the exposed mucosal surface of the stoma and are termed "stomal granulomas" (Fig. 28.6). Histologically they resemble inflammatory polyps. They occur more commonly with long than with short stomas and were commoner with the old rubber appliance bags than with the new plastic bags. They are the commonest cause of bleeding from stomas and when the symptoms become severe then excision of the existing stoma and re-fashioning is the treat-

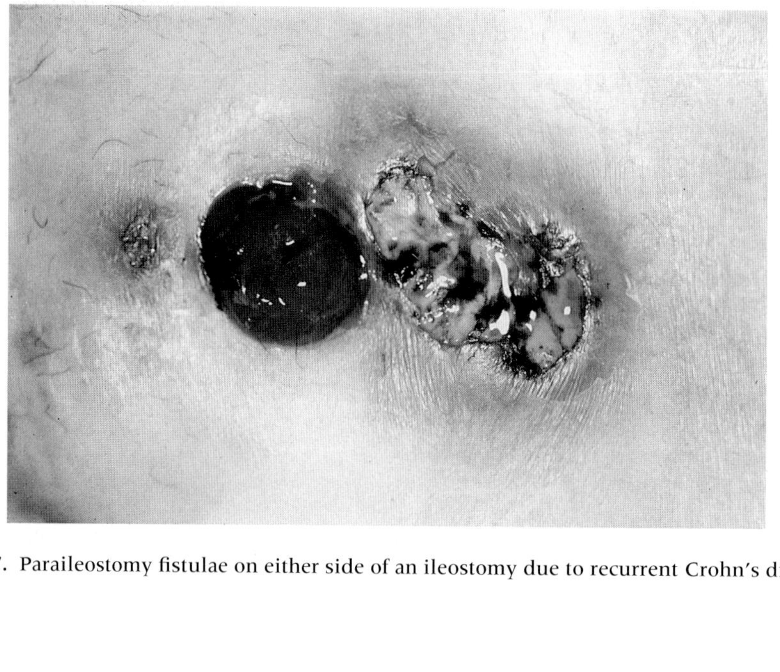

Fig. 28.7. Paraileostomy fistulae on either side of an ileostomy due to recurrent Crohn's disease.

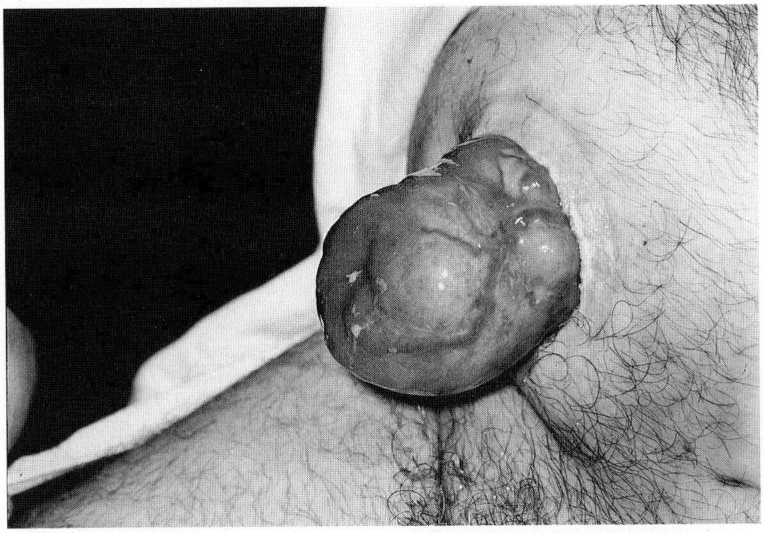

Fig. 28.8. Recurrent Crohn's ulceration on the side of an oedematous stoma.

ment of choice. They can also be cauterized with hot wire cautery or photocoagulation.

Paraileostomy fistula

The commonest cause of paraileostomy fistula (Fig. 28.7) is recurrent disease particularly Crohn's disease. Often there is an associated parastomal abscess due to non-removed suture or even non-removed rods. The patient usually presents with systemic symptoms as well as local symptoms secondary to recurrent disease. The treatment of choice is adequate drainage of sepsis and excision of the segment of bowel with fistula and re-siting of stoma.

Malfunction of stoma

This is more important and more serious with ileostomies than with colostomies due to the loss of significant amounts of sodium chloride and water. A high-output ileostomy (more than 1 litre of effluent per day) can result from short bowel syndrome, from stomal stenosis, intra-abdominal sepsis and small bowel obstruction and also from recurrent Crohn's disease (Fig. 28.8). The diagnosis of ileostomy diarrhoea from partial obstruction can be difficult; if an ileostomy stenosis is suspected, a digital examination is often helpful whereas more proximal causes can be diagnosed by a retrograde ileogram (Fig. 28.9) or by flexible endoscopy.

Ileostomy diarrhoea occurs due to the accumulation of osmotically active particles in the intestinal lumen resulting in a concentration gradient which attracts water into the lumen (Hill 1990). Excessive luminal fluid distends the bowel and initiates contractions resulting

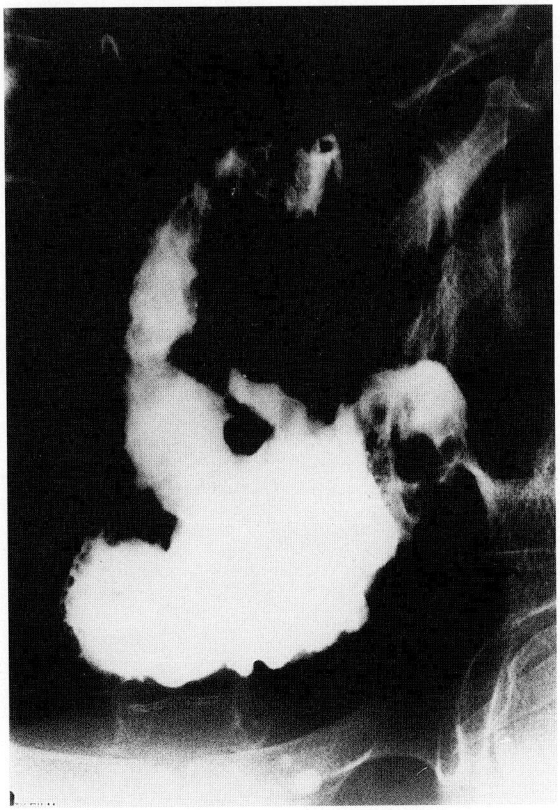

Fig. 28.9. Retrograde ileogram showing a fistula due to recurrent Crohn's disease.

in watery diarrhoea. Ileostomy diarrhoea can also occur due to recurrent Crohn's disease or malabsorption of nutrients. The nutrients of a malfunctioning stoma consists of fluid and electrolyte replacement and occasionally when a mechanical cause for the malfunction is identified, operative treatment may be necessary.

References

Carlstedt A, Fasth S, Hulten L, Nordgren S, Palselius I (1987) Long-term ileostomy complications in patients with ulcerative colitis and Crohn's disease. Int J Colorect Dis 2:22–25.

Gallagher ND, Harrison DD, Skyring AP (1962) Fluid and electrolyte disturbances in patients with long established ileostomies. Gut 3:219

Goldblatt MS, Corman ML, Haggit RC, Coller JA, Veidenheimer MC (1977) Ileostomy complications requiring revision. Lahey Clinic experience 1964–1973. Dis Colon Rectum 20:209–214

Hill G (1990) Ileostomy function. In: 1990 Allan RN, Keighley MRB, Alexander-Williams J, Hawkins CF (eds) Inflammatory bowel disease, 2nd edn. Churchill livingstone, Edinburgh, pp 93–99

Kramer P (1966) The effect of varying sodium loads on the ileal excreta of human ileotomised subjects. J Clin Invest 45:1710

Kurchin A, Ray JE, Bluth EI et al. (1984) Cholelithiasis in ileostomy patients. Dis Colon Rectum 27:585

Ritchie JK (1971) Ileostomy and excisional surgery for chronic inflammatory disease of the colon: a survey of one hospital region. I. Results of complications of surgery. Gut 12:528

Weaver RM, Alexander-Williams J, Keighley MRB (1988) Indications of outcome of reoperation for ileostomy complications in inflammatory bowel disease. Int J Colorect Dis 3:38–42

29 Follow-Up in Inflammatory Bowel Disease

R.N. Allan

Ulcerative colitis and Crohn's disease are uncommon conditions, so that most hospital doctors and family practitioners see few such patients. A follow-up clinic provides a focus for them and the accummulated experience provides the background for rational and consistent advice and care. The resources of medical and surgical follow-up can be linked to stoma care, first class radiology, histopathology and laboratory services. The provision of out-patient and in-patient services in adjacent areas familiarises the patient with the available in-patient facilities which they may need in the future.

Some patients are fortunate and run an uncomplicated course. Most have intermittent exacerbations of their disease, often with unusual but associated complications where appropriate selection of dietary, medical or surgical treatment may be difficult.

Characterisation of the patient group. Patients with ulcerative colitis or Crohn's disease pose a wide variety of problems masquerading under these two specific labels.

All patients subject to review should be characterised in more precise terms so that critical analytical evaluation can be undertaken of symptoms and signs at each follow-up visit.

Patients with ulcerative colitis should be characterised according to extent of disease (proctitis, left-sided disease, extensive disease or total colitis). Each of these groups can then be further subdivided according to the pattern of their symptoms: asymptomatic, chronic intermittent, chronic persistent and the small but important group of patients with severe acute colitis.

Patients with Crohn's disease are grouped according to the site and extent of macroscopic disease and the presence or absence of local complications such as fibrous stricture, abscess or fistula formation. The possibility of other complications including anaemia, malnutrition, fluid and electrolyte imbalance or associated disorders such as peptic ulcer, gall stones or renal stones must also be considered.

Patients' records. The records of each patient are headed by a problem sheet, summarising these features, including previous surgical treatment, the present site and extent of disease, associated complications and current therapy.

Laboratory data. Biochemical, haematological, endoscopic, radiology and pathology data are filed separately to ensure ready access to this important information.

Documentation. The file also includes sequential out-patient follow-up records and a separate area for filing correspondence in date order.

Out-patient visits. Each out-patient follow-up visit opens with a brief review of the problem sheet, previous visit notes, correspondence and recent laboratory data, so that the nature of the patient's previous problems can be categorised to provide the background to evaluate current symptoms.

Symptoms. The patient's symptoms can then be summarised, characterised and the likely cause ascribed, given the particular background. Thus, patients with proctitis are likely to have diarrhoea, urgency and rectal bleeding; the patient with distal ileal disease recurrent obstuctive symptoms; and the patient with extensive colitis diarrhoea, malaise and lethargy. The frequency, duration and severity can all be assessed and symptoms may be quantified for clinical trials with one of the indices of disease activity.

Physical signs. Abnormal physical signs are uncommon, but include fever, tachycardia evidence of weight loss, abdominal mass or perianal disease.

Laboratory evaluation of disease activity. There are a number or readily available laboratory indices for evaluating disease activity in addition to symptoms and signs.

Anaemia occurs from a variety of causes including bone marrow depression in the severely ill patient, overt bleeding or malabsorption of either iron, vitamin B_{12} or folate. Measurement of serum albumin is helpful since a low level indicates a source of protein loss in the gut, usually associated with extensive colitis, or depression of albumin synthesis in the liver in the severely ill patient.

Measurement of acute phase proteins is also valuable. The ESR reflecting increased fibrinogen release from the liver is variably elevated in active inflammatory bowel disease. C-reactive protein (CRP) or serum orosomucoids are better indices of disease activity in these disorders.

Grouping of patients according to symptoms and laboratory indices. The symptomatic patient with normal indices usually has symptoms from mechanical problems such as fibrous stricture in distal ileal Crohn's disease. The symptomatic patient with abnormal laboratory indices has severe or extensive disease which may well need either further evaluation or treatment.

Radiological assessment. Once the initial diagnosis has been established, the frequency and nature of radiological evaluation is determined by the nature and severity of new symptoms.

Thus the asymptomatic patient is unlikely to need further assessment, except perhaps for the individual with extensive colitis entering a surveillance programme for colorectal cancer when a further barium enema examination or colonoscopy would be appropriate.

The frequency of investigation is determined by the severity of symptoms and the rate of change. Radiological investigation may be required frequently in the early years following the diagnosis of Crohn's disease when the macroscopic site and extent of disease can change rapidly. The need for re-evaluation becomes less frequent with time for both ulcerative colitis and Crohn's disease.

Endoscopic evaluation. Endoscopy is primarily used to assess the severity of mucosal inflammation, to explain the nature of new symptoms such as diarrhoea and bleeding and to confirm during an exacerbation that the symptoms are due to the underlying disease. Endoscopic assessment complements the symptoms, signs and laboratory indices in determining the appropriate therapy and detects complications such as carcinoma, particularly in patients with longstanding colitis. Upper gastrointestinal endoscopy may be appropriate in patients suspected of having peptic ulcer.

Evaluation of medical therapy. Most patients are fit and well either without medication or with maintenance therapy alone. Except for maintenance therapy in ulcerative colitis, medical treatment is only needed for the symptomatic patient. At each visit the physician must decide whether the present regime and dose is appropriate or whether alternative therapy is required either alone or in combination with other drugs.

Medical surgical collaboration. Some patients, particularly those with perianal or distal ileal Crohn's disease and those with extensive Crohn's colitis, have persistent or recurrent symptoms despite medical treatment and need to be considered for surgical treatment. It is particularly appropriate for these patients to have a medical and surgical review at the same visit so that they can be considered by the medical and surgical teams for the planning of appropriate management.

Stoma care. The stoma care clinic should also be held concurrently so that patients in whom surgical treatment, including a stoma, is being considered can be counselled. The problems of any stoma patients can be discussed with the stoma therapist and resolved. The role of the stoma nurse has been extended recently to include the counselling of patients who are being considered for pouch operations for the surgical treatment of ulcerative colitis.

Newly diagnosed patients. For newly diagnosed patients, the follow-up clinic provides an excellent opportunity to explain the nature of their disorder both to them and their families, the possible medical and surgical treatment involved, the prognosis and the likely impact on their work and family life.

These newly diagnosed patients are also encouraged to contact the clinic between regular review appointments should any unexpected problems arise, which overcomes the problem of a disorder characterised by unexpected exacerbations and remissions.

Symptomatic patients. For the symptomatic patient each follow-up visit is an opportunity to assess the nature of their symptoms and signs, to indicate or amend treatment and arrange appropriate laboratory, radiological and endoscopic investigations. A clear distinction has to be drawn between organic and functional symptoms.

Asymptomatic patients. For asymptomatic individuals the follow-up clinic is a useful occasional point of contact with the reassurance of direct access between appointments, should the need arise.

Special problems. The follow-up clinic enables the identification of patients with special problems, particularly pregnancy, patients with longstanding ulcerative colitis for screening and complications such as hepatobiliary disorders and other extra-intestinal manifestations.

Consistent advice. The follow-up clinic should provide consistent informed advice to counter often misleading, although well-intentioned advice from family, friends, newspapers and journals, who offer a myriad of alternative solutions and generate many unnecessary anxieties.

Published literature. The follow-up clinic is a useful source of the excellent publications from the NACC and Ileostomy Association which further contributes to the receipt of consistent advice.

Frequency of follow-up. Most patients need only be reviewed once or twice each year at most and patients who have been asymptomatic for several years can be added to an annual mailing list and encouraged to contact the clinic in the interim should their symptoms recur.

Communication. The number of follow-up visits can be minimised by outlining alternative strategies to the family practitioner if symptoms persist or recur. Regular correspondence after each visit provides not only consultant advice for the management of the individual patient, but demonstrates the Unit's interest in these particular problems.

Graduate training. A regular follow-up clinic for inflammatory bowel disease provides an important focus for training of graduates in general medicine and gastroenterology. The natural history and prognosis of a wide range of problems in inflammatory bowel disease can be appreciated within the course of a few months and appropriate management discussed. This clinical training allied to regular meetings of the medical and surgical teams to discuss specific problems provides an excellent training programme.

Clinical research. Regular review of all patients with inflammatory bowel disease enables each centre to collate data on out-patients with similar problems and to determine their medical and surgical treatment and long-term prognosis. Appropriate management of different groups of patients can be analysed and published. Individual patients can be identified for inclusion in controlled drug trials and other studies.

The way ahead. Extending the annual mailing list to include patients with relatively few symptoms should enable the clinic to focus on those individuals with persistent symptoms and yet maintain contact with the whole group.

Much of the clinical information is already entered into a computer database and it should be possible within the next few years to record most of the clinical data in this way and enable on-line communication to the family practitioner.

Conclusions. An appropriately organised follow-up clinic should minimise the number of patients requiring in-patient care and yet identify those few individuals where in-patient care is essential.

It should also minimise morbidity by appropriate medical and surgical treatment and the provision of consistent advice.

One out-patient session each week for medical and surgical patients with inflammatory bowel disease with 3500 out-patient attendances per year enables us to look after 1000 patients with ulcerative colitis and a similar number with Crohn's disease. It seems little enough to offer to patients, usually young adults, who are unlucky enough in the prime of life to develop either ulcerative colitis or Crohn's disease.

Subject Index